AF606486

Ø 180 67Ø Ø13

WITHDRAWN
DE MONTFORT UNIV

ADVANCES IN

Pharmacology and Chemotherapy

VOLUME 19

ADVISORY BOARD

ADVANCES IN

Pharmacology and Chemotherapy

EDITED BY

Silvio Garattini

Istituto di Ricerche Farmacologiche "Mario Negri"
Milano, Italy

A. Goldin

National Cancer Institute
Bethesda, Maryland

F. Hawking

Commonwealth Institute of Helminthology
St. Albans, Herts., England

I. J. Kopin

National Institute of Mental Health
Bethesda, Maryland

Consulting Editor

R. J. Schnitzer

Mount Sinai School of Medicine
New York, New York

VOLUME 19—1982

ACADEMIC PRESS

A Subsidiary of Harcourt Brace Jovanovich, Publishers

New York London

Paris San Diego San Francisco São Paulo Sydney Tokyo Toronto

ACADEMIC PRESS, INC.
111 Fifth Avenue, New York, New York 10003

United Kingdom Edition published by
ACADEMIC PRESS, INC. (LONDON) LTD.
24/28 Oval Road, London NW1 7DX

LIBRARY OF CONGRESS CATALOG CARD NUMBER: 61–18298

ISBN 0–12–032919–0

PRINTED IN THE UNITED STATES OF AMERICA

82 83 84 85 9 8 7 6 5 4 3 2 1

CONTENTS

Contributors to This Volume ix

Chloroethylnitrosourea Cancer Chemotherapeutic Agents

Robert J. Weinkam and Huey-Shin Lin

I. Introduction 1
II. Development of New Chloroethylnitrosoureas 1
III. Chemistry 5
IV. Reactive Intermediates 9
V. Active Species 13
VI. Mechanism of Cytotoxicity 15
VII. Biodisposition 20
VIII. Chemicobiological Interactions 26
IX. Conclusion 27
References 28

The Interaction of Cancer Chemotherapy Agents with Mononuclear Phagocytes

Alberto Mantovani

I. Introduction 35
II. Effects of Chemotherapeutic Agents on Mononuclear Phagocytes 37
III. Effects of Chemotherapeutic Agents on Tumor-Associated Macrophages (TAM) 56
IV. Antitumor Efficacy and Modulation of Mononuclear Phagocytes 57
V. Concluding Remarks 61
References 62

Mebendazole and Related Anthelmintics

Hugo Van den Bossche, Frans Rochette, and Christian Hörig

I. Introduction 67
II. Chemistry and Pharmacology 69
III. Benzimidazole Carbamates in Veterinary Medicine 82
IV. Benzimidazole Carbamates in Human Medicine 109

V. Conclusion 118
References 119

Chemotherapy of Human Intestinal Helminthiasis: A Review with Particular Reference to Community Treatment

D. Stürchler

I. Summary 129
II. Introduction 130
III. The Parasites 131
IV. The Human Host 136
V. The Drugs 138
VI Therapeutic Intervention 147
References 151

Development of Radiosensitizers: A Medicinal Chemistry Perspective

V. L. Narayanan and William W. Lee

I. Introduction 155
II. General Background 156
III. Structure Activity/Toxicity Determinants 163
IV. Medicinal Chemistry of Electron-Affinic Radiosensitizers 173
V. Summary and Perspectus for the Future 198
References 200

The Effects of Antineoplastic Therapy on Growth and Development in Children

Udo Bode and Allen Oliff

I. Introduction 207
II. Antineoplastic Therapy 209
III. Central Nervous System Toxicity 215
IV. Endocrine Organ Toxicity 229
V. Skeletal Growth 236
VI. Psychosocial Development 237
VII. Concluding Remarks 239
References 239

Biological Properties of ICRF-159 and Related Bis(dioxopiperazine) Compounds

Eugene H. Herman, Donald T. Witiak, Kurt Hellmann, and Vaman S. Waravdekar

I. Historical 249
II. Chemistry and Structure–Activity Relationships 250
III. Biological Characteristics 260
IV. Radiosensitization 268
V. Pharmacology 269
VI. Toxicology 270
VII. Clinical 274
VIII. Interactions of ICRF Compounds with Other Agents 278
IX. Prospective Views 286
References 286
Note Added in Proof 290

Index 291

CONTRIBUTORS TO THIS VOLUME

Numbers in parentheses indicate the pages on which the authors' contributions begin.

UDO BODE (207), *Universitaetskinderklinik, Adenauerallee 119, 53 Bonn, Federal Republic of Germany*

KURT HELLMANN (249), *Imperial Cancer Research Fund, Lincoln's Inn Fields, London WC2A 3PX, England*

EUGENE H. HERMAN (249), *Division of Drug Biology, Food and Drug Administration, Washington, D.C. 20204*

CHRISTIAN HÖRIG (67), *Research Laboratories, Janssen Pharmaceutica, B-2340 Beerse, Belgium*

WILLIAM W. LEE (155), *SRI International, Menlo Park, California 94025*

HUEY-SHIN LIN (1), *Department of Medicinal Chemistry and Pharmacognosy, School of Pharmacy and Pharmacal Sciences, Purdue University, West Lafayette, Indiana 47907*

ALBERTO MANTOVANI (35), *Istituto di Ricerche Farmacologiche, "Mario Negri," 20157 Milan, Italy*

V. L. NARAYANAN (155), *Division of Cancer Treatment, National Cancer Institute, Bethesda, Maryland 20205*

ALLEN OLIFF (207), *Laboratory of Tumor Virus Genetics, National Cancer Institute, Bethesda, Maryland 20205*

FRANS ROCHETTE (67), *Research Laboratories, Janssen Pharmaceutica, B-2340 Beerse, Belgium*

D. STÜRCHLER (129), *Swiss Tropical Institute, Medical Department, CH-4051 Basel, Switzerland*

HUGO VAN DEN BOSSCHE (67), *Research Laboratories, Janssen Pharmaceutica, B-2340 Beerse, Belgium*

[1]Present address: Memorial Sloan Kettering Cancer Center, New York, New York 10021.

VAMAN S. WARAVDEKAR (249), *Office of the Director, National Cancer Institute, National Institutes of Health, Bethesda, Maryland 20205*

ROBERT J. WEINKAM (1), *Department of Medicinal Chemistry and Pharmacognosy, School of Pharmacy and Pharmacal Sciences, Purdue University, West Lafayette, Indiana 47907*

DONALD T. WITIAK (249), *Division of Medicinal Chemistry, College of Pharmacy, Ohio State University, Columbus, Ohio 43210*

ADVANCES IN PHARMACOLOGY AND CHEMOTHERAPY, VOL. 19

Chloroethylnitrosourea Cancer Chemotherapeutic Agents

ROBERT J. WEINKAM AND HUEY-SHIN LIN

Department of Medicinal Chemistry and Pharmacognosy
School of Pharmacy and Pharmacal Sciences
Purdue University
West Lafayette, Indiana

I. Introduction . . . 1
II. Development of New Chloroethylnitrosoureas . . . 1
III. Chemistry . . . 5
IV. Reactive Intermediates . . . 9
V. Active Species . . . 13
VI. Mechanism of Cytotoxicity . . . 15
VII. Biodisposition . . . 20
VIII. Chemicobiological Interactions . . . 26
IX. Conclusion . . . 27
References . . . 28

I. Introduction

Chloroethylnitrosoureas have proven to be highly effective cancer chemotherapeutic agents that are in common clinical use. Although the most widely used analog in this class of agents, BCNU, was introduced in the mid 1960s, efforts to develop new compounds with selective sites of action and reduced toxicity have continued to the present day. Along with these developments, studies into the mechanisms of activation and action have been reported and attempts have been made to identify the active species responsible for the antitumor activity and toxicity of this class of drug. Biodistribution and metabolism studies have also been conducted in order to reveal the fate of these chemically reactive agents. Many recent reports have resolved questions concerning the activation of these agents and revealed that activity may be influenced by unusually complex structurally specific interactions. These aspects of the literature on chloroethylnitrosoureas have been reviewed in detail in this article.

II. Development of New Chloroethylnitrosoureas

The chloroethylnitrosoureas are among the earliest and most significant anticancer agents that have been developed by the National Cancer Insti-

ISBN 0-12-032919-0

tute. The evolution of these compounds was initiated by the observation that 1-methyl-1-nitroso-3-nitroguanidine (MNNG), synthesized in 1947 (McKay and Wright, 1947), had weak activity against systemic leukemia L1210 (Greene and Greenberg, 1960). Since MNNG was used as a reagent for the generation of diazomethane in organic synthesis, other progenitors of diazomethane were investigated for antitumor activity.

1-Methyl-1-nitrosourea (MNU) was developed at Southern Research Institute as the first active compound in the nitrosourea series (Johnson *et al.,* 1963). Interestingly, this agent showed activity against both intraperitoneal (ip) and intracerebral (ic) implanted L1210 cells (Skipper *et al.,* 1961). This observation stimulated further studies and many *N*-alkyl-*N*-nitrosourea congeners have been synthesized and evaluated for antitumor activity. MNNG and MNU are now used as experimental carcinogens (Sugimura *et al.,* 1966; Magee and Barnes, 1967).

Most of the early work on these agents has been done at the Southern Research Institute where synthesis and activity of *N*-nitrosoureas, RN(NO)CONHR′, and *N*,*N*″-dinitrosobiureas, RN(NO)CONHCON-(NO)R″, were reported in 1963 (Johnson *et al.,* 1963). 1,3-Bis(2-chloroethyl)-1-nitrosourea (BCNU) was found to be the most active member of this series and was the first agent to be used clinically. Other nitroso derivatives of biureas, biuretes, and carboximides were synthesized and tested for activity against ip L1210 (Johnston and Oplinger, 1967). Some of these compounds showed significant activity but were less effective than BCNU. Continued efforts to improve activity emphasized compounds having the 1-(2-haloethyl)-1-nitrosourea structure, XCH_2CH_2N-(NO)CONHR, where X = Cl or F and R is varied. Screening of these compounds for activity against ip and ic implanted L1210 mouse leukemia indicated that the more active compounds contained 2-haloethyl or cycloaliphatic R groups (Johnston *et al.,* 1966). The 2′-chloroethylene unit is essential, as extended homologs such as 3-chloropropylene are inactive (Lown and McLaughlin, 1979a). 1-(2-Chloroethyl)-3-cyclohexyl-1-nitrosourea (CCNU) and 1-(2-chloroethyl)-3-(4-methylcyclohexyl)-1-nitrosourea (MeCCNU) are members of this series (Johnston *et al.,* 1977). BCNU, CCNU, and MeCCNU are the three chloroethylnitrosoureas that are in noninvestigational clinical use. Extensive reviews of the clinical and experimental antitumor activity of these compounds have been published (Carter *et al.,* 1972, Schabel, 1976). Additional 1-(2-chloroethyl)-1-nitroso analogs (Scheme 1) having alicyclic and heterocyclic substituents were prepared (Johnston *et al.,* 1971; Kameya *et al.,* 1978; Arakawa and Shimizo, 1975). Several analogs had a higher therapeutic index, ED_{50}/LD_{10}, than BCNU when tested against L1210 (Johnston *et al.,* 1971) but were less effective against ic implanted 9L tumors (Levin and

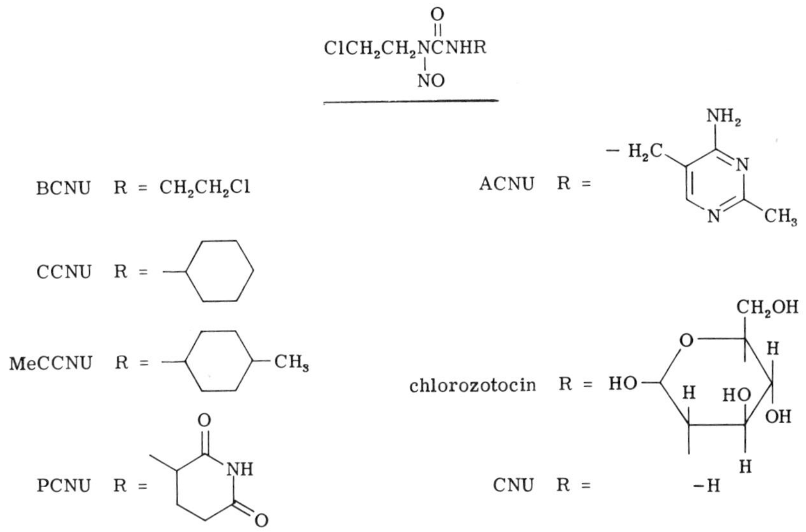

$$ClCH_2CH_2N(NO)C(=O)NHR$$

BCNU R = CH_2CH_2Cl

CCNU R = cyclohexyl

MeCCNU R = 4-methylcyclohexyl (CH_3)

PCNU R = 2,6-dioxo-3-piperidyl (O, NH, O)

ACNU R = $-H_2C$–(4-amino-2-methyl-5-pyrimidinyl) (NH_2, N, N, CH_3)

chlorozotocin R = HO–(glucopyranose ring: O, CH_2OH, H, HO, OH, H)

CNU R = –H

SCHEME 1. 1-(2-Chloroethyl)-1-nitrosoureas.

Kabra, 1974). The heterocyclic chloroethylnitrosourea, 1-(2-chloroethyl)-3-(2,6-dioxo-3-piperidyl)-1-nitrosourea (PCNU) (Johnston *et al.*, 1966), was more active than CCNU and BCNU in this assay. Another heterocyclic analog, 1-(2-chloroethyl)-3-(4-amino-2-methyl-5-pyrimidinyl)-methyl-1-nitrosourea (ACNU), has been found to be active against murine L1210 (Nogourney *et al.*, 1978; Arakawa and Shimizo, 1975). Both PCNU and ACNU have recently been introduced into preliminary clinical trials (Stewart *et al.*, 1980; Wooley *et al.*, 1981). Bifunctional and hydroxyalkyl chloroethylnitrosoureas were found to have significant activity against Walker carcinoma 256 in rats (Fiebig *et al.*, 1977). The water-soluble hydroxyalkyl compounds were more effective than BCNU against subcutaneous tumor but less effective against ic inoculated cells. Attempts have been made to alter the organ specificity of these agents by preparing chloroethylnitrosourea analogs of estrogenic steroids (Lam *et al.*, 1979), prolactin inhibiting ergolenes (Crider *et al.*, 1979), phensuximide (Crider *et al.*, 1980a), pyridine and piperidine (Crider *et al.*, 1980b), or by the combination of a chloroethylnitrosourea with a colchicine derivative (Lin *et al.*, 1980).

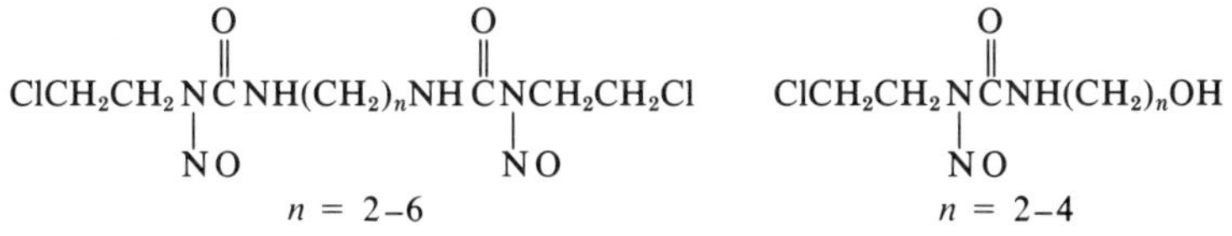

$$ClCH_2CH_2N(NO)C(=O)NH(CH_2)_nNHC(=O)N(NO)CH_2CH_2Cl \quad n = 2\text{–}6$$

$$ClCH_2CH_2N(NO)C(=O)NH(CH_2)_nOH \quad n = 2\text{–}4$$

Most of the above compounds are lipophilic agents that are active against CNS tumors. An impetus toward the development of water-soluble analogs was provided by the discovery of streptozotocin, a naturally occurring methylnitrosourea antitumor antibiotic (Herr *et al.*, 1960; Lewis *et al.*, 1960; Vavra *et al.*, 1960) containing a glucopyransose substituent (Herr *et al.*, 1967; Hardegger *et al.*, 1969). The synthetic 2-chloroethyl analog, chlorozotocin, is active against murine L1210 (Anderson *et al.*, 1975) and displays reduced bone marrow toxicity. Other

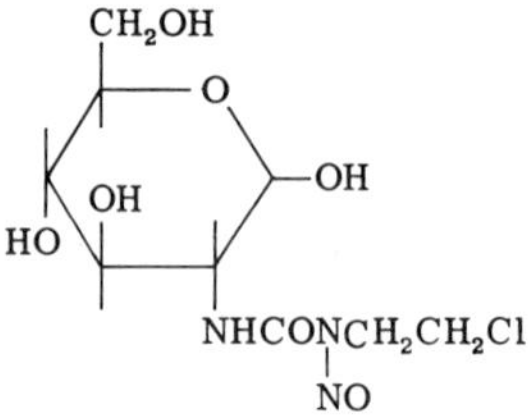

Chlorozotocin 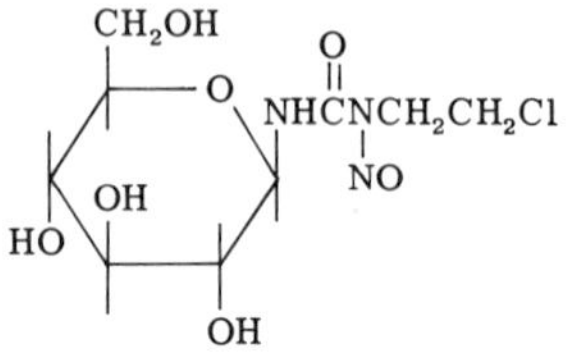 GANU

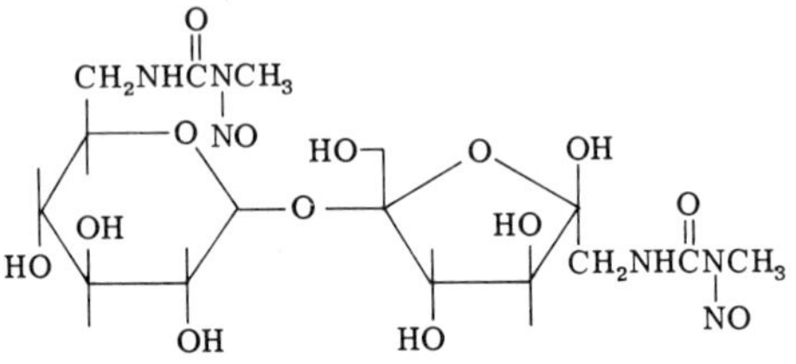

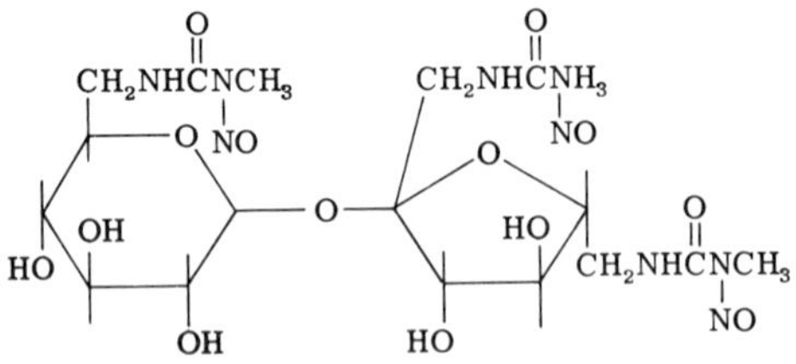

derivatives have been synthesized in an effort to reduce bone marrow toxicity such as GCNU, a tetraacetyl derivative of chlorozotocin which produces a 2-fold increase in life span of an LD_{10} dose without leukopenia side effects (Schein *et al.*, 1973). Placement of the nitrosourea group on the C-1 position of glucose give 1-(2-chloroethyl)-3(β-D-glucopyrenosyl)-1-nitrosourea (GANU) which also shows minimum myelosuppression (Fox *et al.*, 1977). Some sucrose derivatives have been synthesized based on the finding (Bakay, 1970) that sucrose penetrates tumor cell membranes but not normal brain cells. Methylnitrosourea derivatives 6,6′-dideoxyl-6,6′-di(3-methyl-3-nitrosourido)sucrose and 1,6,6′-trideoxy-1,6,6′-tri(3-methyl-3-nitrosourido)sucrose showed activity against both L1210 leukemia and epindymoblastoma brain tumor in mice (Almquist and Reist, 1977). Water-soluble cyclopentane tetrols and cyclohexane tetrol chloroethylnitrosourea analogs also show activity against L1210 that is comparable to BCNU (Swami *et al.*, 1979a,b).

Methyl and chloroethylnitrosourea derivatives of 3′-amino- and 5′-aminothymidines have been found to be more active against L1210 than BCNU (Lin *et al.*, 1978). Ribose-containing chloroethylnitrosoureas have shown activity against Friend leukemia (Larnicol *et al.*, 1977; Montero *et al.*, 1977) and the *p*-nitrophenyl ester derivative is under clinical investigation because of its superior therapeutic index and reduced hemotoxicity (Mori *et al.*, 1980).

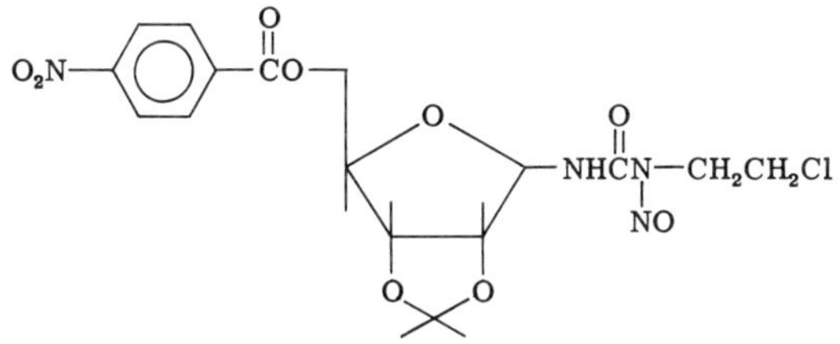

The synthesis and testing of nitrosourea analogs led Johnston and coworkers (Johnston *et al.*, 1963, 1967) to the conclusion that the 1-(2-haloethyl)-1-nitrosourea moiety was the basis for antitumor activity and that modification of the N-3 substituent could effectively alter *in vivo* antitumor activity. This idea has been followed for almost all of the nitrosourea analogs prepared to date. The intact chloroethylnitrosourea structure does not possess antitumor activity, however, and must be converted to reactive alkylating and carbamoylating species. Consequently, the chemical reactions of chloroethylnitrosoureas are important determinants of biological activity. For this reason, there has been considerable interest in the reactions of alkylnitrosoureas and especially of BCNU and CCNU.

III. Chemistry

The stability of chloroethylnitrosoureas is pH dependent. These compounds are very unstable at pH above 8 and have half-lives of less than 5 minutes at 37°C. Stability increases at lower pH and reaches a maximum at pH 4 to 5 with half-lives of 400 to 500 minutes. In highly acidic solutions, pH < 2, they decompose very rapidly and may survive for only a few seconds (Loo *et al.*, 1966). The pH dependence suggests that alkylnitrosoureas undergo both acid (pH < 4) and base (pH > 5) catalyzed mechanisms of decomposition (Fig. 1).

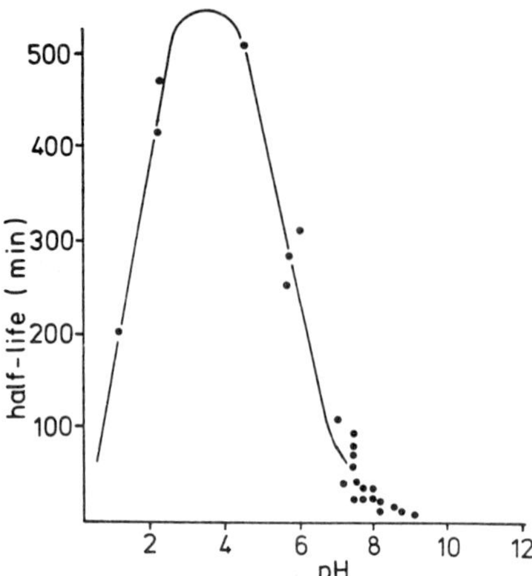

FIG. 1. The pH dependence of chloroethylnitrosourea half-lives at 25°C. Small changes in the pH 7.0 to 7.5 region may significantly alter the stability of these agents.

In very acidic solutions, nitrous acid is liberated rapidly in a proton catalyzed reaction. As a consequence, nitrosoureas may be analyzed colorimetrically by measuring liberated nitrous acid (Loo and Dion, 1965). At pH 3–5, the rate of decomposition increases as the pH decreases (Loo *et al.*, 1966) which was found to be characteristic of general acid catalysis (Chatterji *et al.*, 1978).

$$ClCH_2CH_2N(NO)C(=O)NHR \xrightarrow[HOH]{H^+} ClCH_2CH_2NHC(=O)NHR + HONO$$

There are conflicting reports on the dependence of base catalyzed BCNU reaction kinetics in buffer (Loo *et al.*, 1966; Laskar and Ayres, 1977; Chatterji *et al.*, 1978), salt effects (Loo *et al.*, 1966), and specific hydroxide ion catalysis (Laskar and Ayres, 1977; Chatterji *et al.*, 1978), although the decomposition reaction appears to occur by a mechanism that involves general base catalysis (Chatterji *et al.*, 1978). These contradictions and similar disagreements on the amounts of products formed appear to be due to the extreme dependence of these reactions on pH.

Three different mechanisms have been proposed for the base-induced decomposition of nitrosoureas. An early study by Applequist and McGreer (1960) of the alkoxide-induced decomposition of 1-cyclobutyl-1-nitrosourea implied that the initial step involved ethoxide ion attack on the carbonyl group. This mechanism was rejected by Jones and

$$\text{cyclobutyl-N(NO)C(=O)NH}_2 \xrightarrow{\text{EtO}^-} [\text{cyclobutyl-N=NO}^-] + \text{EtOC(=O)NH}_2$$

Muck who proposed ethoxide attack on the nitroso nitrogen based on the fact that ethyl carbamate could not be detected as a reaction product (Jones and Muck, 1966; Muck and Jones, 1966). They further supported

$$\text{RN(NO)C(=O)NH}_2 \xrightarrow{\text{EtO}^-} [\text{R(CONH}_2\text{)N-N(OEt)O}^-] \rightarrow \text{RN=NOEt} + \text{NO}^- + \text{HOCN} \quad \text{or} \quad \text{RN=NOH} + \text{EtO}^- + \text{HOCN}$$

this proposal by isolating the analogous triazene from the reaction of alkynitrosoureas in pyrolidine (Jones *et al.*, 1966). Hecht and Kozarich (1973) proposed an alternate mechanism involving initial proton abstraction at the urea nitrogen. When one considers the acidity of a nitrosourea, pK_a 8–9 (Garrett *et al.*, 1965; Garrett, 1960) proton transfer appears to be a facile first step although the decomposition to azohydroxide and isocyanate analogs may be concerted with proton abstraction. Disubstituted nitrosoureas (Muck and Jones, 1966) including 1-(2-chloroethyl)-3,3-dimethyl-1-nitrosourea (Colvin *et al.*, 1974) are much more stable than the monoalkylated analogs. This suggests that the proton on N-3 is necessary for facile conversion of alkylnitrosoureas to alkylating and carbamoylating intermediates and that the 1-(2-chloroethyl)-1-nitrosourea structure does not readily undergo alternate reactions.

$$\text{RN(NO)C(=O)NH}_2 \xrightarrow{\text{RO}^-} \text{RN(NO)C(=O)NH}^+ + \text{HOR} \rightarrow \text{RN=NO}^- + \text{HNCO} \rightarrow \text{RN=NOH} + {}^-\text{OCN}$$

The products formed from the reactions of chloroethylnitrosoureas in neutral aqueous solutions appear to result from the initial alkylating and isocyanate intermediates (Montgomery *et al.*, 1967). Quantitative analysis of products formed from the reaction of BCNU at pH 7.4, 37°C, for 2 hours accounts for 85% of starting material (Colvin *et al.*, 1974; Montgomery *et al.*, 1975; Weinkam and Lin, 1979). 2-Chloroethanol (31% of theoretical yield) and acetaldehyde (16%) are major products resulting from the alkylating intermediate. Vinylchloride (4%) and 1,2-dichloroethane (<2%) are minor products. 2-Chloroethylisocyanate reacts in water to

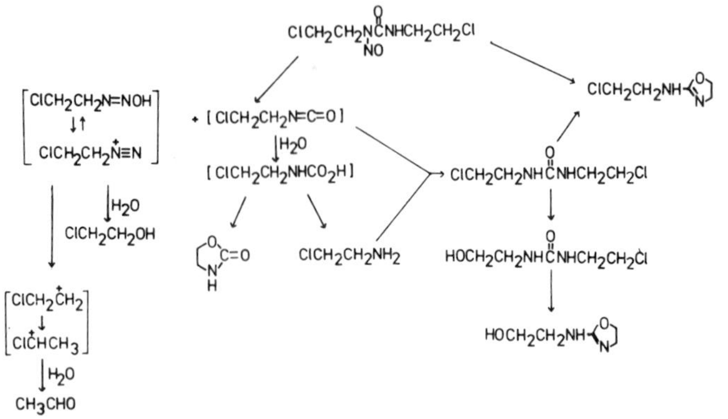

SCHEME 2. The chemical reaction products formed from BCNU at 37°C in pH 7.4 aqueous buffer after approximately 2 hours.

give 2-oxazolidone (33%) by cycloelimination of HCl and 2-chloroethylamine (14%) through decarboxylation. If the initial BCNU concentration is above 1 m*M* a significant amount of 1,3-bis(2-chloroethyl)urea (10%) is formed by condensation of 2-chloroethylamine and isocyanate. This urea cyclizes to give 2-(2-chloroethylamino)-2-oxazoline (11%) which can also be formed in low yield directly from BCNU (4%). These reactions are shown in Scheme 2.

The decomposition of CCNU has also been studied under the same conditions and is similar to that of BCNU (Reed *et al.*, 1975; Montgomery

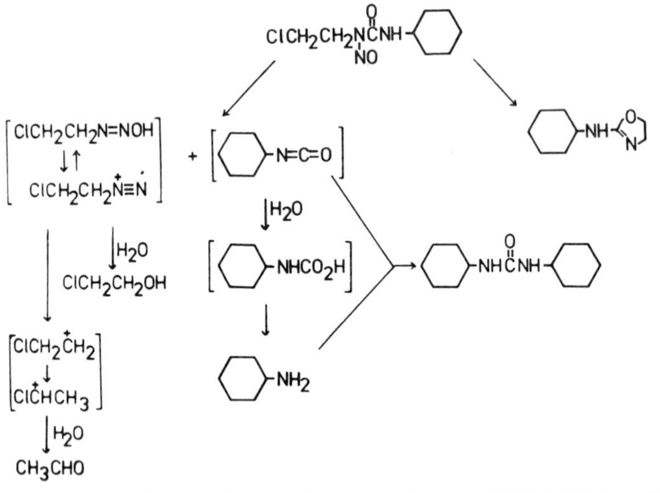

SCHEME 3. The chemical reaction products formed from CCNU at 37°C in pH 7.4 aqueous buffer after approximately 2 hours.

et al., 1975; Weinkam and Lin, 1979). 2-Chloroethanol (22–30%) and acetaldehyde (6–12%) are formed as major products along with small amounts of vinylchloride (1–3%) and ethylene (1–3%). Cychohexylamine (38%) is formed from cyclohexylisocyanate. Dicyclohexylurea (1–2%), 1-(2-chloroethyl)-3-cyclohexylurea (3–6%), and 2-(cyclohexylamino)-2-oxazoline (3–6%) are also formed (Scheme 3). It should be noted that the reactions of these compounds lead almost exclusively to the formation of alkylating and isocyanate intermediates. Similar findings have been made with other alkylnitrosoureas (Boivin and Boivin, 1951).

IV. Reactive Intermediates

Chloroethylnitrosoureas are known to be alkylating agents and to form ureas by carbamoylation of amines. It is clear that the carboylating activity results from the alkylisocyanate formed from the N-3 side of the molecule, however, the nature of the alkylating species has long been the subject of discussion. Skinner and co-workers (1960) suggested that the biological effects of MNNG, the first alkylnitroso compound found to have antitumor activity, were due to the formation of diazomethane during decomposition. It was subsequently assumed that the active species generated from alkylnitrosoureas under physiological conditions were also diazoalkanes (Garrett *et al.*, 1965). *N*-Alkyl-*N*-nitrosoamides (Jones and Muck, 1966), *N*-alkyl-*N*-nitrosoureas (Muck and Jones, 1966), *N*-alkyl-*N*-nitrosocarbamates (Gutsche and Johnson, 1955), and *N*-alkyl-*N*-nitrosourethanes (Bollinger *et al.*, 1950) do in fact liberate diazoalkanes under strongly basic conditions. However, no evidence for the presence of diazoalkanes could be found when these compounds were reacted in a neutral aqueous solution. Data consistent with formation of a methyldiazonium ion were reported for MNNG (Sussmuth *et al.*, 1972), MNU (Lijinsky *et al.*, 1972; Lawley and Shaw, 1973), and *N*-ethyl-*N*-nitrosourea (Lawley and Warren, 1975) with labeled ^{14}C, ^{3}H, or ^{2}H on the alkyl groups. Aqueous decomposition of these compounds gave alkylation products with the same ratio of isotopes as the parent compounds. These studies were extended by Brundrett *et al.* (1976) who reacted deuterated BCNU, 1,3-bis(1,1-dideuterio-2-chloroethyl)-1-nitrosourea, at pH 7.4 and isolated 2-chloroethanol containing two deuteriums while one would have been lost if 2-chlorodiazoethane were an intermediate.

Decomposition of BCNU and CCNU gives 2-chloroethanol, acetaldehyde, and vinylchloride as products. The relative amounts of these compounds are pH dependent. The existence of a variety of reactive intermediates has been postulated to explain these observations. Early work noted that acetaldehyde was formed rather than 2-chloroethanol which led to the suggestion that a vinyl carbocation was a reactive intermediate (Montgomery *et al.*, 1967). Later, Colvin and co-workers (1974) identified 2-chloroethanol, acetaldehyde, vinylchloride, and 1,2-dichloroethane as neutral reaction products from [^{14}C]BCNU. The product distribution was similar to that of the reaction of 2-chloroethylamine and nitrous acid in aqueous solution which suggested that a chloroethyl carbocation was an intermediate. The same intermediate was proposed for the reactions of CCNU and MeCCNU (Reed *et al.*, 1975). A reinvestigation of the decomposition of six chloroethylnitrosoureas in distilled water and aqueous buffer led Montgomery *et al.* (1975) to propose the vinyl carbocation as the precursor to acetaldehyde in addition to the presence of a chloroethyl carbocation intermediate.

More conclusive evidence on the nature of the active alkylating intermediate(s) was determined through the use of deuterium-labeled BCNU (Brundrett *et al.*, 1976). The deuterium distribution in the product acetaldehyde was inconsistent with the intermediacy of the vinyl carbocation but was explained by the rearrangement of $ClCH_2CH_2+$ to Cl^+CHCH_3 followed by addition to HO^- and loss of HCl. Further, the major alkylation product, 2-chloroethanol, was formed largely (90%) without rearrangement of the deuterium atoms. This suggested that 2-chloroethanol was formed via S_N2 attack of water on the intact azohydroxide. It, therefore, appears that the initial alkylation intermediate is the chloroethylazohydroxide, which is kinetically indistinguishable from the 2-chloroethyldiazonium ion, and that some fraction of the 2-chloroethylazohydroxide dissociates to the carbocation which may rearrange via hydride ion migration (Scheme 2). The S_N2 character of primary alkylazohydroxide reactions was also shown by the fact that nitrosative deamination of 1-deuteriobutylamine occurs with over 80% inversion of configuration (Streitwieser and Schaeffer, 1957) and over 66% of the 3-chloro-2-butanols formed from the reactions of 1,3-bis(threo-3-chloro-2-butyl)-1-nitrosourea and the erythro isomer had the inverted configuration (Brundrett and Colvin, 1977). The intermediate that leads to formation of stable alkylation products with macromolecules is the 2-chloroethylazohydroxide or diazonium ion (Scheme 4).

Another structure, 1,2,3-oxadiazolidine, has been proposed as an alkylating intermediate in order to explain the pH dependence of acetaldehyde formation (Chatterji *et al.*, 1978) and the presence of 2-hydroxyethyl products of DNA alkylations (Tong and Ludlum, 1978; Lown and McLaughlin, 1979b). Such an intermediate may form as a consequence of the nucleophilicity of the nitroso group (Michejda and

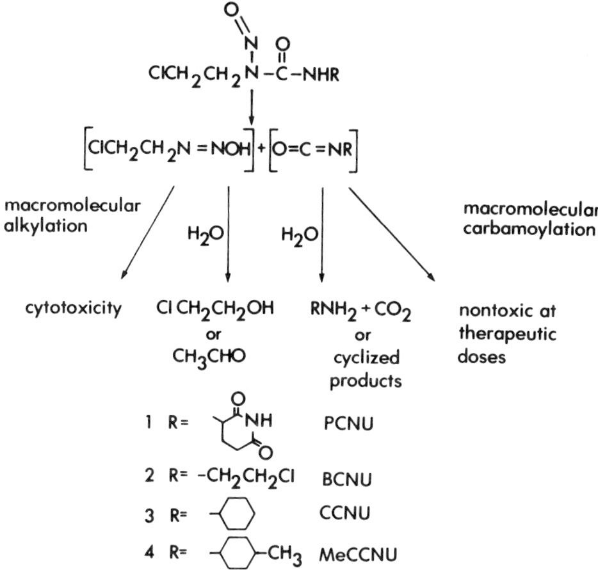

SCHEME 4. Chemical activation of chloroethylnitrosoureas leads to the formation of alkylating and carbamoylating species. The 2-chloroethylating intermediate is common to all agents in this class and appears to be the species responsible for observed anticancer and cytotoxic effects.

Koepke, 1978), however, an expected aqueous decomposition product, ethylene glycol (Behr, 1962), could not be detected as a BCNU reaction product at pH 7.4 (Weinkam and Lin, 1979). This intermediate is formed during reactions in more acidic solution (Brundrett, 1980).

Three parameters, lipophilicity, alkylating activity, and carbamoylating activity, have been considered to be possible determinants of chloroethylnitrosourea antitumor effects and toxicity (Wheeler *et al.*, 1974). The rationale behind the design and synthesis of new chloroethylnitrosourea analogs has included attempts to optimize these parameters in work that largely preceded an understanding of the mechanism of action of these agents. Most early studies investigated the relation between lipophilicity and antitumor activity. A quantitative structure activity correlation of 23 nitrosourea analogs showed an optimal partition coefficient, log *P* (octanol/water), of 0.6 using a 75% increase in lifespan of ic inoculated L1210-bearing mice as an activity endpoint. Maximum toxicity, LD_{10}, was observed for compounds with log *P* (octanol/water) 0.4 (Hansch *et al.*, 1972). This suggestion that activity and toxicity may be separated on the basis of lipid solubility was not varified in other test systems. Fourteen compounds tested against Lewis lung carcinoma in mice found an optimal log *P* (octanol/water) of 0.83 (Montgomery *et al.*, 1974). Neither electronic nor steric parameters could be correlated with activity. About 80 nitrosoureas were evaluated using an activity end-point of 50% cure rate of ip implanted L1210 leukemia and LD_{10} as a toxicity endpoint (Montgomery, 1976). Both of these correlation curves peak between log *P* (octanol/water) 0.63 and 0.75. These studies disclose that specific structural features lack unusual significance (Hansch *et al.*, 1980) and that rather unpredictable effects on antitumor activity may be observed. For example, phenyl substituents on the structure $ClCH_2CH_2N(NO)CONHR$ are inactive and the presence of a carboxyl group one carbon removed from N-3 produces compounds that are less active than analogs having a greater separation. Cycloalkanes are more active than acyclic analogs (Montgomery, 1976). In general, compounds that are most active against Lewis lung carcinoma were most active against other solid tumors, indicating that the structural characteristics necessary for activity against solid tumors are fairly general (Montgomery *et al.*, 1977a). Some of the differences in antitumor activity *in vivo* have been explained by investigations of metabolism and other interactions in which the structure of the parent compound is a significant factor.

Alkylating and carbamoylating activity as well as lipophilicity have been suggested as important determinants of haloethylnitrosourea antitumor activity and toxicity (Wheeler *et al.*, 1974). Decomposition of nitrosoureas leads to the formation of equivalent amounts of an alkylating species, 2-chloroethylazohydroxide, and a carbamoylating species, an alkylisocyanate. 2-Chloroethylazohydroxide is a highly reactive intermediate and probably does not survive long enough to penetrate cell membranes. The same alkylating species is, of course, formed from all of the active chloroethylnitrosourea analogs. Formation of these reactive species appears to be the major route of decomposition for all of the alkylnitrosoureas that have been studied. (Colvin *et al.*, 1974; Montgomery *et al.*, 1975; Reed *et al.*, 1975; Brundrett *et al.*, 1976; Weinkam and Lin, 1979; Lown and McLaughlin, 1979b). Alkylating activity is measured as the absorbance of a chromophore formed on alkylation of 4-(*p*-nitrobenzyl)pyridine (Friedman and Bolger, 1961) at pH 6, 37°C for 2 hours as described by Wheeler *et al.* (1974). Since the half-lives of alkylnitrosoureas at pH 6 are near 2 hours (Garrett *et al.*, 1965), alkylating activity measured in this way reflects, primarily, the rate of decomposition under these conditions (Panasci *et al.*, 1977) plus any differences that may exist in the yield of alkylating species formed during the decomposition reaction. It is not clear that the alkylating activity measured at pH 6 is comparable to that at pH 7.4 since BCNU and CCNU are known to yield equal amounts of alkylation products at pH 7.4 (Colvin *et al.*, 1974;

Montgomery *et al.*, 1975; Reed *et al.*, 1975; Weinkam and Lin, 1979) while CCNU alkylating activity is reported to be 33 to 38% of BCNU (Wheeler *et al.*, 1974; Panasci *et al.*, 1977).

Alkylisocyanates are formed along with alkylating species during chloroethylnitrosourea decomposition but differ from the alkylating species in that they possess significant stability in neutral aqueous solution. 2-Chloroethylisocyanate has a half-life of 17 seconds and cyclohexylisocyanate of 115 seconds (Hilton *et al.*, 1978). Carbamoylating activity is measured as the urea formed with the amino functions of [^{14}C]lysine at pH 7.4 for 6 hours (Wheeler *et al.*, 1974). Since over 75% of even slowly reacting chloroethylnitrosoureas decompose within 6 hours under these conditions, this measurement provides a reasonable reflection of the probability that the isocyanate will react with lysine, analogous to the suspected toxic reaction, or undergo competitive intramolecular cyclization or reactions with solvent water.

An initial study of 17 compounds indicated that carbamoylating activity contributed to toxicity as reflected in LD_{10} and therapeutic index while alkylating activity was a greater factor in determining single ip ED_{99}, the dose required to kill 99% of ip inoculated L1210 cells in mice. The octanol/water partition coefficient was also a major factor in determining toxicity. However, the correlation coefficients obtained from the regression analysis were poor and no significant correlations could be made (Wheeler *et al.*, 1974). Analysis of active compounds having a wide range of carbamoylating activity showed an inverse relation between alkylating activity or half-life of the chloroethylnitrosourea and LD_{10}, while no correlation was found for carbamoylating activity. None of the three parameters demonstrated a significant correlation with antitumor activity (Panasci *et al.*, 1977; Heal *et al.*, 1979).

V. Active Species

The antitumor activity of 1-chloroethyl-1-nitrosoureas has long been thought to result from covalent binding of alkylating and/or carbamoylating species. The binding of BCNU and CCNU reaction products to cellular macromolecules is well documented. Incubation of leukemia L1210 cells with BCNU labeled with ^{14}C indicated that covalent binding was associated with the protein fraction. When reacted with DNA, nucleohistone or histone radioactivity was largely bound to the histone. Reactions of carbonyl-^{14}C-labeled BCNU with lysine gave a product identified as N^6-(2-chloroethyl carbamoyl)lysine (Bowdon and Wheeler, 1971). Reaction of CCNU with L1210 leukemia cells in mice and with isolated nucleic acids and proteins showed, in each case, that the cyclohexylisocyanate was bound extensively to proteins. Labeled chloroethyl alkylating groups were bound to both nucleic acids and proteins, but to a much lesser extent that of the cyclohexyl moiety (Chang *et al.*, 1972). Similar patterns of BCNU binding were observed for resistant and sensitive TLX 5 lymphoma cells (Conners and Have, 1974).

Carbamoylation of amino acids, peptides, and proteins by CCNU and cyclohexylisocyanate *in vitro* occurs at the α-amino groups of amino acids, terminal amines of peptides and proteins, and at lysine ϵ-amino groups to give stable cyclohexylureas (Wheeler *et al.*, 1975; Schmall *et al.*, 1973). Carbamoylation by 2-chloroethylisocyanate derived from BCNU differs in that the product 2-chloroethylurea can cyclize with loss of HCl to give 2-oxazolin-2-yl groups (Wheeler *et al.*, 1975). *In vivo*, CCNU carbamoylation occurs primarily at lysine-rich histones in L1210 cells (Whoolley *et al.*, 1976), but histone carbamoylation of HeLa cells was not detected at a comparable dose (Tew *et al.*, 1978).

Alkylation reactions occur on both proteins and nucleic acids. Alkylation products 3-hydroxyethyl and 3-N^4-ethanocytidine monophosphate have been isolated from the reaction of BCNU with polycytidine (Kramer *et al.*, 1974) and similar products have been identified for BFNU reactions (Tong and Ludlum, 1974). BCNU reactions with polyquanine give 7-(β-hydroxyethyl)guanine monophosphate (Ludlum *et al.*, 1975). Alkylation of polycytidine is more efficient than that of polyguanine while adenine and uridine polymers are not alkylated (Ludlum *et al.*, 1975). CCNU alkylations of intact HeLa cells occur specifically at the extended euchromatin fraction of the cell genome and preferentially in regions associated with the nucleosomal cores (Tew *et al.*, 1978).

It is clear from these studies that the prevalent covalent binding reactions of chloroethylnitrosourea reaction products involve alkylation of DNA by 2-chloroethyldiazonium ion and carbamoylation of peptide amino functions. Although carbamoylation occurs to a much greater extent than alkylation and isocyanates are known to possess significant toxicity (Baril *et al.*, 1975; Bray *et al.*, 1975; Kann *et al.*, 1975), it has not been established that detectable toxicity results from carbamoylation at doses that result in cytotoxic DNA 2-chloroethylation. Carbamoylating species such as 2-chloroethylisocyanate have been found to inhibit DNA repair (Kann *et al.*, 1980), tubulin polymerization (Brodie *et al.*, 1980), and glutathione reductase (Babson and Reed, 1978).

A number of recent developments convincingly argue against the role of carbamoylation in chloroethylnitrosourea antitumor activity or toxicity and suggest that the chloroethylating intermediate is the only species responsible for activity at cytotoxic doses. Chlorozotocin is an effective antitumor agent that has little carbamoylating activity and relatively low bone marrow toxicity (Panasci *et al.*, 1977). Initially this appeared to support the role of carbamoylation in toxicity (Anderson *et al.*, 1975). However, other sugar-containing chloroethylnitrosoureas such as GANU have been found to have carbomylating activity comparable to BCNU but to have low myelotoxicity (Panasci *et al.*, 1977; Heal *et al.*, 1979). The nonsubstituted analog, 1-(2-chloroethyl)-1-nitrosourea (CNU) does not produce the alkylisocyanate-related toxic effect of inhibiting RNA processing that is caused by BCNU and other N-3 substituted compounds indicating that this agent does not possess intracellular carbamoylating activity or that the carbamoylation product is nontoxic (Kann *et al.*, 1974a). Nevertheless, the compound has *in vitro* cytotoxicity comparable to BCNU (Colvin *et al.*, 1976; Panasci *et al.*, 1977; Brundrett *et al.*, 1979) and the optimal *in vivo* CNU dose is 25% of BCNU (Schabel *et al.*, 1963). The alkylisocyanate effects on RNA processing are observed at doses that are 10-fold higher than required for cytotoxicity, 250 μM BCNU for 50 minutes compared to 25 μM BCNU required to kill 90% of L1210 cells over the same incubation period. Hilton and co-workers calculated the peak isocyanate concentration formed during BCNU or CCNU decomposition in cell culture medium and then showed that no L1210 cell toxicity occurred at these concentrations (Hilton *et al.*, 1978).

As discussed below, the cytotoxic activity of chloroethylnitrosoureas BCNU, CCNU, MeCCNU, PCNU, CNU, and chlorozotocin has been analyzed in terms of the amount of active alkylating species formed during exposure of cell to the drug. This removes the apparent differences in activity due to different rates of conversion to active species and the chloroethylnitrosoureas are found to have identical cytotoxic activity in cell culture (Weinkam and Deen, 1982). This is consistent with the fact that these compounds are chemically converted to an identical chloroethyldiazonium ion and the resulting macromolecular alkylation is independent of the structure of the N-3 substituent. There is no apparent effect due to the different carbamoylating species and different levels of carbamoylating activity of these agents.

VI. Mechanism of Cytotoxicity

In cell culture, the chloroethylnitrosourea in the culture medium partitions into the cell and reacts to form active chloroethylating intermediates. The half-lives of chloroethylnitrosoureas are between 1.5 and 5 minutes for CNU (Heal *et al.*, 1979; Brundrett *et al.*, 1979) and 30 and 90 minutes for substituted analogs (Panasci *et al.*, 1977; Heal *et al.*, 1979).

Partitioning of small molecules into isolated cells in suspension is very fast. Significant intracellular concentrations (0.1 to 1 m*M*) can be attained in 1 to 5 seconds by molecules with log *P* (octanol/water) between 4 and 0 (von Bahr *et al.*, 1974; Weinkam, unpublished) so that intracellular drug concentration reaches equilibrium before significant amounts of drug react in the extracellular medium. As the cell volume is relatively small in cell

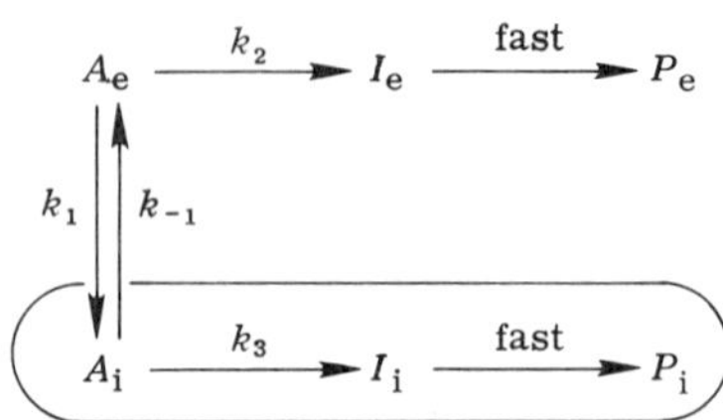

culture assays (0.1%), the intracellular concentration will approach the initial concentration of drug added to medium. Chloroethylnitrosoureas are not cytotoxic agents but must be converted to alkylating species by a decomposition reaction so that cytotoxicity is not determined by initial parent drug concentration, A_0, but by the amount of drug that decomposes to active intermediate during the period that the cells are incubated with the agent (Weinkam and Deen, 1982). More specifically, since the active chloroethylazohydroxide is very short lived and does not survive long enough to partition into the cell, cytotoxicity is related to the amount of alkylating species formed within the cell

$$\Delta A = A_0(e^{-k_3 t_1} - e^{-k_3 t_2})$$

where t_1 and t_2 are the start and end of the incubation period. The intracellular decomposition rate constants, k_3, for BCNU, CCNU, MeCCNU, and PCNU have been calculated from the time course of loss of activity and found to be equal to the respective k_2 values, the measured decomposition rate in cell culture medium or aqueous buffer (Hilton *et al.*, 1978). Consequently, the concentration decrease of added drug during the incubation period, ΔA, equals the moles/liter of active intermediate formed and the number of alkylation events that have occurred.

When analyzed in this way, the cytotoxicity produced by different initial drug concentrations and different incubation periods can be compared by calculating the respective values of ΔA. No difference has been found between the 9L cell kill produced from equal values of ΔA obtained during incubation periods ranging from 5 minutes to 4 hours, which indicates that toxicity is produced by an accumulation of alkylation reactions (Fig. 2) (Weinkam and Deen, 1982). These data are consistant with the observation that repair of sublethal damage does not occur in this cell line (Ber-

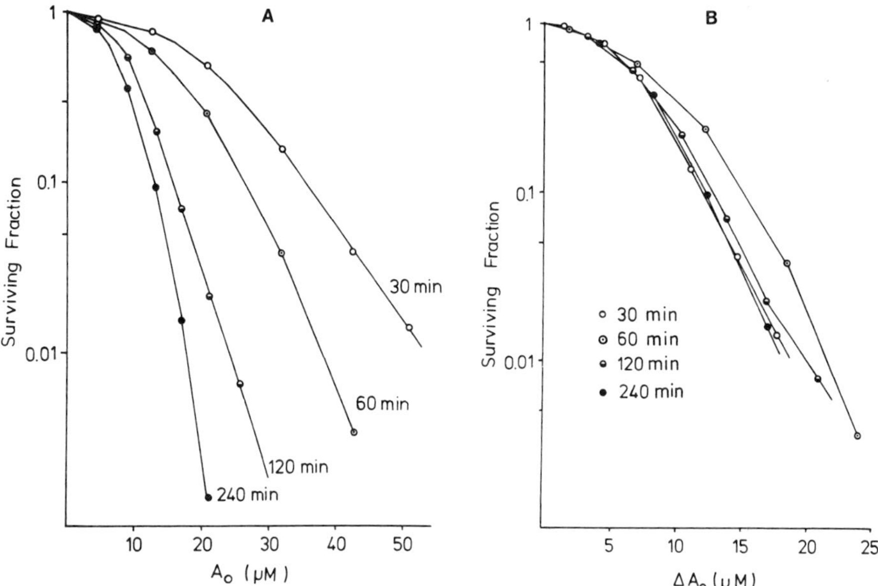

FIG. 2. Survival curves obtained from the incubation of 9L cells with various initial BCNU concentrations, A_0, for 30, 60, 120, and 240 minutes (A) and the same cell survival data plotted against the concentration of BCNU converted to active chloroethylating species during the incubation intervals (B). There is no significant difference in the activity of BCNU for these treatment intervals (data from Weinkam and Deen, 1982).

trand *et al.*, 1980) and suggests that the frequency of alkylation is not a significant factor influencing toxicity. Interestingly, 9L cell toxicity produced by BCNU, CCNU, MeCCNU, and PCNU are identical. The data of H. E. Kann (1978) for L1210 cell toxicity of BCNU, CCNU, chlorozotocin, and CNU (Fig. 3A) may be analyzed using the values for decomposition rates (Wheeler, 1976) and shows that these four compounds also have equal activity (Fig. 3B). Similar results have been obtained with P388 cells (Weinkam and Dolan, 1982). An explanation for the equal cytotoxicity of these agents is that they are all converted to the same active chloroethylating species that reacts randomly with sensitive macromolecules within the cell, that is, the structure of the parent chloroethylnitrosourea does not influence the site of alkylation. This would occur if the activation reaction occurred as a first-order reaction in aqueous medium and did not involve macromolecular interactions.

It may be estimated from the 9L cell volume (Deen and Hoshino, 1978) and the above considerations that cytotoxicity caused by 2-chloroethyl-

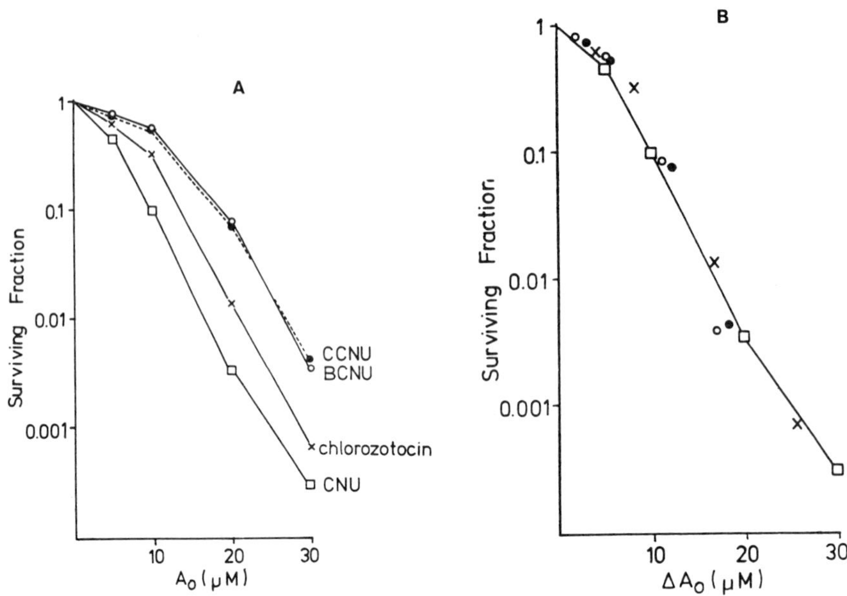

FIG. 3. Survival curves obtained from the incubation of L1210 cells with various initial concentrations, A_0, of BCNU, CCNU, chlorozotocin, and CNU for 60 minutes (A) and the same cell survival data plotted against the concentration of agents converted to chloroethylating species during the exposure interval (B). The half-lives of Table I may be used to show that 62, 55, 86, and 100% of these agents are activated in 60 minutes, respectively. There is no significant difference in the cytotoxic activity of these four agents (data from Kann, 1978).

ation involves an accumulation of between 2×10^6 alkylation events/cell at the lower limit of toxicity (<2% cells killed) and 25×10^6 events/cell for 99.9% cell kill (1 to 12×10^{-18} mole/cell). Approximately 10% of alkylation events lead to chloroethylation of cellular macromolecules (calculated from the data of Tew *et al.*, 1978, and Cheng *et al.*, 1972).

Chemical activation is also consistent with the observed synergistic effect of hyperthermia on chloroethylnitrosourea activity *in vivo* (Thuning *et al.*, 1980) and in cell culture (Twentyman *et al.*, 1978; Hahn, 1979; Weinkam and Dolan, 1982). The effect of temperature appears to be due to an increase in the rate of activation (Weinkam and Dolan, 1982).

As has been pointed out before (Drewinko *et al.*, 1979), many rapidly dividing cell lines are equally sensitive to the effects of chloroethylnitrosoureas. The ED_{90} values expressed as ΔA (μM) between 20 and 70 μM have been reported for L1210 mouse leukemia (Ewing and Kohn, 1977), EMT6 mouse mammary (Twentyman, 1978), 9L mouse brain tumor (Weinkam and Deen, 1982; Wheeler *et al.*, 1975), CHO hamster ovary

(Tobey and Cressman, 1975), HA1 hamster ovary (Hahn *et al.,* 1974), DON hamster fibroblast (Bhuyan *et al.,* 1972), and human colon carcinoma cells (Drewenko *et al.,* 1979).

It has been difficult to identify a target macromolecule that, following 2-chloroethylation, initiates the cytotoxic process, if indeed there is a single process. In view of the facts that toxicity results from low levels of alkylation and is common to a variety of cell lines, it is reasonable to believe that nucleic acids are target molecules. Cell toxicity could then result from DNA cross-linking (Kohn, 1977; Tong and Ludlum, 1981) or nucleic acid strand breaks (Erikson *et al.,* 1977; Hilton *et al.,* 1977) in a variety of cell types. As yet undiscovered membrane interactions or inactivation of sensitive enzymes could lead to cell death but these are less likely to be common features of several cell types or to be independent of the parent molecular structure.

Evidence has been obtained for several cytotoxic mechanisms that involve nucleic acids: (1) inhibition of DNA synthesis by the inhibition of nucleotidyl transferase (Wheeler and Bowden, 1968), (2) inhibition of DNA synthesis by the inhibition of DNA polymerase II (Baril *et al.,* 1975), (3) DNA cross-linking following 2-chloroethylation with subsequent displacement of the chloro group (Kohn, 1977; Thomas *et al.,* 1978; Ewig and Kohn, 1978; Lown and McLaughlin, 1979b; Tong and Ludlum, 1979, 1980), (4) regulation of ribosomal RNA synthesis and processing to inhibit protein synthesis and thus inhibit cell growth (Walker and Gehan, 1972; Penman *et al.,* 1976; Kann *et al.,* 1974a), (5) DNA strand breaks (Erickson *et al.,* 1977; Hilton *et al.,* 1977), and (6) inhibition of repair of DNA strand breaks (Kann *et al.,* 1974b; Erickson *et al.,* 1978a,b; Fornace *et al.,* 1978). It is not surprising that a wide range of biological effects is produced by these agents since the intermediates formed from chloroethylnitrosoureas are highly reactive and would therefore react nonselectively. The overall toxicity could be a summation of these effects but clarification of this point is complicated by the fact that these experiments, often for good technical reasons, are conducted at effective doses that are higher than that required to cause cytotoxicity.

The quantitative response of several lines of cultured cells measured as rapidly dividing asynchronous populations are similar, $\Delta A = 20\text{–}70\ \mu M$ at ED_{90}, with the exception of certain human cell lines with $\Delta A = 140\ \mu M$ at ED_{90} (Drewinko *et al.,* 1979; Erickson *et al.,* 1978b; Thomas *et al.,* 1978) and resistant L1210 leukemia (Wheeler *et al.,* 1980). The range of ΔA is comparable to the normal variation in assays using a single cell line (Weinkam and Deen, 1982) and those caused by periodic changes in serum used to supplement culture media (Hahn *et al.,* 1974). Rapidly dividing and stationary phase cells are equally sensitive for most cell types. This applies to EMT6 mouse mammary (Twentyman, 1978), mouse blastocytoma (Hegeman, 1973), HA1 hamster ovary (Hahn, 1974), hamster embryo (Thatcher and Walker, 1969), and human colon carcinoma (Drewinko *et al.*, 1979) and lymphoma cells (Drewinko *et al.*, 1976) while stationary phase CHO hamster ovary (Tobey and Chrissman, 1975) and L1210 mouse leukemia cells (Bhuyan *et al.*, 1972) are reported to be more sensitive to the effects of chloroethylnitrosoureas than are rapidly dividing cells. These drugs appear to be cell cycle nonspecific agents but there is evidence that they are more toxic at late G_1 or early S phases of hamster fibroblast or ovary cells (Bhuyan *et al.*, 1972; Barranco and Humphrey, 1971; Drewinko *et al.*, 1979); BCNU, CCNU, and MeCCNU cause arrest of cells in the G_1 phase of the cell cycle (Tobery and Chrissman, 1975). Progression through early phases was normal and the G_2 phase was slow (Tobey, 1975) which may indicate that DNA synthesis reaches completion (Bono, 1976). The ornithine decarboxylase inhibitor α-difluoromethylornithine, which inhibits polyamine biosynthesis, has a potentiating effect on the antitumor activity of BCNU (Marton *et al.*, 1981; Hung *et al.*, 1981).

VII. Biodisposition

The distribution of chloroethylnitrosoureas, particularly BCNU, CCNU, and MeCCNU, has many of the characteristics expected of chemically labile, lipophilic compounds. Distribution into all tissues occurs in the relatively short period that the parent drug circulates within the body (Wheeler *et al.*, 1965; Oliverio *et al.*, 1970; Levin *et al.*, 1978). Nevertheless, pharmacokinetic parameters and antitumor activity may be affected by specific interactions such as metabolism, protein binding catalyzed chemical degradation, and lipid partitioning so that each chloroethylnitrosourea analog has a unique biodistribution pattern.

The study of chloroethylnitrosourea pharmacokinetics has been complicated by the lack of chemically specific and sensitive analytical methods. Early studies using radioisotope-labeled analogs provided preliminary data in animals and man as summarized by Oliverio (1976). Interpretation of these data is complicated by the rapid rate at which these compounds are chemically converted to a variety of products, many of which have much longer half-lives than the parent drug. The thermal lability of chloroethylnitrosoureas makes gas chromatographic methods unsuitable. Liquid chromatography, which can be used to separate and quantify both parent drugs (Montgomery *et al.*, 1977b; Reed, 1975; Weinkam *et al.*, 1980a) and metabolites (Montgomery *et al.*, 1977b;

Lin and Weinkam, 1981), lacks the sensitivity required to measure circulating plasma concentrations following a therapeutic dose. Colorimetric analyses based upon conversion of the nitrosourea to nitrous acid have sensitivity near the required range but lack specificity (Loo and Dion, 1965) as do polarographic methods (Bartosek *et al.*, 1978). Direct sample insertion chemical ionization mass spectrometry has been used in a pharmacokinetic study of BCNU but is not suited for use with other analogs (Weinkam *et al.*, 1978). Recently, however, a gas chromatographic method based on conversion of chloroethylnitrosoureas to methylcarbamates has been found to be suitable for pharmacokinetic studies and may be used for the analysis of BCNU, CCNU, MeCCNU, PCNU, ACNU, and hydroxylated CCNU metabolites (Weinkam and Liu, 1982).

The biodisposition of the lipophilic nitrosoureas has been studied most frequently, although only BCNU has been investigated in detail. BCNU and CCNU are distributed throughout the body (Oliverio *et al.*, 1970; DeVita *et al.*, 1967; Levin *et al.*, 1978a; Castronovo *et al.*, 1980). Both drugs appear in the CSF immediately after iv administration (Oliverio, 1976; Walker and Hilton, 1976), however both the parent drug and the biological activity are rapidly lost. The half-life for intact BCNU in plasma is less than 5 minutes in dogs, monkeys, and man (DeVita *et al.*, 1967) and 15 minutes for CCNU (Oliverio *et al.*, 1970; Hilton and Walker, 1975). The biological half-life of BCNU activity against L1210 cells in mice is between 15 and 30 minutes while the half life of CCNU extends up to 90 min (Chirigos *et al.*, 1965; Klein *et al.*, 1968).

The pharmacokinetic parameters of BCNU have been determined in normal and phenobarbital-pretreated rats following iv and ip administration (Levin *et al.*, 1979). Peak plasma concentrations of 10 μg/ml were obtained after 14 mg/kg iv doses. The clearance of BCNU in phenobarbital-pretreated animals was significantly greater than normal. This was especially true following ip administration, where induction resulted in a 90% decrease in area under the plasma clearance curve, 206 $\pm$ 106 to 20 $\pm$ 23 μg minute-kg. Significantly, induction also produced a 100% reduction in BCNU activity against ic 9L tumors, T/C $\times$ 100 for 14 mg/kg ip drops from 213 to 100 (Levin *et al.*, 1979). This effect was correlated with an increase in the rate of *in vitro* rat liver homogenate metabolism (Levin *et al.*, 1979) which leads almost exclusively to the formation of the inactive metabolite, 1,3-bis(2-chloroethyl)urea (BCU) (Lin and Weinkam, 1981). Hill and co-workers have reported this same reaction in mouse (Hill *et al.*, 1975; Hill, 1976).

The pharmacokinetics of BCNU plasma clearance has also been studied in man (Levin *et al.*, 1978b). Peak plasma concentrations of 1 to 5 μg/ml were observed after an average dose of 95 mg/m^2 via a 40-minute infusion.

The initial rapid elimination phase was complete within 10 minutes to give plasma concentrations of less than 0.5 μg/ml which were then cleared in a slow phase extending up to 3 hours. The rapid disappearance of BCNU appears to be due to a combination of partitioning into tissue lipids, as expected for a lipophilic drug, and chemical decomposition in serum. BCNU is much less stable in plasma, $t_{1/2}$ 12 to 15 minutes, than in aqueous solution at pH 7.4, 37°C, $t_{1/2}$ 50 minutes (Levin *et al.*, 1978b).

Large interindividual variations in BCNU plasma concentration and clearance were observed within this patient population that could not be explained by differences in body weight, fat, or blood flow. There is as yet no evidence that BCNU is metabolically deactivated in man but the possible deleterious interaction with phenobarbital remains a significant question as a large fraction of brain tumor patients are treated with this agent prior to BCNU chemotherapy.

CCNU clearance curves have been reported in rats following a 30 mg/kg iv dose (Hilton and Walker, 1975). A peak plasma concentration of 70 μg/ml decays to 15 μg/ml in 10 minutes and this concentration is slowly cleared by 60 minutes. A similar clearance pattern was observed using radiolabeled CCNU (Oliverio *et al.*, 1970). CCNU is removed from plasma as rapidly as BCNU but a major CCNU clearance pathway appears to involve metabolic hydroxylation of the cyclohexyl group (May *et al.*, 1974; Hill *et al.*, 1975; Hilton and Walker, 1975) to give products that retain antitumor properties (Johnston *et al.*, 1975). Radioactivity from labeled CCNU and MeCCNU appeared in patient plasma within 10 minutes of a 30 to 100 mg/kg oral dose although intact drug could not be detected (Sponzo *et al.*, 1973).

PCNU plasma clearance has also been determined in man (Levin *et al.*, 1981) and rats following 22.5 mg/kg iv doses (Weinkam and Liu, 1980). Peak plasma concentrations of 20 to 50 μg/ml were observed to fall to 5 μg/ml in 10 minutes. Slow clearance proceeded to eliminate the drug by 3.5 hours.

The clearances of BCNU, CCNU, and PCNU are similar (Levin *et al.*, 1981), however, chloroethylnitrosoureas are not biologically active molecules so that comparable pharmacokinetics does not imply comparable antitumor activity. It is clear that the parent chloroethylnitrosourea must distribute to the tumor locus and therefore the drug must be present in plasma at a concentration and duration sufficient to permit this to occur. As pointed out by Levin (1980), physical properties of the drug, lipophilicity, and size, as well as characteristics of the tumor, size, vascularization, blood flow, and capillary permeability, will determine the amount of drug reaching the tumor from a given plasma concentration.

The antitumor activity resulting from the drug that enters the tumor will be related to the rate at which the agent is converted to active chloroethylating intermediate. Studies with 9L tumor and other tissue homogenate 100,000 *g* supernate fractions indicate that this rate is comparable to the decomposition rate in aqueous buffer for BCNU, CCNU, and PCNU (Weinkam, unpublished).

Antitumor activity is, therefore, determined by a balance between the high plasma concentrations and the slow clearance required for diffusion into the tumor and rapid conversion and consequent short life time required to generate active intermediate. Antitumor activity is also determined by the many chemicobiological interactions that affect the fate of chloroethylnitrosoureas outside of the tumor. These include tissue distribution and protein binding (Oliverio *et al.*, 1970), which are known pharmacokinetic factors. There is little evidence that intact lipophilic chloroethylnitrosoureas are excreted although this might be a factor for water-soluble analogs. Metabolism and serum-catalyzed reactions discussed below may influence antitumor activity.

BCNU, as well as MNU (Hill *et al.*, 1975), MNNG (Sugimura *et al.*, 1973), and 1-*n*-butyl-1-nitrosourea (Hashimoto and Tada, 1973), are metabolically denitrosated *in vitro* by liver homogenate preparations (Hill *et al.*, 1975; Hill, 1976; Lin and Weinkam, 1980). In mouse liver microsomal metabolism, this NADPH dependent reaction, K_m 1.7 mM, V_{max} 0.4 nM/mg/minute, is inhibited by carbon monoxide and BCNU was found to inhibit nicotine oxidation, K_i 0.15 mM. This suggests that denitrosation reaction is catalyzed by cytochrome P-450 (Hill *et al.*, 1975). In rat liver 9000 *g* supernate metabolism, BCNU disappearance, K_m 0.6 mM, V_{max} 1.7 nM/mg/minute, is enhanced by phenobarbital pretreatment, K_m 0.6 mM, V_{max} 4.2 nM/mg/minute (Levin *et al.*, 1979). The metabolic product, BCU, is formed at a rate, 54 ± 23 nM/mg/10 minutes, that is comparable to the rate of BCNU disappearance, 56 ± 11 nM/mg/10 minutes, while BCU is subject to further metabolism, 32 nM/mg/10 minutes (Lin and Weinkam, 1981). The increased rate of BCNU metabolism induced by phenobarbital administration in rats is sufficient to significantly increase BCNU clearance and reduce antitumor activity (Levin *et al.*, 1979).

Evidence has been presented that BCNU is a substrate for glutathione-S-transferase in mouse liver homogenate. At optimum conditions, the reaction has a K_m 0.6 mM and V_{max} 0.8 nM/mg/minute. Product analysis by field desorption mass spectrometry gave m/e = 532 and 534 suggesting the structure, $K_2GSCH_2CH_2NHCONHCH_2CH_2Cl$ (Hill, 1976). This reaction was not observed in rat liver preparations, however (Lin, 1980).

In the mouse, the liver was the primary site of metabolism; lung tissue homogenate had 30% of the activity of liver and no significant activity was detected in kidney, spleen, brain, muscle or intestine (Hill, 1976). BCNU metabolites formed *in vivo* have not been identified and BCU was not present in the urine of patients following BCNU therapy (Lin and Weinkam, 1981). These results indicate that BCNU is a substrate for hepatic denitrosation. The rate of this deactivation reaction, at least in phenobarbital-induced animals, may be competitive with chemical degradation *in vivo* and may significantly reduce the antitumor activity of this chloroethylnitrosourea analog.

CCNU, in contrast to BCNU, is metabolized solely by hydroxylation on the cyclohexyl ring (May *et al.*, 1974; Hill *et al.*, 1975; Hilton and Walker, 1975). The *in vitro* rat liver microsomal reaction is dependent on O_2 and NADPH (May *et al.*, 1974) and may be induced by phenobarbital pretreatment but not by 3-methylcholanthrene (Reed and May, 1975). Normal rat microsomal metabolism of CCNU has K_m 0.4 mM, V_{max} 43 nM/mg/minute which is increased by phenobarbital induction to K_m 0.24 mM, V_{max} 68 nM/mg/minute (Hilton and Walker, 1975). CCNU also gives a type I cytochrome P-450 binding spectrum, K_S 40 μM, that is similar to that of cyclohexane, K_S 740 μM (May *et al.*, 1974) suggesting, along with the above information, that CCNU as well as BCNU is a cytochrome P-450 substrate. This is further supported by the observation that BCNU inhibits CCNU metabolism *in vitro* (Lin and Weinkam, 1981).

All of the CCNU metabolites formed in microsomal incubations are products of monohydroxylation on the cyclohexane ring. Five of the six possible axial and equatorial isomers have been identified (May *et al.*, 1974, 1975; Hilton and Walker, 1975b; Montgomery *et al.*, 1977b). There is some disagreement about the distribution of products but 77% of metabolized CCNU has been identified as *cis*-4-hydroxy, 53%; *trans*-4-hydroxy, 3%; *cis*-3-hydroxy, trace; *trans*-3-hydroxy, 30%; and *trans*-2-hydroxy, 14% (Hilton and Walker, 1975b). Phenobarbital pretreatment changes the distribution of CCNU hydroxylation with increases primarily in the *cis*-4-hydroxy and *trans*-4-hydroxy metabolites so that *cis*-4-hydroxy CCNU accounts for 77% while *trans*-3-hydroxy CCNU is 11% of products (May *et al.*, 1975; Reed and May, 1975). Deuteration of the cyclohexyl ring also changes the distribution of hydroxylation (Farmer *et al.*, 1978).

Ring hydroxylated products are also formed *in vivo* in rats and man. Metabolites isolated from plasma 20 minutes after administration of 5 mg CCNU/kg to rats were *cis*-4-hydroxy, 54%; *trans*-4-hydroxy, 8%, *cis*-3-hydroxy, 4%; *trans*-3-hydroxy, 23%; and *trans*-2-hydroxy, 8%. During this period, 96% of the CCNU was metabolized (Hilton and Walker,

1975b). In addition to ring hydroxylation, thioacetic acid has been identified as a major urinary product from [^{14}C]chloroethyl-CCNU (Reed and May, 1975). Phenobarbital also altered the distribution of hydroxylated metabolites *in vivo*. Two minutes after CCNU administration, *cis*-4-hydroxy CCNU was the major metabolite, 62%, along with significant amounts of *trans*-3-hydroxy CCNU, 21% (Hilton and Walker, 1975). Only *cis*-4-hydroxy and *trans*-4-hydroxy CCNU were isolated from human plasma (Hilton and Walker, 1975b).

CCNU is rapidly metabolized to hydroxylated products that retain the chloroethylnitrosourea group intact. As a consequence, much of the observed CCNU antitumor activity may be due to its metabolites (Wheeler *et al.*, 1977). The hydroxylated CCNU metabolites have been synthesized (Johnston *et al.*, 1975) and the antitumor activity was found to be comparable to CCNU itself (Wheeler *et al.*, 1977; Heal *et al.*, 1978). These results are consistent with the fact that no decrease in CCNU antitumor activity was observed following phenobarbital pretreatment (Levin *et al.*, 1979).

MeCCNU is metabolized by ring hydroxylation as well as by denitrosation although MeCCNU metabolism in mouse liver homognates is much slower than CCNU metabolism (Hill *et al.*, 1975). Hydroxylation occurs on the methyl group, 34% on the cyclohexyl ring, 20% at the cis and trans-3 and cis-4 positions, and on the 2-chloroethyl moiety, 0.5% as well as by denitrosation 24%. The rate of ring hydroxylation was enhanced by phenobarbital pretreatment (Reed and May, 1978; May *et al.*, 1979). Chemical, physical, and metabolic properties of some chloroethylnitrosoureas are listed in Table I.

TABLE I

CHEMICAL AND CHEMICOBIOLOGICAL PROPERTIES OF CHLOROETHYLNITROSOUREA ANTITUMOR AGENTS

Compound	$t_{1/2}$(min)[a]	log P (octanol/water)	$t_{1/2}$(serum, min)[a]	Metabolism D-denitrosation H-hydroxylation
CNU	5	—	—	—
BCNU	49	1.5	14	D
CCNU	53	2.8	34	H
MeCCNU	60	3.3	22	D/H
PCNU	26	0.37	27	D
ACNU	34–75	0.39	—	—
Chlorozotocin	21	−1.02	—	—

[a] Half-life measured at pH 7.4, 37°C in aqueous buffer or human serum.

VIII. Chemicobiological Interactions

The metabolism studies of BCNU and CCNU suggest that chloroethylnitrosoureas may be susceptible to alternative cytochrome P-450 catalyzed reactions. Metabolic denitrosation and consequent deactivation appears to be a slow reaction that will occur, especially in phenobarbital-induced animals, if other more facile reactions are not possible. The cyclohexyl group of CCNU appears to serve as a site of hydroxylation that leads to the formation of biologically active metabolites. The addition of the methyl group in MeCCNU blocks the favored site of hydroxylation and switches metabolism toward denitrosation and deactivation (May *et al.*, 1979). Other chloroethylnitrosourea analogs may also be substrates for cytochrome P-450 denitrosation as indicated by the decrease in PCNU antitumor activity following phenobarbital induction (Levin *et al.*, 1979).

Chloroethylnitrosoureas are also subject to protein binding catalyzed chemical degradation (Weinkam *et al.*, 1980b). The increased rate of reaction of BCNU, CCNU, and MeCCNU in serum has been related to isolated serum protein fractions and purified albumin-catalyzed reactions. This reaction may be saturated at high drug concentrations, 1 to 1 mole ratio, and the catalysis may be inhibited by highly protein bound agents such as salicyclic acid and dodecanoic acid. Covalent binding of [^{14}C]ethylene-BCNU reaction products to albumin is very efficient and only reaction products derived from 2-chloroethylazohydroxide and isocyanate could be detected. PCNU is not subject to protein catalyzed reaction which may be due in part to less than optimal lipophilicity or to structurally related binding interactions. Since the serum reaction rates are comparable to clearance and metabolism rates, it appears that this affects the antitumor activity and toxicity of lipophilic chloroethylnitrosoureas by causing a significant fraction of these agents to react to active intermediates in serum rather than at the tumor locus. Drugs that bind strongly to proteins may also alter the pharmacologic effects of these agents, but this has not been investigated.

Protein-catalyzed degradation of lipophilic chloroethylnitrosoureas is also inhibited by normal concentrations of serum lipoproteins (Weinkam *et al.*, 1980a) and phospholipids (Maker *et al.*, 1978). In this case, inhibition is caused by partitioning of the chloroethylnitrosourea into serum lipids. MeCCNU, the most lipophilic analog, is most strongly affected by this interaction while the stability of PCNU is unchanged by alterations in lipoprotein concentrations. Partitioning of lipophilic chloroethylnitrosoureas into lipoproteins and normal variations in lipoprotein levels may influence the biodisposition of these agents.

IX. Conclusion

The high antitumor activity and continued clinical success that chloroethylnitrosoureas possess have stimulated continuing efforts to develop new analogs and to understand the pharmacologic activity and biodistribution of commonly used agents such as BCNU and CCNU. New chloroethylnitrosourea analogs with good antitumor activity and occasionally with reduced toxicity have been synthesized. Quantitative structure–activity relationships have not proven to be successful predictors of antitumor activity. Neither lipophilicity, alkylating activity, carbamoylating activity, nor chemical reactivity consistently correlates with *in vivo* antitumor activity. The rather unpredictable influence of structure on activity is apparently due to specific interactions that influence the biodistribution and chemical activation of these agents.

Chemical studies show that the 2-chloroethylnitrosoureas are converted to 2-chloroethylazohydroxide or diazonium ions in aqueous solution. This species is formed in apparently high yield from all of the analogs of this class although the rates of reaction differ. This alkylating species is apparently responsible for cytotoxic activity through macromolecular alkylation including DNA cross-linking. No convincing evidence has been reported for any significant activity of the associated chemical degradation products, alkylisocyanates, at cytotoxic doses. The activities of a wide range of chloroethylnitrosoureas in cell culture are identical when related to the amount of 2-chloroethylalkylating intermediate generated during exposure of cells.

In spite of the identical activity in cell culture, these compounds display a wide range of activities *in vivo*. Several factors have been identified that control biodistribution. Lipophilicity is, of course, a major factor influencing absorption and distribution from plasma to the tumor locus. In addition, chloroethylnitrosoureas are subject to two competitive cytochrome P-450 metabolic pathways: deactivating denitrosation and hydroxylation that generates products retaining antitumor activity. The metabolic pathway depends on the substituents on the N-3 position of the 1-(2-chloroethyl)- 1-nitrosourea moiety. Some analogs are also decomposed through a serum protein-catalyzed chemical degradation reaction and lipophilic analogs may partition into serum lipoproteins to a significant extent. The rate of chemical reaction to active alkylating intermediate would also determine antitumor activity. These factors, which are summarized in Scheme 5, and presumably others as yet undiscovered, influence biodistribution and activity in a manner that would not be predictable using quantitative structure–activity methods.

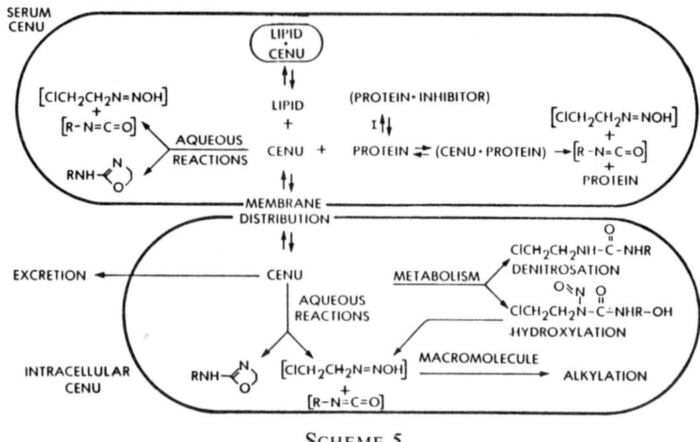

SCHEME 5.

REFERENCES

Almquist, R. G., and Reist, E. J. (1977). *J. Med. Chem.* **20,** 1246–1250.

Anderson, T., McMenamin, M., and Schein, P. S. (1975). *Cancer Res.* **35,** 761–765.

Applequist, D. E., and McGrier, D. E. (1960). *J. Am. Chem. Soc.* **82,** 1965–1969.

Arakawa, M., and Shimizo, F. (1975). *Gann* **66,** 149–154.

Babson, J. R., and Reed, D. J. (1978). *Biochem. Pharmacol.* **83,** 754–757.

Bakay, L. (1970). *Brain* **93,** 699–706.

Baril, B. E., Baril, E. F., Laszlo, J., and Wheeler, G. P. (1975). *Cancer Res.* **35,** 1–5.

Barranco, S. C., and Humphrey, R. M. (1971). *Cancer Res.* **31,** 191–195.

Bartosek, I., Daniel, S., and Sykara, S. (1978). *J. Pharm. Sci.* **67,** 1160–1163.

Behr, L. C. (1962). *In* "The Chemistry of Heterocyclic Compounds" (R. H. Wiley, ed.), pp. 235–244. Wiley, New York.

Bertrand, M., Deen, D. F., Hoshino, T., and Knebel, K. (1980). *Cancer Treat. Rep.,* in press.

Bhuyan, B. K., Scheidt, L. G., and Fraser, T. J. (1972). *Cancer Res.* **32,** 398–407.

Boivin, J. L., and Boivin, P. A. (1951). *Can. J. Chem.* **29,** 478–482.

Bollinger, F. W., Hayes, F. N., and Siegel, S. (1950). *J. Am. Chem. Soc.* **72,** 5592–5596.

Bono, V. H. (1976). *Cancer Treat. Rep.* **60,** 699–702.

Bowdon, B. J., and Wheeler, G. P. (1971). *Proc. Am. Assoc. Cancer Res.* **12,** 67.

Bray, D. A., DeVita, V. T., Adamson, R. H., and Oliverio, V. T. (1971). *Cancer Chemother. Rep.* **55,** 215–220.

Brodie, A. E., Babson, J. R., and Reed, D. J. (1980). *Biochem. Pharmacol.* **29,** 652–654.

Brundrett, R. B., and Colvin, M. (1977). *J. Org. Chem.* **42,** 3538–3541.

Brundrett, R. B., Cowens, J. W., Colvin, M., and Jardin, I. (1976). *J. Med. Chem.* **19,** 958–961.

Brundrett, R. B., Colvin, M., White, E. H., McKee, J., Hartman, P. E., and Brown, D. L. (1979). *Cancer Res.* **39,** 1328–1333.

Carter, S. K., Schabel, F. M., Broder, L. E., and Johnston, T. P. (1972). *Adv. Cancer Res.* **16,** 273–332.

Castronovo, F. P., Potsaid, M. S., and Kpiwada, S. (1980). *Cancer Res.* **40,** 3473–3476.

Chatterji, D. C., Greene, R. F., and Gallelli, J. F. (1978). *J. Pharm. Sci.* 1527–1532.

Cheng, C. J., Jujimura, S., and Grunberger, D. (1972). *Cancer Res.* **32,** 22–27.
Chirigos, M. A., Humphres, S. R., and Goldin, A. (1965). *Cancer Chemother. Rep.* **49,** 15–19.
Colvin, M., Cowens, J. W., Brundrett, R. B., Kramer, B. S., and Ludlum, D. B. (1974). *Biochem. Biophys. Res. Commun.* **60,** 515–520.
Colvin, M., Brundrett, R. B., Cowens, W., Jardin, I., and Ludlum, D. B. (1976). *Biochem. Pharmacol.* **25,** 695–699.
Conners, T. A., and Have, J. R. (1974). *Br. J. Cancer* **30,** 477–481.
Crider, A. M., Lu, C. K. L., Floss, H. G., Cassady, J. M., and Clemens, J. A. (1979). *J. Med. Chem.* **22,** 32–35.
Crider, A. M., Kolezynski, T. M., and Yates, K. M. (1980a). *J. Med. Chem.* **23,** 324–326.
Crider, A. M., Lamey, R., Floss, H. G., Cassady, J. M., and Bradner, W. J. (1980b). *J. Med. Chem.* **23,** 848–851.
Deen, D. F., and Hoshino, T. (1978). *Am. Lab.* **10,** 115–119.
DeVita, V. T., Denham, C., Davidson, J. D., and Oliverio, V. T. (1967). *Clin. Pharmacol. Ther.* **8,** 566–577.
Drewinko, B., Loo, T. L., and Gottlieb, J. A. (1976). *Cancer Res.* **36,** 511–515.
Drewinko, B., Barlogie, B., and Freireich, E. J. (1979). *Cancer Res.* **39,** 2630–2636.
Erickson, L. C., Bradley, M. O., and Kohn, K. W. (1977). *Cancer Res.* **37,** 3744–3750.
Erickson, L. C., Bradley, M. O., and Kohn, K. W. (1978a). *Cancer Res.* **38,** 672–677.
Erickson, L. C., Osieka, R., and Kohn, K. W. (1978b). *Cancer Res.* **38,** 802–808.
Ewig, R. A., and Kohn, K. W. (1977). *Cancer Res.* **37,** 2114–2122.
Ewig, R. A., and Kohn, K. W. (1978). *Cancer Res.* **38,** 3197–3203.
Farmer, P. B., Foster, A. B., Jarman, M., Oddy, M. R., and Reed, D. J. (1978). *J. Med. Chem.* **21,** 514–516.
Fiebig, H. H., Eisenbrand, G., Zeller, W. J., and Deutsch-Wenzel, T. (1977). *Eur. J. Cancer* **13,** 937–945.
Fornance, A. J., Kohn, K. W., and Kann, H. E. (1978). *Cancer Res.* **38,** 1064–1069.
Fox, P. A., Panasci, L. C., and Schein, P. S. (1977). *Cancer Res.* **37,** 783–787.
Friedman, O. M., and Boger, E. (1961). *Anal. Chem.* **33,** 906–910.
Garrett, E. R. (1960). *J. Am. Assoc. Sci. Ed.* **49,** 767–769.
Garrett, E. R., Goto, S., and Stubbins, J. F. (1965). *J. Pharm. Sci.* **54,** 119–122.
Greene, M. O., and Greenberg, J. (1960). *J. Cancer Res.* **20,** 1166–1170.
Gutsche, C. D., and Johnson, H. E. (1955). *J. Am. Chem. Soc.* **77,** 109–113.
Hagemann, R. F., Schenken, L. L., and Lesher, S. (1973). *J. Natl. Cancer Inst.* **50,** 467–474.
Hahn, G. (1979). *Cancer Res.* **39,** 2264–2268.
Hahn, G. M., Gordon, L. F., and Kukjiam, S. D. (1974). *Cancer Res.* **34,** 2373–2377.
Hansch, C., Smith, N., Engle, R., and Wood, H. (1972). *Cancer Chemother. Rep.* **56,** 443–456.
Hansch, C., Leo, A., Schmidt, C., and Jow, P. U. C. (1980). *J. Med. Chem.* **23,** 1095–1101.
Hardegger, E., Meier, A., and Stoos, A. (1969). *Helv. Chem. Acta* **52,** 2555–2265.
Hashimoto, Y., and Tada, K. (1973). *In* "Topics of Chemical Carcinogenesis" (W. Nakahara, S. Takayama, T. S. Sugimura, and S. Odashama, eds.), pp. 501–509. University Park Press, Baltimore.
Heal, J. M., Fox, P. A., Dowkas, D., and Schein, P. S. (1978). *Cancer Res.* **38,** 1070–1074.
Heal, J. M., Fox, P., and Schein, P. S. (1979). *Biochem. Pharmacol.* **28,** 1301–1306.
Hecht, S. M., and Kozarich, J. W. (1973). *J. Org. Chem.* **38,** 182–186.
Herr, R. R., Eble, T. E., Bergy, M. E., and Jahnke, H. K. (1960). *Antibiot. Annu.* 1959–1960, 236–240.
Herr, R. R., Jahnke, H. K., and Arguodelis, A. D. (1967). *J. Am. Chem. Soc.* **89,** 4808–4809.

Hill, D. L. (1976). *Proc. Am. Assoc. Cancer Res.* **17,** 52.

Hill, D. L., Kirk, M. C., and Struck, R. F. (1975). *Cancer Res.* **35,** 296–301.

Hilton, J., and Walker, M. D. (1975a). *Biochem. Pharmacol.* **24,** 2153–2158.

Hilton, J., and Walker, M. D. (1975b). *Proc. Am. Assoc. Cancer Res.* **16,** 103.

Hilton, J., Bowie, D. L., Gutin, P. H., Zito, D. M., and Walker, M. D. (1977). *Cancer Res.* **37,** 2262–2266.

Hilton, J., Maldarelli, F., and Sargent, S. (1978). *Biochem. Pharmacol.* **27,** 1359–1363.

Hung, D. T., Deen, D. F., Seidenfeld, J., and Marton, L. J. (1981). *Cancer Res.* **41,** 2783–2785.

Johnston, T. P., and Opliger, P. S. (1967). *J. Med. Chem.* **10,** 675–681.

Johnston, T. P., McCaleb, G. S., and Montgomery, J. A. (1963). *J. Med. Chem.* **6,** 669–681.

Johnston, T. P., McCaleb, G. S., Opliger, P. S., and Montgomery, J. A. (1966). *J. Med. Chem.* **9,** 892–911.

Johnston, T. P., McCaleb, G. S., Opliger, P. S., and Montgomery, J. A. (1971). *J. Med. Chem.* **14,** 600–614.

Johnston, T. P., McCaleb, G. S., and Montgomery, J. (1975). *J. Med. Chem.* **18,** 634–637.

Johnston, T. P., McCaleb, G. S., Clayton, S. D., Frye, J. L., Krauth, C. A., and Montgomery, J. A. (1977). *J. Med. Chem.* **20,** 279–290.

Jones, W. M., and Muck, D. L. (1966). *J. Am. Chem. Soc.* **88,** 3798–3803.

Jones, W. M., Muck, D. L., and Tandy, T. K. (1966). *J. Am. Chem. Soc.* **88,** 68–74.

Kamiya, S., Miyahara, M., Saeyoshi, S., Suzuki, J., and Odashima, S. (1978). *Chem. Pharm. Bull.* **26,** 3884–3888.

Kann, H. E. (1978). *Cancer Res.* **38,** 2363–2366.

Kann, H. E., Kohn, K. W., and Widerlite, L. (1974a). *Cancer Res.* **34,** 1982–1988.

Kann, H. E., Kohn, K. W., and Lyles, J. M. (1974b). *Cancer Res.* **34,** 398–402.

Kann, H. E., Schott, M. A., and Petkas, A. (1980). *Cancer Res.* **40,** 50–55.

Klein, I., Gang, M., and Tyrer, D. D. (1968). *Chemotherapy* **13,** 28–41.

Kohn, K. W. (1977). *Cancer Res.* **37,** 1450–1454.

Kramer, B. S., Fenselau, C. C., and Ludlum, D. B. (1974). *Biochem. Biophys. Res. Commun.* **56,** 783–788.

Lam, H.-Y. P., Begleiter, A., Goldenberg, G. J., and Wong, C.-M. (1979). *J. Med. Chem.* **22,** 200–202.

Larnicol, N., Auggery, Y., Jasmin, C., Montero, J. L., and Imbach, J. L. (1977). *Biomedicine* **26,** 176–181.

Lasker, P. A., and Ayres, J. W. (1977). *J. Pharm. Sci.* **66,** 1073–1078.

Lawley, P. D., and Shah, S. A. (1973). *Chem.-Biol. Interact.* **7,** 115–119.

Lawley, P. D., and Warren, W. (1975). *Chem.-Biol. Interact.* **11,** 55–59.

Levin, V. A. (1980). *J. Med. Chem.* **23,** 682–684.

Levin, V. A., and Kabra, P. (1974). *Cancer Chemother. Rep.* **58,** 787–792.

Levin, V. A., Kabra, P. M., and Freeman-Dove, M. A. (1978a). *Cancer Chemother. Pharmacol.* **1,** 233–242.

Levin, V. A., Hoffman, W., and Weinkam, R. J. (1978b). *Cancer Treat. Rep.* **62,** 1305–1312.

Levin, V. A., Stearns, J., Byrd, A., Finn, A., and Weinkam, R. J. (1979). *J. Pharmacol. Exp. Ther.* **208,** 1–6.

Levin, V. A., Liu, J., and Weinkam, R. J. (1981). *Cancer Res.* **41,** 3475–3477.

Lewis, C., and Barbiers, A. R. (1960). *Antibiot. Annu.* 1959–1960, 247–253.

Lijinsky, W., Garcia, H., Keifer, L., Loo, J., and Ross, A. E. (1972). *Cancer Res.* **32,** 893–898.

Lin, H.-S. (1979). Ph.D. Dissertation, School of Pharmacy, University of California, San Francisco.

Lin, H.-S., and Weinkam, R. J. (1981). *J. Med. Chem.* **24,** 761–763.
Lin, T. S., Fischer, P. H., Shiau, G. T., and Prusoff, W. H. (1978). *J. Med. Chem.* **21,** 130–133.
Lin, T.-S., Shiau, G. T., and Prusoff, W. H. (1980). *J. Med. Chem.* **23,** 1440–1442.
Loo, T. L., and Dion, R. L. (1965). *J. Pharm. Sci.* **54,** 809–810.
Loo, T. L., Dion, R. L., Dixon, R. L., and Rall, D. P. (1966). *J. Pharm. Sci.* **55,** 492–500.
Lown, J. W., and McLaughlin, L. W. (1979a). *Biochem. Pharmacol.* **28,** 2123–2128.
Lown, J. W., and McLaughlin, L. W. (1979b). *Biochem. Pharmacol.* **28,** 2115–2121.
Ludlum, D. B., Kramer, B. S., Wong, J., and Fensilau, C. C. (1975). *Biochemistry* **14,** 5480–5484.
McKay, A. F., and Wright, G. F. (1947). *J. Am. Chem. Soc.* **69,** 3028–3032.
Magee, P. N., and Barnes, J. M. (1967). *Adv. Cancer Res.* **10,** 163–185.
Maker, H. S., Syral, H. H., and Lehrer, G. M. (1978). *J. Natl. Cancer Inst.* **60,** 1055–1059.
Marton, L. J., Levin, V. A., Hervatin, S. J., Koch-Weser, J., McCann, P. P., and Sjoerdsma, A. (1981). *Cancer Res.* **41,** 4426–4431.
May, H. E., Boose, R., and Reed, D. J. (1974). *Biochem. Biophys. Res. Commun.* **57,** 426–433.
May, H. E., Boose, R., and Reed, D. J. (1975). *Biochemistry* **14,** 4723–4727.
May, H. E., Kohlhepp, S. J., Boose, R. B., and Reed, D. J. (1979). *Cancer Res.* **39,** 762–772.
Michejda, C. J., and Koepke, S. R. (1978). *J. Am. Chem. Soc.* **100,** 1959–1960.
Montero, J. L., Moruzzi, A., Oiry, J., and Imbach, J. L. (1977). *Eur. J. Med. Chem.* **12,** 397–401.
Montgomery, J. A. (1976). *Cancer Treat. Rep.* **60,** 651–664.
Montgomery, J. A., James, R., McCaleb, G. S., and Johnston, T. P. (1967). *J. Med. Chem.* **10,** 668–672.
Montgomery, J. A., Mayo, J. G., and Hansch, C. (1974). *J. Med. Chem.* **17,** 477–480.
Montgomery, J. A., James, R., McCaleb, G. S., Kirk, M. C., and Johnston, T. P. (1975). *J. Med. Chem.* **18,** 586–590.
Montgomery, J. A., McCaleb, G. S., Johnston, T. P., Mayo, J. G., and Laster, W. R. (1977a). *J. Med. Chem.* **20,** 291–295.
Montgomery, J. A., Johnston, T. P., Thomas, H. J., Piper, J. R., and Temple, C. (1977b). *Adv. Chromatogr.* **15,** 169–195.
Mori, K. J., Jasmin, C., Hayat, M., MacDonald, J. S., and Mathe, G. (1980). *Cancer Res.* **40,** 4282–4286.
Muck, D. L., and Jones, W. M. (1966). *J. Am. Chem. Soc.* **88,** 74–77.
Nagourney, R. A., Fox, P. A., and Schein, P. S. (1978). *Cancer Res.* **38,** 65–68.
Oliverio, V. T. (1976). *Cancer Treat. Rep.* **60,** 703–707.
Oliverio, V. T., Vietzke, W. M., Williams, M. K., and Adamson, R. H. (1970). *Cancer Res.* **30,** 1330–1337.
Panasci, L. C., Green, D., Nagourney, R., Fox, P., and Schein, P. S. (1977). *Cancer Res.* **37,** 2615–2618.
Penman, M., Huffman, P., and Kumar, A. (1976). *Biochemistry* **15,** 2661–2665.
Reed, D. J., and May, H. E. (1975). *Life Sci.* **16,** 1263–1270.
Reed, D. J., and May, H. E. (1978). *Biochemistry* **60,** 989–995.
Reed, D. J., May, H. E., Boose, R. B., Gregory, K. M., and Beilstein, M. A. (1975). *Cancer Res.* **35,** 568–572.
Schabel, F. M. (1976). *Cancer Treat. Rep.* **60,** 665–699.
Schabel, F. M., Johnston, T. P., McCaleb, G. S., Montgomery, J. A., Laster, W. R., and Skipper, H. E. (1963). *Cancer Res.* **23,** 725–733.

Schein, P. S., McMennamin, M. G., and Anderson, T. (1973). *Cancer Res.* **33,** 2005–2009.
Schmall, B., Cheng, C. J., Fujimura, S., Gersten, N., Greenberger, D., and Weinstein, B. (1973). *Cancer Res.* **33,** 1921–1924.
Skinner, W. A., Gram, H. F., Greene, M. O., Greenberg, J., and Baker, B. R. (1960). *J. Med. Pharm. Chem.* **2,** 299–304.
Skipper, H. E., Schabel, F. M., Trader, M. W., and Thompson, J. R. (1961). *Cancer Res.* **21,** 1154–1164.
Sponso, R. W., DeVita, V. T., and Oliverio, V. T. (1973). *Cancer* **31,** 1154–1159.
Stewart, D. J., Benjamen, B. S., Leavens, M., Valdivie, S. M., Burgess, M. A., and Bodey, G. P. (1980). *Cancer Res.* **40,** 3750–3754.
Streitwieser, A., and Schaeffer, B. (1957). *J. Am. Chem. Soc.* 2288–2294.
Sugimura, T., Nagao, M., and Okada, Y. (1966). *Nature (London)* **210,** 962–963.
Sugimura, T., Tawachi, T., Kogure, K., Nagao, M., Tanaka, N., Fugimura, S., Takayama, S., Shimosata, Y., Naguchi, M., Kuwabara, N., and Yomada, T. (1973). *In* "Topics in Chemical Carcinogenesis" (W. Nakahara, S. Takayama, T. Sugimura, and S. Odashima, eds.), pp. 105–117. University Park Press, Baltimore.
Süssmuth, R., Haerlin, R., and Lingens, F. (1972). *Biochem. Biophys. Acta* **269,** 276–282.
Swami, T., Tadano, K.-C., and Bradner, W. T. (1979a). *J. Med. Chem.* **22,** 314–316.
Swami, T., Machenami, T., and Hesamatsu, T. (1979b). *J. Med. Chem.* **22,** 247–250.
Tew, K. D., Sudhaker, S., Schein, P. S., and Smulson, M. E. (1978). *Cancer Res.* **38,** 3371–3378.
Thatcher, D. J., and Walker, I. G. (1969). *J. Natl. Inst. Cancer Res.* **44,** 363–367.
Thomas, C. B., Osieka, R. O., and Kohn, K. W. (1978). *Cancer Res.* **38,** 2448–2454.
Thuning, C. A., Bakir, N. A., and Warren, J. (1980). *Cancer Res.* **40,** 2726–2729.
Tobey, R. A. (1975). *Nature (London)* **254,** 245–247.
Tobey, R. A., and Chressman, H. A. (1975). *Cancer Res.* **35,** 460–470.
Tong, W. P., and Ludlum, D. B. (1978). *Biochem. Pharmacol.* **27,** 77–81.
Tong, W. D., and Ludlum, D. B. (1981). *Cancer Res.* **41,** 380–382.
Twentyman, P. R. (1978). *Cancer Res.* **38,** 2395–2400.
Twentyman, P. R., Morgan, J. E., and Donaldson, J. (1978). *Cancer Treat. Rept.* **62,** 439–443.
Vavra, J. J., Deboer, C., Dietz, A., Hanka, L. J., and Sokolski, W. T. (1960). *Antibiot. Annu.* 1959–1960, 230–235.
von Bahr, C., Vadi, H., Grundin, R., Moldeus, P., and Orrenius, S. (1974). *Biochem. Biophys. Res. Commun.* **59,** 334–339.
Walker, M. D., and Gehan, E. A. (1972). *Proc. Amer. Asoc. Cancer Res.* **13,** 67.
Walker, M. D., and Hilton, J. (1976). *Cancer Treat. Rep.* **60,** 725–728.
Weinkam, R. J., and Deen, D. F. (1982). *Cancer Res.* **42,** 1008–1014.
Weinkam, R. J., and Dolan, M. E. (1982). *Proc. Am. Assoc. Cancer Res.* **23,** 163.
Weinkam, R. J., and Lin, H.-S. (1979). *J. Med. Chem.* **22,** 1193–1198.
Weinkam, R. J., and Liu, T.-Y. (1982). *J. Pharm. Sci.* **71,** 153–157.
Weinkam, R. J., Wen, J. H. C., Furst, D. E., and Levin, V. A. (1978). *Clin. Chem.* **34,** 45–49.
Weinkam, R. J., Finn, A., Levin, V. A., and Kane, J. P. (1980a). *J. Pharmacol. Exp. Ther.* **214,** 318–323.
Weinkam, R. J., Liu, T.-Y., and Lin, H.-S. (1980b). *Chem. Biol. Interact.* **21,** 167–177.
Wheeler, G. P. (1976). *Am. Chem. Symp. Ser.* **30,** 87–119.
Wheeler, G. P., and Bowden, B. J. (1968). *Cancer Res.* **28,** 52–59.
Wheeler, G. P., Bowden, B. J., and Herrer, T. C. (1964). *Cancer Chemother. Rep.* **42,** 9–12.
Wheeler, G. P., Bowdon, B. J., Grimsley, J. A., and Lloyd, H. H. (1974). *Cancer Res.* **34,** 194–200.

Wheeler, G. P., Bowdon, B. J., and Struck, R. F. (1975a). *Cancer Res.* **35,** 2974–2984.
Wheeler, K. T., Tel, N., Williams, M. E., Sheppard, S., Levin, V. A., and Kabra, P. M. (1975a). *Cancer Res.* **35,** 1464–1469.
Wheeler, G. P., Johnston, T. P., Bowdon, B. J., McCaleb, G. S., Hill, D. J., and Montgomery, J. A. (1977). *Biochem. Pharmacol.* **26,** 2331–2336.
Wheeler, G. P., Alexander, J. A., and Adamson, D. J. (1980). *Cancer Res.* **40,** 3723–3727.
Wooley, P., Dion, R. L., Kohn, K. W., and Bono, V. H. (1976). *Cancer Res.* **36,** 1470–1474.
Wooley, P. V., Rahman, A., Korsmeyer, S. J., Smith, F. P., and Schein, P. S. (1981). *Cancer Res.* **41,** 3896–3900.

The Interaction of Cancer Chemotherapy Agents with Mononuclear Phagocytes

ALBERTO MANTOVANI

Istituto di Ricerche Farmacologiche "Mario Negri"
Milan, Italy

I. Introduction 35
II. Effects of Chemotherapeutic Agents on Mononuclear Phagocytes 37
A. Glucocorticosteroids 37
B. Antimetabolites 41
C. Alkylating Agents 44
D. Intercalating Agents 48
E. Agents Affecting the Cytoskeleton 52
F. Overview 54
III. Effects of Chemotherapeutic Agents on Tumor-Associated Macrophages (TAM) 56
IV. Antitumor Efficacy and Modulation of Mononuclear Phagocytes 57
V. Concluding Remarks 61
References 62

I. Introduction

Cells of the monocyte–macrophage lineage represent a primitive first line of defense, maintained and refined in evolution. In addition, in higher organisms, phagocytic cells have become integrated into subsequently evolved specialized mechanisms of defense, while retaining their basic role of primary line of resistance. Cooperation between lymphoid cells and macrophages occurs at different levels in the genesis of immune reactions and, in inflammatory sites, they play important roles in the expression of cell-mediated immune reactions (Nelson, 1976). The role played by macrophages in resistance against infectious agents is well recognized (Nelson, 1976). In addition, the capacity of cells of the monocyte–macrophage lineage to kill eukaryotic cells, neoplastic cells in particular either "spontaneously" (Mantovani *et al.*, 1980b) or following *in vivo* or *in vitro* activation (Evans and Alexander, 1976; Keller, 1976; Hibbs, 1976) has suggested the possibility that these elements act as a primitive mechanism of surveillance against nascent neoplasia (Evans and Alexander, 1976; Keller, 1976; Hibbs, 1976). Macrophages infiltrate experimental and human tumors (Evans, 1967, 1972, 1976; Carr, 1977; Wood and Gollahon,

ISBN 0-12-032919-0

1977; Lauder *et al.*, 1977; Svennevig *et al.*, 1979) but their role *in vivo* in the control of established malignancy and metastasis remains to be defined (Evans, 1976).

In addition to expressing different heterogeneous functions, populations of cells belonging to the mononuclear phagocyte system are not homogeneous, but vary from site to site and within a given site as well (see for review Walker, 1976). Macrophages can be identified in virtually every anatomic compartment and there are regional differences in their biochemistry, morphology, and function. Such differences are particularly prominent when widely differing milieus, such as the lung alveoli and the peritoneal cavity, are considered (Walker, 1976). For instance we found that human alveolar macrophages have defective natural tumoricidal activity and defective responsiveness to interferon (IFN) when compared to blood monocytes or peritoneal exudate macrophages (Bordignon *et al.*, 1980). Similarly, when the interaction with natural killer (NK) cells was studied, human alveolar macrophages, unlike blood monocytes, peritoneal macrophages, and milk macrophages, were found capable to inhibit NK activity, and evidence suggested that suppression by mononuclear phagocytes could play a role in determining the low levels of NK cytotoxicity of unseparated lung cells (Bordignon *et al.*, 1981).

The maturation stage along the macrophage lineage critically affects the expression of some functions by mononuclear phagocytes and therefore is a further source of heterogeneity within the lineage (Territo and Cline, 1976). For instance both in humans and in rodents, monocytes or young monocyte-derived macrophages are efficient effectors of tumoricidal activity whereas resident tissue macrophages or "old" macrophage-derived epithelioid and giant cells are poor mediators of this reactivity (Ruco and Meltzer, 1978; Poste and Kirsh, 1979; Mantovani *et al.*, 1980b).

Cytotoxic agents used in the medical treatment of neoplasia have profound effects on host immunity and affect mononuclear phagocytes. Inhibition of host defense mechanisms is generally considered an important determinant of infections occurring concomitantly with the use of cytotoxic chemotherapy. Moreover, modulation of host defense mechanisms could also be relevant to the antitumor efficacy of drugs. On the one hand, it has been suggested that interference with immunity is an intrinsic limiting factor in the efficacy of anticancer agents: according to this view, chemotherapeutic drugs would be "self defeating" (Schwartz, 1968). On the other hand, evidence has accumulated that several cancer chemotherapeutic agents (e.g., cyclophosphamide and adriamycin) do not cause a nonspecific generalized inhibition of immune responsiveness, but have selective effects on host defense mechanisms (Spreafico and Anaclerio, 1977; Spreafico and Mantovani, 1981). Therefore, the relationship between antitumor efficacy and modulation of host resistance might be more complicated than expected on the somewhat simplistic assumption that chemotherapeutic agents act as pure depressants of immunity and that no substantial differences exist among antitumor drugs in their interaction with host defence mechanisms.

The depressive and, at least under certain experimental conditions, stimulatory activity of chemotherapeutic agents on specific immunity has been repeatedly reviewed (Spreafico and Anaclerio, 1977; Makinodan *et al.,* 1970; Bach, 1975; Haskell, 1977). These reviews provide the framework for the examination, to be performed here, of the effects of these compounds on mononuclear phagocytes. The effects of antitumor drugs on macrophage functions have been only marginally examined, even though mononuclear phagocytes could play an important role in the regulation of growth of primary tumors and metastasis. In this article, I will at first analyze in detail the effect of different antitumor drugs on various aspects of mononuclear phagocyte function. Given the variety of functions which can be performed by mononuclear phagocytes and the appreciable heterogeneity existing within the macrophage series it is not surprising that different xenobiotics can exhibit differences in their interaction with the mononuclear phagocyte system and have substantial selectivity in their effects on different cells or functions. The effect of anticancer chemotherapeutic agents on tumor-associated macrophages has been the object of limited investigation and available data will be discussed in the second part of this article. Finally, I will examine the relationship between interaction with cells of the monocyte–macrophage series and antineoplastic efficacy, with emphasis on the antitumor efficacy of combined chemoimmunotherapy approaches with immunomodulatory compounds with macrophage stimulatory properties.

II. Effects of Chemotherapeutic Agents on Mononuclear Phagocytes

A. Glucocorticosteroids

Glucocorticosteroids are widely used in the treatment of diverse human pathology including neoplastic diseases, and their effects on mononuclear phagocytes have been analyzed extensively. Early studies directed at providing a better understanding of the immunosuppressive activity of corticosteroids led to the concept that there are remarkable differences in susceptibility to these drugs among various species (reviewed by Claman, 1972). It was shown that hamster, mouse, rat, and rabbit are species sensitive to corticosteroids, whereas ferret, monkey, guinea pig, and man are rather resistant. The idea of a different species sensitivity was largely based on studies where parameters such as the lymphoid–organ weights and the total lymphocyte numbers are investigated. However, more recent reports clearly showed that a potent selective immunodepressive effect of glucocorticosteroids on certain cell subsets can also be observed in strains considered steroid-resistant (Claman, 1972; Jeter and Seebohm, 1952; Bovornkitti *et al.*, 1960; Fauci and Dale, 1974). Among other cell subpopulations, the monocyte–macrophage series was shown to be profoundly affected by corticosteroids; Table I summarizes selected effects of these compounds on mononuclear phagocytes. Werb and co-workers (1978) have demonstrated the presence of glucocorticoid-binding saturable macromolecules in monocytes, macrophages, and a tumor line (P388 D1) with macrophage properties. The dissociation constant of the receptors was within physiological ranges and the specificity and affinity correlated with biological function.

The effect of glucocorticosteroids on the kinetics of promonocytes, monocytes, and macrophages was investigated by Thompson and van Furth (1970, 1973) in the mouse, a corticosteroid-sensitive species. They found that administration of glucocorticosteroids induces a rapid decrease (within 3–6 hours) in the number of circulating monocytes. The duration of this effect was dependent on both the kind and the dose of the compound administered. In fact, after a single injection of 25 μg of water-soluble dexamethasone sodium sulfate, the monocytes reappeared in the circulation within 12 hours. Injection of 15 mg of insoluble hydrocortisone acetate, which formed a subcutaneous depot releasing the steroid, re-

TABLE I

SELECTED EFFECTS OF GLUCOCORTICOIDS ON MONONUCLEAR PHAGOCYTES

Parameter	Effect	Reference
Monocyte production	Slightly reduced	Thompson and van Furth (1973)
Monocyte release from the bone marrow	Reduced	Thompson and van Furth (1973)
Monocyte entry into sites of inflammation	Reduced	Blussé van Oud Alblas *et al.* (1981a)
Responsiveness to chemotactic factors	Reduced (man)	Rinehart *et al.* (1974)
	Unaffected (guinea pig)	Wahl *et al.* (1975)
Responsiveness to MIF	Reduced	Balow and Rosenthal (1973); Wahl *et al.* (1975)
Phagocytosis	Unaffected	Gadeberg *et al.* (1975)
Tumor cytotoxicity	Reduced	Hibbs (1974); Keller (1974)

sulted in prolonged monocytopenia lasting at least 14 days. In the same study, hydrocortisone did not affect the number of macrophages already present in the peritoneal cavity, but the transit of mononuclear phagocytes from the circulation into the peritoneal cavity was arrested. When an inflammatory response in the peritoneal cavity of hydrocortisone-treated mice was induced by injection of newborn calf serum, the increase in the number of monocytes in the circulation and in the peritoneal cavity was suppressed. Since no lytic action of steroids on the mononuclear phagocytes could be demonstrated, it was hypothesized that monocytopenia after hydrocortisone administration could be due to diminished production of monocytes in the bone marrow, as a result of a cytostatic action on their direct precursor cells, or to inhibition of the release of monocytes from the bone marrow. Thompson and van Furth (1973) showed that glucocorticosteroids do not induce decreased mitotic activity of the promonocytes and cause only a moderate reduction of monocyte production. Since the release of monocytes from the bone marrow was found to be influenced by hydrocortisone, it was concluded that this drug interferes with the release of newly formed monocytes from the bone marrow, resulting in a prolonged permanence of these cells in this compartment. Similarly to the above mentioned results obtained in the mouse, a great fall in circulating monocytes (4–6 hours) after glucocorticoids was reported by Fauci and Dale (1974) who administered both 100 and 400 mg of hydrocortisone to normal volunteers. Based on the results obtained, these investigators also concluded that the dramatic depletion of circulating monocytes is likely due to a redistribution of cells out of the circulation into other body compartments.

The effects of glucocorticosteroids on the kinetics of pulmonary macrophages were investigated by Blussé van Oud Alblas *et al.* (1981a,b) in mice. Following the administration of a depot of hydrocortisone acetate the monocyte influx into normal lungs was reduced to 14% of normal, and local production to 7%. To compensate for a reduced influx of monocytes and for a virtually abolished local production, the efflux of pulmonary macrophages was decreased to 12% of normal with an overall increase of the turnover time (Blussé van Oud Alblas *et al.*, 1981b). Hydrocortisone also inhibited the accumulation of macrophages into inflamed pulmonary tissue (Blussé van Oud Alblas *et al.*, 1981a).

Since monocytes and macrophages are important for the development and expression of cellular immunity, the capability of corticosteroids to compromise the recruitment of these cells into inflammatory sites was investigated further in an attempt to better clarify the mechanisms at the basis of the depression of delayed type reactivities caused by steroids (Claman, 1972; Jeter and Seebohm, 1952; Casey and McCall, 1971; Balow and Rosenthal, 1973; Weston *et al.,* 1973). Employing macrophage migration inhibition assays, Casey and McCall (1971) showed that methylprednisolone-treated rabbits previously immunized with Bacillus Calmette Guérin (BCG) had impaired development of delayed hypersensitivity to purified protein derivative (PPD). This observation was then confirmed and extended by Balow and Rosenthal (1973), who reported that hydrocortisone and dexamethasone, but not desoxycorticosterone, estrogens, testosterone, and progesterone, inhibit macrophage migration in guinea pigs. Interestingly, glucocorticosteroids blocked the macrophage responsiveness to migration inhibitory factor (MIF) but did not affect the production of this lymphokine. Wahl *et al.* (1975) also found that glucocorticosteroid blocked the responsiveness of macrophages to MIF, but production of this lymphokine by lymphocytes was also compromised by these agents. Macrophage responsiveness to aggregation factor was completely inhibited by *in vitro* addition of 10^{-3} cortisol but the capability of producing this factor by lymphoid cells was not affected (Weston *et al.,* 1973). Responsiveness of human monocytes to a chemotactic lymphokine was inhibited by hydrocortisone (Rinehart *et al.,* 1974). At variance with this observation in humans Wahl *et al.* (1975) reported that steroids rendered guinea pig macrophages unresponsive to MIF but not to lymphocyte-derived chemotactic factor. Thus it can be concluded that corticosteroids render macrophages refractory to certain lymphokines. Hydrocortisone is a known membrane stabilizing agent (Weissman and Dingle, 1961), and functional membranes are thought to be important for normal lymphokines responsiveness (reviewed in Cohen *et al.,* 1979). The defective membrane functionality after corticosteroid could account for the lack of response to lymphokines of macrophages from steroid-treated animals (Casey and McCall, 1971; Balow and Rosenthal, 1973; Weston *et al.,* 1973).

In addition to causing monocytopenia, to inhibiting recruitment of mononuclear phagocytes at sites of inflammation, and to suppressing responsiveness to lymphokines, glucocorticoids interfere with various macrophage functions such as production of plasminogen activator and of prostaglandins (Bray and Gordon, 1976; Vassalli *et al.,* 1976). Using murine macrophage cell lines Ralph and co-workers (1978) found that glucocorticoids did not inhibit the baseline production of myeloid colony-stimulating activity, phagocytosis, and killing of antibody-coated erythrocytes and tumor cells. In contrast, they observed marked suppression of these functions when they were stimulated by bacterial lipopolysaccharide or by tuberculin purified protein derivative (Ralph *et al.,* 1978).

Mononuclear phagocytes are thought to play an important role in the defense mechanisms activated in the host by bacterial infections and tumors. Therefore several investigators have performed studies directed to elucidate the effect of corticosteroids on monocyte and macrophage functions in animals bearing infections (North, 1971) and tumors (Hibbs, 1974; Keller, 1974; Schultz *et al.,* 1978b; Cameron and Churchill, 1981). North (1971) reported that a single 2.5 mg dose of cortisone acetate given at the beginning of the infection with *Listeria monocytogenes* in mice delays and suppresses blood monocyte accumulation at the infective foci in tissues. The defective macrophage recruitment at the site of infection could contribute to suppression by corticosteroids of resistance to a wide range of bacterial infections (Germuth, 1956). Although phagocytosis does not seem to be affected by corticosteroids (Gadeberg *et al.,* 1975) glucocorticoids decreased the bactericidal and fungicidal activity of mononuclear phagocytes (Rinehart *et al.,* 1975).

The results obtained by investigating the *in vitro* effects of macrophages on tumor cells clearly indicate that glucocorticosteroid can directly interfere with killing mechanisms. In fact, hydrocortisone and other steroids were observed to reduce the cytostatic and cytotoxic activity of *in vivo* (Hibbs, 1974) and *in vitro* (Keller, 1974; Schultz *et al.,* 1978b) activated mouse and rat macrophages against several tumor cell lines. Furthermore, human macrophage-mediated cytotoxicity against tumor cells was reported to be affected by hydrocortisone added to the *in vitro* cultures (Cameron and Churchill, 1981). Since it has been shown that macrophage–target cell interaction is associated with the fusion of the two plasma membranes and the transfer of lysosomes from the macrophage to the target cell (Hibbs, 1974; Chambers and Weiser, 1969), it was suggested that transfer of lysosomes may be a killing mechanism.

Hydrocortisone could block the lysosome transfer (Hibbs, 1974; Keller, 1974; Schultz *et al.,* 1978b; Cameron and Churchill, 1981) through the stabilization of cell membranes (Weissman and Dingle, 1961). It is of interest in this context that *in vivo* treatments with cortisone acetate abolishes the nonspecific protection induced by *Corynebacterium parvum* in mice bearing the P815 mastocytoma (Scott, 1975).

B. Antimetabolites

Azathioprine (AZA) is widely used in clinical practice as an immunosuppressant and its interaction with mononuclear phagocytes has been studied extensively. This discussion will focus on AZA and its thiopurine analog 6-mercaptopurine (6MP) because little information is available concerning other antimetabolites and this will be briefly mentioned. AZA is rapidly transformed *in vivo* into its parent compound, 6-MP (Elion and Hutchings, 1975), and has to some extent similar immunosuppressive properties (Berenbaum, 1971; Spreafico *et al.,* 1973).

Treatment with relatively low doses of thiopurines resulted in a profound monocytopenia in various animal species (Hurd and Ziff, 1968; Latta and Gentry, 1958; Page *et al.*, 1962; Borel and Schwartz, 1964; Ziff *et al.*, 1970; Zweiman and Phillips, 1970; Spiegelberg and Miescher, 1963; Gassman and Van Furth, 1975; Van Furth *et al.*, 1975). The mechanisms responsible for the reduction in monocyte counts following treatment with AZA were extensively investigated by Van Furth and co-workers (Gassmann and Van Furth, 1975; Van Furth *et al.*, 1975). These investigators found a decreased mitotic activity of promonocytes during AZA treatment in mice; however, the labeling index of promonocytes exposed to AZA increased and a higher percentage of these cells were tetraploid. Therefore it was concluded that AZA arrests the cell cycle of the promonocytes late in the DNA synthesis phase or in the postsynthesis (G_2) phase, thus preventing mitosis. During acute inflammation the cell cycle time of bone marrow promonocytes decreased and monocyte production increased: relatively low doses of AZA (3 mg/kg) abolished this response elicited by inflammatory stimuli. Moreover, while in untreated mice 40% of the monocytic cells leaving the circulation entered the site of inflammation, this fraction was reduced to 10% in AZA-treated mice. It is of interest in this connection that Phillips and Zweiman (1973) showed that high concentrations of 6MP directly affected macrophage migration in guinea pigs. Similarly, *in vitro* exposure to AZA or to amethopterin inhibited the response of rabbit macrophages to MIF (Pekarek *et al.*, 1976). Interestingly enough, production of MIF by lymphocytes was not markedly affected by AZA in rabbits and baboons (Pekarek *et al.*, 1976; Brown *et al.*, 1976).

The *in vivo* clearance of carbon particles, colloidal gold, bovine serum albumin (BSA), or ^{51}Cr-labeled erythrocytes was not appreciable affected by AZA treatment, unless hepatotoxic doses were used (Schwartz and Andre, 1960; Kaufman and McIntosh, 1971; Winkelstein *et al.*, 1971; Gadeberg *et al.*, 1975). While these reports suggest that thiopurines do not affect phagocytosis, Phillips and Zweiman (1973) found a decrease of phagocytosis of ^{14}C-labeled particles and of latex in guinea pigs, as well as an impaired spreading capacity on glass.

Antibody-dependent cellular cytotoxicity (ADCC) mediated by macrophages was not inhibited by AZA in mice (Purves, 1975): if anything AZA-treated mice exhibited enhanced macrophage-mediated ADCC. In contrast, in the same series of experiments Purves (1975) reported a selective impairment of ADCC mediated by nonadherent K cells.

While the antibody-dependent cytocidal activity of macrophages was not inhibited by AZA, direct antibody-independent tumoricidal activity of peritoneal macrophages was drastically reduced following *in vivo* exposure to AZA (Mantovani *et al.*, 1980a). Suppression of direct macrophage-mediated cytotoxicity was observed using both untreated or BCG-stimulated effector cells (Mantovani *et al.*, 1980a). Since monocytes or young monocyte-derived macrophages have cytotoxic activity on tumor cells (Mantovani *et al.*, 1979b, 1980a,b; Tagliabue *et al.*, 1979) and better responsiveness (in terms of cytotoxicity) to lymphokine supernatants (Ruco and Meltzer, 1978; Poste and Kirsch, 1979) it was speculated that AZA inhibited macrophage-mediated tumoricidal activity by interfering with the supply of young bone marrow-derived mononuclear phagocytes, endowed with appreciable cytotoxic capacity (Mantovani *et al.*, 1980a).

In conclusion (Table II), it is well established that thiopurines cause a profound monocytopenia even at low doses by interfering with the cell cycle of promonocytes. As far as mature macrophages are concerned, different effects were reported for different cell functions.

Phagocytosis and antibody-dependent cellular cytotoxicity generally are not inhibited by these drugs. In contrast, there are indications that entry of monocytes of sites of inflammation and responsiveness of mononuclear phagocytes to MIF is inhibited by exposure to thiopurines. Similarly, *in vivo* treatment with AZA was found to inhibit the direct tumoricidal activity of mouse macrophages. The latter effect might in part be related to an impaired production of lymphokine-responsive young mononuclear phagocytes, and, in part, to impaired responsiveness to activating lymphokines by analogy with results obtained with MIF.

The subcellular basis for the interaction of thiopurines with the mononuclear phagocyte system is not entirely clear. These agents have antiproliferative activity by blocking *de novo* purine synthesis and interconversion and thus inhibiting DNA, RNA, and protein synthesis (Elion and Hutchings, 1975). While the antiproliferative activity can account for effects on monocyte production, it remains unclear whether it can represent

TABLE II

SELECTED EFFECTS OF THIOPURINES (AZA OR 6MP) ON MONONUCLEAR PHAGOCYTES

Parameter	Effect	Reference
Monocyte production	Block at the promonocyte	Van Furth *et al.* (1975)
Monocyte entry into sites of inflammation	Reduced	Van Furth *et al.* (1975)
Migration	Reduced	Phillips and Zweiman (1973)
Phagocytosis	Unaffected	Gadeberg *et al.* (1975)
Antibody-dependent cytotoxicity	Unaffected or enhanced	Purves (1975)
Tumor cytotoxicity	Reduced	Mantovani *et al.* (1980a)

the sole basis for effects such as the inhibition of monocyte entry at sites of inflammation and inhibition of macrophage responsiveness to MIF.

C. Alkylating Agents

The most extensively studied alkylating agent is cyclophosphamide (Cy, Fig. 1, Table III). As illustrated in Fig. 1, this compound, inactive per se, requires metabolic activation at the level of the liver microsomal en-

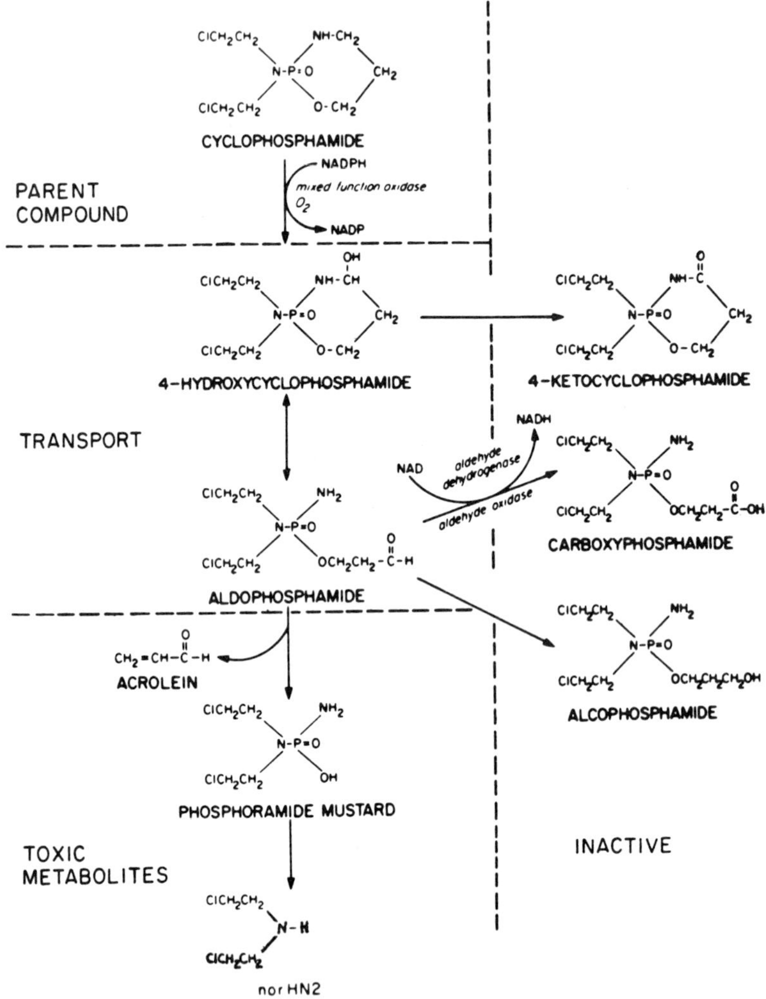

FIG. 1. Metabolism of cyclophosphamide.

TABLE III

SELECTED EFFECTS OF CYCLOPHOSPHAMIDE ON MONONUCLEAR PHAGOCYTES

Parameter	Effect	Reference
Monocyte counts	Reduced	Evans *et al.* (1980)
Phagocytosis	Unaffected or enhanced	Zschiesche (1972); Buhles and Shifrine (1977)
Antibody-dependent cytotoxicity	Reduced	Hunninghake and Fauci (1976, 1977)
Mitogen-induced cytotoxicity	Reduced	Hunninghake and Fauci (1976, 1977)
Induction (BCG) of tumor cytotoxicity	Unaffected or reduced	Stoychkov *et al.* (1979); Schultz *et al.* (1978a)
Expression of tumor cytotoxicity	Unaffected or enhanced	Mantovani *et al.* (1980a); Stoychkov *et al.* (1979)

zymes (Hohorst *et al.*, 1976; Domeyer and Sladek, 1980). Cyclophosphamide reduces blood monocyte counts in various animal species (Lemmel *et al.*, 1971; Hunninghake and Fauci, 1976; Evans *et al.*, 1980). The relative contribution to this effect of direct destruction of mononuclear phagocytes and of interference with monocyte precursors has not been elucidated. Since at least large doses of Cy rapidly reduce the number of long lasting resident peritoneal macrophages (Zschiesche, 1972; Gadeberg *et al.*, 1975; Mantovani *et al.*, 1980a), it appears likely that at least high doses of this compound can be cytotoxic on mature mononuclear phagocytes. Therefore in this respect Cy appears to differ from AZA, which only affects monocyte production, without killing mature macrophages (Gassmann and Van Furth, 1975; Van Furth *et al.*, 1975). In addition to reducing peritoneal macrophage counts, treatment with high doses of Cy caused morphological alterations in macrophages, with increase in size, heavy vacuolization, and appearance of giant cells (Gadeberg *et al.*, 1975).

While there are data suggesting that Cy can inhibit the production of MIF by lymphocytes (Balow *et al.*, 1975, 1977), it is unclear whether this cytotoxic agent can affect the responsiveness of macrophages to lymphokines. Pekarek *et al.* (1976) showed that spleen macrophages exposed *in vitro* to extremely high levels of Cy had somewhat impaired responsiveness to MIF. However, the drug was used as such, in the absence of liver microsomal enzymes: given the need for metabolic activation of this agent, the interpretation of this observation remains unclear.

High doses of various alkylating agents, but not Cy, impaired reticuloendothelial function as assessed by particle clearance (Zschiesche,

1972). Following Cy administration, Gadeberg *et al.* (1975) reported impaired *in vitro* phagocytosis of bacteria by peritoneal macrophages but after long-term Cy treatment, Buhles and Shifrine (1977) noted an increased phagocytosis by murine macrophages.

The effect of Cy on ADCC mediated by mononuclear phagocytes from different anatomical sites has been extensively studied by Fauci and co-workers in guinea pigs (Balow *et al.*, 1975, 1977; Hunninghake and Fauci, 1977).

In vitro exposure to serum from Cy-treated guinea pigs, presumably containing active metabolites, caused a transient depression of the capacity of blood mononuclear cells to mediate ADCC and mitogen-induced cytotoxicity against erythrocytes (Balow *et al.*, 1977). Monocytes can play a role in both reactivities, but their relative contribution was not analyzed in this study (Balow *et al.*, 1977).

The effect of *in vivo* exposure to Cy on antibody or mitogen-dependent lysis of red cells was critically affected by the schedule of administration. Using doses causing similar levels of monocytopenia and leukopenia, a single treatment with a large dose of Cy did not affect the antibody or mitogen-dependent cytotoxicity of blood mononuclear cells or alveolar macrophages (Hunninghake and Fauci, 1976, 1977). In contrast repeated daily drug administrations caused a significant impairment of these effector functions in blood or lung alveoli (Hunninghake and Fauci, 1976, 1977).

The effect of Cy on direct macrophage cytotoxicity was studied in mice using cytolysis (Mantovani *et al.*, 1980a) or cytostasis (Schultz *et al.*, 1978a; Stoychkov *et al.*, 1979) assays. Unlike AZA and 5-(3,3-dimethyl-1-trazenyl)-1*H*-imidazole-4-carboxamide (DTIC), Cy did not interfere with the expression of tumoricidal activity by normal or BCG-stimulated mouse peritoneal macrophages (Mantovani *et al.*, 1980a). Using a cytostasis assay, Chirigos and co-workers (Schultz *et al.*, 1978a; Stoychkov *et al.*, 1979) reported enhanced growth inhibitory capacity of Cy-treated macrophages. When the effect of Cy on activation of macrophages by various agents was studied, high concentrations of Cy (300 mg/kg) did not interfere with the augmentation of cytostatic activity by Pyran copolymer or glucan (Schultz *et al.*, 1978a). In contrast Cy given concomitantly with BCG decreased macrophage-mediated cytostasis measured 6 days later in one study (Schultz *et al.*, 1978a), but this was not confirmed in a subsequent investigation (Stoychkov *et al.*, 1979).

The apparent discrepancy between the latter finding (Schultz *et al.*, 1978a) and the above mentioned observations in a cytolysis assay (Mantovani *et al.*, 1980a) is probably related to the different timing of Cy administration relative to the activating stimulus (BCG). Schultz *et al.* (1978a) gave Cy on the same day as BCG, and the drug, which causes monocytopenia (Evans *et al.*, 1980), might have interfered either with the recruitment in the peritoneal cavity of lymphokine-responsive monocytes (Tagliabue *et al.*, 1979; Ruco and Meltzer, 1978; Poste and Kirsh, 1979), or with the lymphokine production by lymphocytes, this agent inhibiting MIF (Balow *et al.*, 1975, 1977; Winkelstein *et al.*, 1973). In contrast, in our studies, by giving Cy 8 days after BCG, we evaluated the effect of this agent on the expression of cytotoxic activity (Mantovani *et al.*, 1980a). In support of this hypothesis, adriamycin (AM) did not affect the expression of cytotoxicity by normal or activated macrophages, but it inhibited the induction of cytotoxic activity when administered together with *C. parvum* (Mantovani *et al.*, 1977).

The mode of action of Cy in its interaction with mononuclear phagocytes remains in part to be elucidated. While it appears likely that the cytotoxic activity of this agent can account for the monocytopenia, reversible modulation of cytocidal functions (Balow *et al.*, 1977; Hunninghake and Fauci, 1976) remains to be explained.

Available information concerning alkylating agents other than Cy is scanty and fragmentary. As already mentioned, nitrogen mustard-containing benzimidazole derivatives inhibited at high concentrations reticuloendothelial function (Zschiesche, 1972). A similar effect was observed with chlorambucil, but it was attributed to defective serum opsonic activity (Megirian, 1965; Megirian *et al.*, 1968).

A large number of nitrosourea analogs are now available, but the interaction of these compounds with macrophage-mediated host defense mechanisms has received limited attention (Ghaffar *et al.*, 1978; Saijo *et al.*, 1980). Following *in vivo* administration of antitumorally active doses which profoundly reduced T or B cell responses in mouse spleen (Ghaffar *et al.*, 1978), antibody-dependent cytotoxicity of red cells, mediated to a large extent by macrophages, was not appreciably modified by 1,3-bis(2-chloroethyl)-1-nitrosourea (BCNU) or by 1-(2-chloroethyl)-3-(-4-methylcyclohexyl)-1-nitrosourea (MeCCNU).

In rats, *in vivo* administration of 1-(4-amino-2-methyl-pyrimidyl)-methyl-3-(2-chloroethyl)-3-nitrosourea (ACNU) inhibited the spontaneous tumoricidal activity of peritoneal macrophages and this reduction was reversed by BCG (Saijo *et al.*, 1980).

One interesting aspect of nitrosoureas is their effect on target cell susceptibility to mononuclear phagocytes. Nathan *et al.* (1980) reported that macrophage-mediated cytolysis was augmented by exposing tumor target cells to BCNU, an effect related to inhibition of the glutathione redox cycle.

DTIC causes a profound and long lasting suppression of immune responsiveness in mice (Vecchi *et al.*, 1976a). This agent also inhibited macrophage-mediated cytotoxicity (Mantovani *et al.*, 1980a).

cis-Platinum diammine dichloride (DDP) is an antitumor agent active in humans (Einhorn and Williams, 1979). Kleinerman and co-workers investigated the effect of this agent on the *in vitro* generation of human monocyte cytotoxicity against red blood cells. *In vitro* exposure to DDP or to AM augmented the generation of cytotoxicity by directly affecting killer monocytes (Kleinerman *et al.*, 1980a,b; Kleinerman and Muchmore, 1981). Unlike DDP and the anthracycline AM, L-phenylalanine mustard (L-PAM) augmented the generation of monocytes cytotoxic against red cells by interfering with suppressor lymphocytes too (Kleinerman and Muchmore, 1981). These *in vitro* observations with DDP appeared to have some bearing on *in vivo* conditions inasmuch as ovarian cancer patients responding to DDP-containing regimens showed enhanced generation of monocytes lytic against erythrocytes (Kleinerman *et al.*, 1980a,b).

In a series of studies we investigated the tumoricidal activity of macrophages from ascitic ovarian tumors treated with chemotherapy (Mantovani *et al.*, 1980b). The direct cytostatic or cytolytic activity of tumor-associated macrophages was not appreciably affected by treatment with Cy, alone or in combination with other antitumor agents such as AM and DDP. Similarly, the levels of antibody-dependent macrophage-mediated cytostasis were not appreciably modified by the chemotherapy protocols employed in these studies (unpublished data). The limitations inherent to these studies in humans (e.g., lack of time course or dose–response experiments) caution against drawing definite conclusions, but these observations tentatively suggest that in humans as well as in mice, Cy, alone or in combination with AM, DDP, or hexamethylmelamine, does not inhibit the expression of macrophage-mediated tumoricidal activity.

D. Intercalating Agents

The anthracycline antibiotics AM and daunomycin (DM) are the intercalators most extensively investigated for their effects on cells of the monocyte–macrophage lineage (Table IV). No direct information is available concerning the effects of these agents on macrophage precursors. Mature peritoneal macrophages were relatively resistant to the cytotoxic activity of AM, when exposed to the drug *in vitro* or *in vivo* (Mantovani, 1977; Mantovani *et al.*, 1976a,b, 1977, 1979a,c,d, 1980a,b; Stoychkov *et al.*, 1979; Orsini *et al.*, 1977). Following *in vivo* administration of the drug, the relative proportion of spleen mononuclear phagocytes was increased, as assessed by counting phagocytic-adherent cells (Mantovani *et al.*,

TABLE IV

SELECTED EFFECTS OF ADRIAMYCIN ON MONONUCLEAR PHAGOCYTES

Parameter	Effect	Reference
Monocyte counts	Reduced	Mantovani (unpublished data)
Phagocytosis	Unaffected	Facchinetti *et al.* (1978)
Antibody-dependent cytotoxicity	Unaffected	Mantovani *et al.* (1976b)
Induction (*C. parvum*) of tumor cytotoxicity	Reduced or enhanced[a]	Mantovani *et al.* (1977)
Expression of tumor cytotoxicity	Unaffected or enhanced	Mantovani (1977); Mantovani *et al.* (1980a); Stoychkov *et al.* (1979)
Generation of cytotoxic T lymphocytes[b]	Enhanced	Orsini *et al.* (1977, 1980)
T and B lymphocyte colonies[b]	Enhanced	Orsini and Henderson (1979, 1980)

[a] The effect of AM on the induction of augmented tumor cytotoxicity by *C. parvum* was dependent on the relative time of administration of the two compounds.
[b] Alteration of these lymphocyte functions by AM was macrophage dependent.

1976a) or histologically (Orsini *et al.*, 1977). The increased percentage of splenic macrophages was attributed to a preferential killing of T and B cells (Mantovani *et al.*, 1976a). DM was, both *in vitro* and *in vivo*, somewhat more toxic than AM for murine macrophages (Mantovani, 1977; Facchinetti *et al.*, 1978). *In vitro* exposure to AM did not affect macrophage phagocytosis whereas DM reduced the phagocytic capacity of peritoneal macrophages (Facchinetti *et al.*, 1978).

Several reports have dealt with effects of anthracyclines on macrophage cytolytic or cytostatic activity on tumor cells (Mantovani, 1977; Mantovani *et al.*, 1977, 1979a,c, 1980a; Stoychkov *et al.*, 1979). AM did not inhibit macrophage-mediated cytostatic or cytolytic activity expressed spontaneously or induced by BCG or *C. parvum* (Mantovani, 1977; Mantovani *et al.*, 1977, 1979a,c, 1980a; Stoychkov *et al.*, 1977). In contrast, equitoxic doses of DM caused some inhibition of *C. parvum*-induced cytostasis (Mantovani, 1977).

While these studies showed that AM did not inhibit the cytolytic or cytostatic capacity of murine macrophages, in one report AM was found to induce growth inhibitory capacity in normal peritoneal macrophages (Stoychkov *et al.*, 1979).

Moreover, AM treatment augmented the *in vivo* radioresistant antitumor response mediated by hemopoietic histocompatibility-like mechanisms (Riccardi *et al.*, 1979a). This effect of the drug was abrogated by the antimacrophage agents silica and carrageenan (Riccardi *et al.*, 1979b).

Natural killer (NK) cells, relatively unaffected by pharmacologic doses of AM (Mantovani *et al.*, 1978; Santoni *et al.*, 1980), could also play a role in this type of radioresistant activity.

The effect of AM on the *in vivo* induction of macrophage-mediated cytostasis by *C. parvum* was examined in some detail (Mantovani *et al.*, 1977). Administration of AM around the time of *C. parvum* injection inhibited the induction of cytotoxicity measured 6 to 14 days later (Table V). This was interpreted as an indication of a cytotoxic effect of the drug at the level of proliferating precursors. In contrast, treatment with AM 3 to 7 days prior to *C. parvum* did not interfere with the subsequent induction of cytostasis. Actually, at least in part of the experiments, mice given AM 5 days before *C. parvum* showed an accelerated appearance of enhanced cytostasis possibly as a consequence of rebound proliferation of precursors (Mantovani *et al.*, 1977).

The effects of AM on other aspects of macrophage function, such as ADCC or MIF responsiveness, have been the object of limited attention. As expected on the basis of results discussed so far, AM did not reduce ADCC against chicken red blood cells (Tagliabue and Mantovani, unpublished data) nor against tumor cells (Mantovani *et al.*, 1976b). In studies on the effect of drugs on lymphokines, AM inhibited the production of MIF by murine spleen cells (Tagliabue, unpublished data).

Little information is available on the effects of anthracyclines on cells of the monocyte–macrophage lineage in humans. *In vitro* exposure to AM

TABLE V

EFFECT OF AM ON THE INDUCTION AND EXPRESSION OF MACROPHAGE CYTOSTASIS BY *C. parvum*[a]

AM injected on day	Cytostatic activity on day	
	6	11
—	55	91
−7	50	89
−5	85[b]	88
−1	12[c]	69[c]
+2	NT[d]	50[c]
+11	60	94

[a] CD2F$_1$ mice were given *C. parvum* (0.7 mg iv) on day 0 and 6 or 12 days later spleen macrophage cytostasis was measured at an effector-to-target cell ratio of 50 : 1 in a postlabeling [^{125}I]iododeoxyuridine uptake test (Mantovani, 1977). AM was administered at a dose of 10 mg/kg iv at different times before (−sign) or after (+sign) *C. parvum* treatment.

[b] $p < 0.05$.

[c] $p < 0.01$.

[d] NT, not tested.

augmented the generation in culture of monocytes cytotoxic against erythrocytes. This effect was dependent on direct stimulation of the killer monocyte (Kleinerman and Muchmore, 1981). In our laboratory, we have studied the antibody-dependent or independent tumoricidal activity of tumor-associated macrophages in patients with ascitic ovarian tumors treated with chemotherapy regimens including AM (Mantovani *et al.*, 1980b). Chemotherapy with drug combinations including AM did not reduce antibody-dependent or independent cytotoxicity against tumor cells, thus tentatively suggesting a resistance of human mature mononuclear phagocytes to drug toxicity similar to that observed in mice.

The relative sparing of macrophages by AM, or the augmentation of selected mononuclear phagocyte functions by this agent, has important consequences for the effects of AM on other immune parameters which are macrophage-dependent. At least under selected experimental conditions AM resulted in augmented generation of cytotoxic T lymphocytes and of PHA or LPS-induced lymphocyte colonies (Mantovani *et al.*, 1976b; Orsini *et al.*, 1977, 1980; Orsini and Henderson, 1979, 1980; Ehrke *et al.*, 1978; Tomazic *et al.*, 1980). Several lines of evidence suggested that cells of the monocyte–macrophage lineage play an important role in these drug effects (Mantovani *et al.*, 1976b; Orsini *et al.*, 1977, 1980; Orsini and Henderson, 1979, 1980; Ehrke *et al.*, 1978; Tomazic *et al.*, 1980).

The pharmacologic basis of the effects of anthracycline antibiotics on the immune system has not been elucidated. The kinetics of spleen cell depletion by the anthracyclines AM or DM appeared to be related to the different rates of accumulation of the drugs in this organ (Mantovani *et al.*, 1976a, 1979a; Yesair *et al.*, 1972) and the levels of cellular depletion caused by AM in the peritoneal cavity, spleen, and lymph nodes were inversely related to the drug levels in these organs and to the macrophage concentration at these anatomical sites (Mantovani *et al.*, 1979a). The mechanism through which anthracyclines, DM in particular, can kill nonproliferating macrophages *in vitro* is unclear. In addition to inhibiting DNA template function (Wilson and Jones, 1981), anthracyclines have been suggested to interact with membranes, and this level of action would account for the selectivity of these agents (Schwartz, 1976; Goldman *et al.*, 1978; Young *et al.*, 1981). AM and DM concentrate mainly in the nucleus, but when the cytoplasmic drug concentrations are considered, higher levels of DM than of AM are measured within lysosomes (Noel *et al.*, 1975). A preferential accumulation of DM into lysosomes could account for the greater *in vitro* toxicity of this agent, compared to AM, for lysosome-rich mature macrophages (Mantovani, 1977; Facchinetti *et al.*, 1978). In addition to DNA synthesis, anthracyclines inhibit RNA and, secondarily, protein synthesis (Di Marco, 1978; Young *et al.*, 1981). Protein synthesis is important for the expression of tumoricidal activity by murine and human mononuclear phagocytes (Keller, 1974; Keller *et al.*, 1974; Sharma and Piessens, 1978a; Cameron and Churchill, 1980) and one might speculate that inhibition of macrophage cytostasis by DM was in part related to an effect of this agent at this level, as observed with actinomycin D (Sharma and Piessens, 1978a; Cameron and Churchill, 1980).

E. Agents Affecting the Cytoskeleton

The *Vinca rosea* alkaloids vinblastine and vincristine inhibit the assembly of microtubules (Inoué and Sato, 1967; Bhisey and Freed, 1971; Wilson and Bryan, 1974) and represent useful tools in the cancer chemotherapy armamentarium, being among the most employed drugs for several types of cancer. Among drugs affecting microtubules, colchicine is widely investigated in experimental conditions whereas the *Vinca rosea* alkaloids are clinically useful drugs.

The microtubular system is involved in a variety of macrophage functions; thus several studies have been performed to clarify the interaction between microtubule-disrupting agents and macrophages. Selected information is summarized in Table VI. Employing an antiserum against microtubule proteins to permit visualization of these structures by immunofluorescent light microscopy, Frankel (1976) showed that microtubules of mouse macrophages radiate from a small region at the cell center. After 1 hour in 0.1 μg/ml of colchicine, all the microtubules had depolymerized but large numbers still remained at the cell center. After 2 hours, most of these had also depolymerized. Within 1 hour after removal of the drug, the cells again had normal distribution of the tubules which regrew out from the cytocenter. The microtubule-deprived macrophages generally lose complexity of shape and functional activity. Mouse macrophages after 48 hours of *in vitro* culture revealed a shift in cellular locomotion when colchicine (10^{-5} *M*) or vinblastine (10^{-6} *M*) was added to

TABLE VI

Effects of Microtubule-Disrupting Agents (Colchicine, Vinblastine) on Mononuclear Phagocytes

Parameter	Effect	Reference
Migration	Enhanced	Pick and Abrahamer (1973)
Responsiveness to MIF	Inhibited	Pick and Abraher (1973)
Tumor cytotoxicity	Unaffected	Keller (1974)
	Inhibited	Sharma and Piessens (1978b); Martin *et al.* (1981)

the incubation medium (Bhisey and Freed, 1971). The macrophage movement was changed from a gliding form of locomotion to an induced ameboid form. Since electron microscopy showed that after the disappearance of the microtubules from the cytoplasm of the drug-treated cells, the normal polarization of cytoplasmic organelles was disrupted, Bhisey and Freed (1971) concluded that in the absence of cytoskeletal structures differences in cortical tension may lead to cytoplasmic streaming and consequent ameboid movement. This finding prompted Pick and Abrahamer (1973) to investigate the susceptibility to MIF after treatment with microtubular-disruptive agents. They found that macrophage migration from capillary tubes was enhanced by colchicine and vinblastine. Moreover, drug-treated macrophages were not susceptible to MIF. Therefore it was concluded that integrity of the microtubular cytoskeleton of macrophages is a requisite for inhibition of motility by MIF. In a subsequent report, Pick and Grunspan-Swirzky (1977) showed that deuterium deoxide (D_2O), a microtubule-stabilizing agent (Marsland *et al.,* 1971), blocks spontaneous migration and intensifies MIF responsiveness. These results were recently confirmed by McCarthy *et al.* (1979), who also presented evidence that lumocolchicine, a derivative of colchicine which lacks the antimicrotubular properties of its analog but retains the non-tubulin-associated effects of colchicine on membrane transport (Mizel and Wilson, 1972), does not affect macrophage responsiveness to MIF. Colchicine was also shown to prevent the capability of MIF to induce macrophage refractoriness to adenylate cyclase stimulators such as β-adrenergic agents or prostaglandins (PG) of the E series (Pick and Grunspan-Swirzky, 1977). The refractoriness induced by MIF was increased by D_2O. Thus, the control of MIF responsiveness via cyclic nucleotides (Koopman *et al.,* 1973) seems to involve the microtubules. However, further studies are needed to understand this point better.

To further support the fact that the mitosis inhibitors can affect adenylate cyclase, it was shown in two reports that colchicine (Gemsa *et al.,* 1977) and vinblastine (Remold-O'Donnell and Alpert, 1979) increase the intracellular cyclic AMP levels after the stimulation of macrophages with PGE. Unfortunately, the contradiction between the latter study, where lumocholchicine induced the same effect as colchicine, and the former, where lumocolchicine did not, leaves some doubts about the relationship between microtubules and cyclic nucleotides. An important feature of macrophages is the induction of lysosomal enzymes and the intracellular degradation of materials endocytosed. Colchicine, but not lumocolchicine, inhibited induction of acid phosphatase resulting from both phagocytic and pinocytic stimuli (Pesanti and Axline, 1975). Furthermore, collagenase and elastase secretion by macrophages was enhanced by colchicine and vinblastine, whereas lysozyme secretion was inhibited (Gordon and Werb, 1976).

Effects of microtubule-disruptive agents on certain macrophage membrane reactivities were also shown (Medgyesi *et al.*, 1980; Williams *et al.*, 1977). Vinblastine enhances formation of rosettes with sheep red blood cells coated with IgG_1 type antibodies (Medgyesi *et al.*, 1980) and colchicine promoted concanavalin A capping in alveolar macrophages (Williams *et al.*, 1977).

The effect of microtubule-disrupting agents on macrophage tumoricidal activity has been the object of conflicting reports. Keller (1974) reported that colchicine did not inhibit rat macrophage cytotoxicity. In contrast Sharma and Piessens (1978b) and Martin *et al.* (1981) reported that rat and guinea pig macrophage-mediated tumoricidal activity was reduced by colchicine or vinblastine. Cytochalasin B, while affecting microfilaments (Wessels *et al.*, 1971), did not interfere with the expression of rat macrophage cytotoxicity (Martin *et al.*, 1981), but the tumoricidal activity of guinea pig macrophages was reduced by this compound (Sharma and Piessens, 1978b). Tumor cells exposed to cytochalasin B showed enhanced susceptibility to the cytotoxic capacity of rat macrophages (Martin *et al.*, 1981).

Thus, a variety of macrophage functions can be affected by drugs affecting the cytoskeleton, either at the intracellular level or at the membrane level. This class of drugs has been revealed to be an extremely useful tool to be employed in basic studies directed to understanding the macrophage biology. So far no information is available on the *in vivo* effect of *Vinca rosea* alkaloids on macrophage functions.

F. Overview

Given the variety of functions which can be performed by mononuclear phagocytes and the appreciable heterogeneity existing within the macrophage series, it is not surprising that different xenobiotics can exhibit differences in their interaction with the mononuclear phagocyte system and have substantial selectivity in their effects on different cells or functions. Some chemotherapeutic drugs used in the medical treatment of neoplasia or for immunosuppression (e.g., AZA, Cy, or AM) have been studied to some extent for their effects on the monocyte–macrophage lineage, but even for these xenobiotics the available information on this aspect of their mode of action is generally scanty and fragmentary. Figure 2 is an attempt to summarize the inhibitory effects of selected agents on various facets of mononuclear phagocyte function. It is apparent that different chemotherapeutic drugs differ in their capacity to affect a given function of cells of the monocyte–macrophage lineage. This is clearly

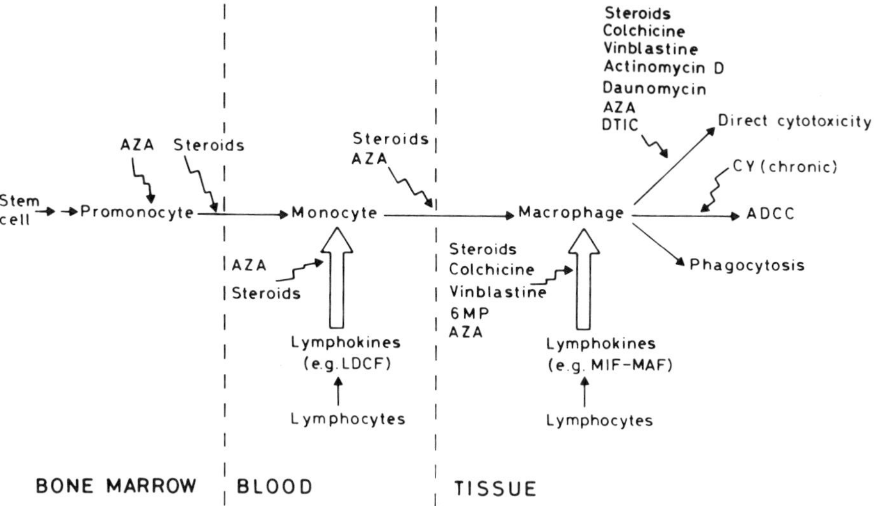

FIG. 2. Selected inhibitory effects of chemotherapeutic drugs on mononuclear phagocytes.

illustrated by the anthracycline antibiotics AM and DM, of which only the latter has considerable toxicity for mature macrophages. When different aspects of the mononuclear phagocyte system are considered, the same drug has different effects depending on the parameter considered: phagocytosis is notably resistant to inhibition by anticancer agents at nontoxic doses.

The effects of chemotherapeutic drugs on the mononuclear phagocyte system are usually inhibitory, but under selected experimental conditions augmentation of function after administration of some of these agents was reported. Table VII summarizes selected stimulatory effects of anticancer

TABLE VII

SELECTED STIMULATORY EFFECTS OF CHEMOTHERAPEUTIC AGENTS ON MONONUCLEAR PHAGOCYTES

Drug	Parameter	Reference
Colchicine	Random migration	Pick and Abrahamer (1973)
Cy	Phagocytosis	Buhles and Shifrine (1977)
AZA	ADCC	Purves (1975)
AM	Tumor cytotoxicity	Stoychkov *et al.* (1979); Mantovani *et al.* (1977)
	Interaction with T cells	Orsini *et al.* (1977, 1980); Orsini and Henderson (1979, 1980)

drugs on mononuclear phagocytes. With the exception of the effect of cytoskeletal-affecting agents on migration, the mechanisms of stimulation of certain mononuclear phagocyte functions by chemotherapeutic drugs remain a matter of speculation. The possibility is that at least some of these effects (e.g., stimulation of cytotoxicity induced by selected schedules of administration of drugs) are related to a rebound increased proliferation after treatment with myelotoxic compounds.

III. Effects of Chemotherapeutic Agents on Tumor-Associated Macrophages (TAM)

The effect of antineoplastic agents on the number and function of macrophages within tumors has been the object of a limited number of studies. Evans and co-workers (Evans, 1977a,b, 1978, 1980; Evans *et al.*, 1980) investigated the effect of AZA, X-irradiation, and Cy on the infiltration of mononuclear phagocytes in murine sarcomas. Treatment with AZA before or after tumor implantation caused a marked reduction in the percentage of TAM (Evans, 1977a). The mechanism of this effect was not fully elucidated but the above described interference of AZA with monocyte production and impairment of macrophage responsiveness to lymphokines could play a role in the reduction of TAM. A reduced accumulation of macrophages in AZA-pretreated tumor-transplanted animals was associated with a reduced growth of a murine sarcoma (Evans, 1977a). This observation, together with data in X-irradiated mice (Evans, 1977b), suggested that tumor-associated macrophages were providing a stimulus for tumor cell proliferation *in vivo* (Evans, 1977a,b). Evans and co-workers (Evans, 1978, 1980; Evans *et al.*, 1980) investigated the effect of antitumorally active doses of Cy on TAM in various murine sarcomas. Drug-induced regression was associated with monocytopenia and, at the tumor site, with an increase of the proportion of mononuclear phagocytes relative to tumor cells. The increased host cell to tumor cell ratio did not prevent recurrence of the sarcomas. An increased percentage of TAM after chemotherapy with Cy was also reported by Szymaniec and James (1976). An increased ratio between TAM and tumor cells was noted during AM-induced tumor regression (Mantovani, unpublished data).

Little information is available concerning the effect of cancer chemotherapeutic agents on the functional status of TAM. Radov *et al.* (1976) briefly mentioned that melphalan did not inhibit the cytotoxic activity of tumor-associated mononuclear cells in a mouse mammary carcinoma. As observed with mouse peritoneal macrophages (Mantovani, 1977), AM did not alter the cytostatic capacity of macrophages from a murine sarcoma (Mantovani, unpublished data). In the course of studies aimed at characterizing TAM from human ascitic or solid ovarian carcinomas, we tested the cytotoxic effector capacity of TAM from carcinomatous effusions before and after treatment with Cy alone or in combination with AM, hexamethylmelamine, or DDP (Mantovani *et al.*, 1980b). In the limited series of subjects tested these chemotherapy regimens did not appreciably inhibit the capacity of human TAM to directly kill tumor cells (Mantovani *et al.*, 1980b) or to mediate ADCC (unpublished data).

IV. Antitumor Efficacy and Modulation of Mononuclear Phagocytes

Although host defense mechanisms have been frequently credited with an important role in determining the antineoplastic efficacy of chemotherapy (Schwartz, 1968), a relative paucity of systematic studies is available in this area. Indications that, for a given drug, the therapeutic activity is the result of cooperation between host resistance and direct tumor cell killing have been obtained through different approaches, by comparing therapeutic efficacy in specifically preimmunized or immunodepressed hosts (Mihich, 1969; Moore and Williams, 1973; Schwartz and Grindey, 1973; Steele and Pierce, 1974; Steele *et al.*, 1974; Radov *et al.*, 1976; Heppner and Calabresi, 1972, 1976; Mantovani *et al.*, 1979c), or in tumor sublines of different immunogenicity (e.g., Mantovani *et al.*, 1979c; Giuliani *et al.*, 1974), or by evaluating therapeutic efficacy in tumors transplanted across minor histocompatibility barriers (e.g., Riccardi *et al.*, 1979a).

In some selected murine experimental systems there is convincing evidence that immune responses may contribute to the antitumor action of selected chemotherapeutic agents. Basically, agents such as Cy, arabinosyl cytosine, melphalan, and AM show reduced efficacy when given to immunosuppressed hosts in selected experimental murine systems (Mihich, 1969; Moore and Williams, 1973; Schwartz and Grindey, 1973; Steele and Pierce, 1974; Steele *et al.*, 1974; Radov *et al.*, 1976; Heppner and Calabresi, 1972, 1976; Mantovani *et al.*, 1979c; Giuliani *et al.*, 1974; Riccardi *et al.*, 1979a). While evidence in these particular models is convincing, one should guard against generalization of these findings. In two studies in murine sarcomas, host immunity was a prerequisite for optimal expression of Cy antitumor efficacy (Moore and Williams, 1973; Steele and Pierce, 1974; Steele *et al.*, 1974). However, in a large series of chemically induced sarcomas, Evans (1978, 1980; Evans *et al.*, 1980) found no correlation between Cy-induced regression and tumor immunogenicity, and immunosuppressed hosts were as responsive as intact mice to chemotherapy. The role of host defense mechanisms in the antitumor activity of AM has been studied in murine solid tumors and leukemias (Schwartz and Grindey, 1973; Mantovani *et al.*, 1979c; Giuliani *et al.*, 1974). While in immunogenic neoplasms impairment of host resistance by various procedures discussed in detail below compromised the antineoplastic efficacy of the drug, in poorly immunogenic tumors no evidence for an appreciable role of host immunity was obtained (Giuliani *et al.*, 1974; Mantovani *et al.*, 1979c).

Therefore, while host resistance appears to contribute to the antitumor activity of selected anticancer agents in some experimental murine tumors, these observations cannot be generalized to other drugs or neoplasms. Even in the experimental models in which indications have been obtained for a role of host immunity in chemotherapeutic efficacy, an analysis of the role played by different populations in the antitumor activity of cancer chemotherapeutic agents is largely lacking. In particular, the relationship, if any, between effects of drugs on various facets of immune responsiveness and participation of different host defense mechanisms to the antitumor action of these drugs remains to be elucidated.

In the last few years we have studied the interaction of anthracycline antibiotics, AM in particular, with host defense mechanisms and we have investigated the relationship, if any, between the immunological and the antitumor efficacy of this compound, alone or in combination with macrophage activators (Mantovani, 1977; Mantovani *et al.*, 1976a,b, 1977, 1978, 1979a,b,c,d, 1980a; Tagliabue *et al.*, 1977).

The lymphomas with greater immunogenicity responded better to AM chemotherapy but not to DM (Mantovani *et al.*, 1979c). In immunogenic tumor models the antineoplastic effectiveness of AM was markedly reduced in thymus-deprived mice or by inhibition of host defense mechanisms with silica and carrageenan, or with DTIC, this drug suppressing thymus-dependent responses (Vecchi *et al.*, 1976a) and macrophage cytotoxicity (Mantovani *et al.*, 1980a) but not NK cytotoxicity and hemopoietic histocompatibility reactions (Mantovani *et al.*, 1978). Using the L1210 Ha leukemia resistant to cytotoxicity of DTIC, suppression with this drug could be applied after tumor transplantation (day 0) and after AM injection (day 1, Table VIII). As illustrated in Table VIII, AM cured up to 80% of L1210 Ha transplanted mice, but suppression by DTIC of host defense mechanisms, including macrophages, as late as 9 days after chemotherapy resulted in progressive tumor growth. Thus as late as 9 days after "curing" the mice with AM, viable tumor cells persisted in the peritoneal cavity, restrained by host defense mechanisms. This observation could be interpreted as an indication of a "dormancy"-like status

TABLE VIII

EFFECT OF IMMUNOSUPPRESSION WITH DTIC AFTER CHEMOTHERAPY ON ANTITUMOR ACTIVITY OF AM IN DTIC-RESISTANT L1210 HA LEUKEMIA[a]

AM	Suppression with DTIC applied on day	MST[b]	D/T[c]
−	—	11	10/10
−	+5	11	10/10
+	—	24	2/10
+	−5	19	10/10[d]
+	+5	20	10/10[d]
+	+10	26	8/10[d]
+	+20	17	2/10

[a] Cells (10^5) of the DTIC-resistant L1210 Ha leukemia line were transplanted ip on day 0 into $CD2F_1$ mice. AM (10 mg/kg iv) was given on day +1 and mice were immunodepressed with 180 mg/kg DTIC ip at different times before or after tumor inoculation.

[b] Median survival time.

[c] Dead with leukemia over total number of transplanted mice.

[d] $p < 0.05$ compared to mice given AM alone.

induced by chemotherapy and maintained by host resistance, possibly by macrophages which, when recovered from "AM-cured" L1210 Ha transplanted mice, showed enhanced cytostatic activity (Mantovani *et al.*, 1979c). Consistent with this hypothesis is the observation that the macrophage toxins silica and carrageenan reduced the antitumor efficacy of AM in these immunogenic tumor models (Mantovani *et al.*, 1979c).

These series of observations were interpreted as evidence that, although AM can markedly inhibit humoral antibody production and cell-mediated responses (Vecchi *et al.*, 1976b), specific immunity was a prerequisite for optimal expression of the antineoplastic effectiveness of this agent, and that the residual host immune responsiveness represented a critical determinant of the ultimate curative efficacy of AM in those particular immunogenic tumor models. Moreover, the data appeared consistent with the possibility, though did not conclusively prove, that sparing of mononuclear phagocytes, possibly activated as a consequence of immune responses to strongly immunogenic tumors, contributed to the antitumor activity of AM (Mantovani *et al.*, 1979c). Results to some extent similar were reported by Radov *et al.* (1976) in a murine carcinoma treated with melphalan. Specific immunity to the tumor was required for optimal antitumor efficacy of chemotherapy and the cytotoxic activity of tumor-associated mononuclear cells was not affected by the drug regimens (Radov *et al.*, 1976).

The results discussed so far indicate that host defense mechanisms, and macrophages in particular, could play a role in the antitumor activity of selected anticancer agents at least in some experimental models. Compounds capable of activating macrophages, such as BCG and *C. parvum*, have limited but significant antitumor efficacy in rodents (see for review Alexander, 1977; Terry and Windhorst, 1978). In various transplanted murine tumors combinations of "immunostimulatory" compounds with cytoreductive chemotherapy have given better therapeutic results than either modality alone (e.g., Fisher *et al.*, 1975a,b, 1976; Tagliabue *et al.*, 1977; Mantovani *et al.*, 1979c). In such combined approaches, whereby chemotherapeutic agents are used in conjunction with macrophage activators, it appears reasonable to hypothesize that the interaction of cytoreductive therapy with macrophages has important consequences for therapeutic results.

Several investigators have observed that the choice of the agent used for chemotherapy is a critical determinant of the antineoplastic effectiveness of chemoimmunotherapy (Fisher *et al.*, 1975a,b, 1976; Tagliabue *et al.*, 1977). The reasons why, in the various models investigated, chemotherapeutic agents having similar cytoreductive efficacy have a different capacity to synergize with nonspecific immunotherapeutic compounds remain largely unclear. With the anthracycline antibiotics AM and DM, better antitumor activity was observed when AM was combined with *C. parvum*, but little therapeutic advantage was obtained when DM was substituted for AM in the chemotherapy arm of the combination (Tagliabue *et al.*, 1977; Mantovani *et al.*, 1979c). It is important to note that the addition of *C. parvum* really increased the therapeutic index of AM, which was employed up to its maximal nontoxic, chemotherapeutically optimal dose (Mantovani *et al.*, 1979c). Too often in experimental chemoimmunotherapy protocols the effectiveness of the combination with a suboptimal dose of the cytotoxic drug is not higher than that of the drug administered alone at its best dosage. Given the greater *in vitro* and *in vivo* toxicity of DM for mature murine macrophages (Mantovani, 1977) the therapeutic "synergism" of AM combined with *C. parvum* was attributed to the relative lack of toxicity for mature mononuclear phagocytes of the latter chemotherapeutic drug (Mantovani, 1977; Facchinetti *et al.*, 1978; Orsini *et al.*, 1977; Stoychkov *et al.*, 1979; Tagliabue *et al.*, 1977; Mantovani *et al.*, 1979c).

The antineoplastic efficacy of chemoimmunotherapy combinations is schedule-dependent and this could in part be related to the time dependency of the effects of chemotherapeutic drugs on mature macrophages or macrophage precursors. As discussed above (Table II), AM did not interfere with the induction of macrophage cytotoxicity by *C. parvum*, provided at least 3–5 days had elapsed before injection of the macrophage activator (Mantovani *et al.,* 1977). Interestingly enough, when different schedules of administration of the AM–*C. parvum* combination were tested for antitumor efficacy in murine lymphomas, a 5-day interval between chemotherapy and treatment with the anaerobic coryneform was found optimal (Mantovani *et al.,* 1977; Tagliabue *et al.,* 1977). Thus, in these murine models and for this chemoimmunotherapy combination, the possibility is that the time dependency of the antitumor activity of combinations of AM and *C. parvum* is a reflection of the interplay of these two agents with cells of the monocyte–macrophage lineage.

V. Concluding Remarks

The studies discussed here indicate that, in rodents, cancer chemotherapeutic drugs can be heterogeneous in terms of their interaction with cells of the monocyte–macrophage lineage. Not only do drugs from different classes have different effects, but even closely structurally related analogs can differ significantly in their effects on mononuclear phagocytes, the anthracycline antibiotics being particularly significant in this respect. The suppressive or at times stimulatory effects of cytotoxic agents can be relatively selective, only or mainly a maturation stage or a cell function being affected. Therefore chemotherapeutic drugs provide useful tools to dissect the mononuclear phagocyte system. Although it appears that the modulation of mononuclear phagocytes by chemotherapeutic drugs is not solely a consequence of cytotoxicity, the cellular mode of action of these agents at this level remains largely elusive and our understanding remains, with a few exceptions, at a descriptive phenomenological level.

In selected experimental models, there is evidence that the cells of the monocyte–macrophage lineage contribute to the antitumor activity of drugs. These observations are confined to specific model systems and drugs, and, although little systematic work has been done in this area, it appears that generalizations and extrapolations in terms of drugs, tumors, or species, are unwarranted.

In spite of a considerable effort, in human neoplasia therapeutic results of immunotherapy approaches, usually applied after cytoreductive chemotherapy, have been by and large disappointing and at best marginal (Alexander, 1977; Terry and Windhorst, 1978). Limited findings in transplanted animals tumors suggest that the antitumor efficacy of combinations of cytoreductive chemotherapy and nonspecific immunomodulators capable of activating macrophages is critically affected by the interaction of chemotherapeutic drugs with mononuclear phagocytes. Therefore it appears conceivable that a better understanding of the effects at this level of cytotoxic agents could provide a basis for a less empirical design of chemoimmunotherapy approaches.

Acknowledgments

This work was supported by a generous contribution from the Italian Association for Cancer Research, Milan, Italy. I thank Drs. S. Garattini, F. Spreafico, A. Tagliabue, and A. Vecchi for discussion and criticism. Miss A. Mancini skillfully typed the manuscript.

References

Alexander, P. (1977). *Cancer* **40** (Suppl. 1), 467–470.

Bach, J. F. (1975). "The Mode of Action of Immunosuppressive Agents." North-Holland Publ., Amsterdam.

Balow, J. E., and Rosenthal, A. S. (1973). *J. Exp. Med.* **137,** 1031–1041.

Balow, J. E., Hurley, D. L., and Fauci, A. S. (1975). *J. Clin. Invest.* **56,** 65–70.

Balow, J. E., Parrillo, J. E., and Fauci, A. S. (1977). *Immunology* **32,** 899–904.

Berenbaum, M. C. (1971). *Clin. Exp. Immunol.* **8,** 1–8.

Bhisey, A. N., and Freed, J. J. (1971). *Exp. Cell Res.* **64,** 419–429.

Blussé van Oud Alblas, A., van der Linden-Schrever, B., and van Furth, R. (1981a). *J. Exp. Med.* **154,** 235–252.

Blussé van Oud Alblas, A., van der Linden-Schrever, B., Mattie, H., and van Furth, R. (1981b). *J. Reticuloendothel. Soc.* **30,** 1–14.

Bordignon, C., Avallone, R., Peri, G., Polentarutti, N., Mangioni, C., and Mantovani, A. (1980). *Clin. Exp. Immunol.* **41,** 336–342.

Bordignon, C., Villa, F., Introna, M., Avallone, R., and Mantovani, A. (1981). *Clin Exp. Immunol.,* in press.

Borel, Y., and Schwartz, R. (1964). *J. Immunol.* **92,** 754–761.

Bovornkitti, S., Kangsadal P., Sathirapat, P., and Oonsombatti, P. (1960). *Dis. Chest* **38,** 51–55.

Bray, M. A., and Gordon, D. (1976). *Br. J. Pharmacol.* **52,** 466–467.

Brown, T. E., Ahmed, A., Filo, R. S., Knudsen, R. C., and Sell, K. W. (1976). *Transplantation* **21,** 27–35.

Buhles, W. C., and Shifrine, M. (1977). *J. Reticuloendothel. Soc.* **21,** 285–297.

Cameron, D. J., and Churchill, W. H. (1981). *Int. J. Immunopharmacol.* **3,** 77–85.

Carr, I. (1977). *In* "The Macrophage and Cancer" (K. James, B. McBride, and A. Stuart, eds.), pp. 364–374. Univ. of Edinburgh Press, Edinburgh.

Casey, W. J., and McCall, C. E. (1971). *Immunology* **21,** 225–231.

Chambers, V. C., and Weiser, R. S. (1969). *Cancer Res.* **29,** 301–317.

Claman, H. N. (1972). *N. Engl. J. Med.* **287,** 388–397.

Cohen, S., Pick, E., and Oppenheim, J. J. (1979). "Biology of the Lymphokines." Academic Press, New York.

Di Marco, A. (1978). *Antimicrob. Agents Chemother.* **23,** 216–227.

Domeyer, B. E., and Sladek, N. E. (1980). *Cancer Res.* **40,** 174–180.

Ehrke, M. J., Tomazic, V., Eppolito, C., and Mihich, E. (1978). *Fed. Proc. Fed. Am. Soc. Exp. Biol.* **37,** 1652.

Einhorn, L. H., and Williams, S. D. (1979). *N. Engl. J. Med.* **300,** 289–291.
Elion, G. B., and Hutchings, G. H. (1975). *In* "Handbook of Experimental Pharmacology. 38/2: Antineoplastic and Immunosuppressive Agents, pt. II" (A. C. Sartorelli and D. G. Johns, eds.), pp. 404–425. Springer-Verlag, Berlin and New York.
Evans, R. (1967). *J. Gen. Virol.* **1,** 363–374.
Evans, R. (1972). *Transplantation* **14,** 468–473.
Evans, R. (1976). *In* "The Macrophage in Neoplasia" (M. A. Fink, ed.), pp. 27–42. Academic Press, New York.
Evans, R. (1977a). *Br. J. Cancer* **35,** 557–566.
Evans, R. (1977b). *Int. J. Cancer* **20,** 120–128.
Evans, R. (1978). *Int. J. Cancer* **21,** 611–616.
Evans, R. (1980). *Am. J. Pathol.* **99,** 667–682.
Evans, R., and Alexander, P. (1976). *In* "Immunobiology of the Macrophage" (D. S. Nelson, ed.), pp. 535–576. Academic Press, New York.
Evans, R., Madison, L. D., and Eidlen, D. M. (1980). *Cancer Res.* **40,** 395–402.
Facchinetti, T., Raz, A., and Goldman, R. (1978). *Cancer Res.* **38,** 3944–3949.
Fauci, A. S., and Dale, D. C. (1974). *J. Clin. Invest.* **53,** 240–246.
Fisher, B., Wolmark, N., Rubin, H., and Saffer, E. (1975a). *J. Natl. Cancer Inst.* **55,** 1147–1153.
Fisher, B., Wolmark, N., Saffer, E., and Fisher, E. (1975b). *Cancer* **35,** 134–143.
Fisher, B., Rubin, H., Saffer, E., and Wolmark, N. (1976). *Cancer Res.* **36,** 2714–2719.
Frankel, F. R. (1976). *Proc. Natl. Acad. Sci. U.S.A.* **73,** 2798–2802.
Gadeberg, O. V., Rhodes, J. M., and Larsen, S. O. (1975). *Immunology* **28,** 59–70.
Gassmann, A. E., and Van Furth, R. (1975). *Blood* **46,** 51–64.
Gemsa, D., Steggeman, L., Till, G., and Resh, K. (1977). *J. Immunol.* **119,** 524–529.
Germuth, F. G. (1956). *Pharmacol. Rev.* **8,** 1–24.
Ghaffar, A., Lichter, W., Wellham, L. L., and Sigel, M. M. (1978). *J. Natl. Cancer Inst.* **60,** 1483–1487.
Giuliani, F., Casazza, A. M., and Di Marco, A. (1974). *Biomedicine* **21,** 435–439.
Goldman, R., Facchinetti, T., Bach, D., Raz, A., and Shinitzky, M. (1978). *Biochim. Biophys. Acta* **512,** 254–269.
Gordon, S., and Werb, Z. (1976). *Proc. Natl. Acad. Sci. U.S.A.* **73,** 872–876.
Haskell, C. M. (1977). *Annu. Rev. Pharmacol. Toxicol.* **17,** 179–195.
Heppner, G. H., and Calabresi, P. (1972). *J. Natl. Cancer Inst.* **48,** 1161–1167.
Heppner, G. H., and Calabresi, P. (1976). *Annu. Rev. Pharmacol. Toxicol.* **16,** 367–379.
Hibbs, J. B. (1974). *Science* **184,** 468–471.
Hibbs, J. B. (1976). *In* "The Macrophage in Neoplasia" (M. A. Fink, ed.), pp. 83–98. Academic Press, New York.
Hohorst, H. J., Draeger, U., Peter, G., and Voelcker, G. (1976). *Cancer Treat. Rep.* **60,** 309–315.
Hunninghake, G. W., and Fauci, A. S. (1976). *J. Immunol.* **117,** 337–341.
Hunninghake, G. W., and Fauci, A. S. (1977). *Clin. Exp. Immunol.* **27,** 555–559.
Hurd, E. R., and Ziff, M. (1968). *J. Exp. Med.* **128,** 785–800.
Inoué, S., and Sato, H. (1967). *J. Cell. Physiol.* **50,** 259–292.
Jeter, W. S., and Seebohm, P. M. (1952). *Proc. Soc. Exp. Biol. Med.* **80,** 694–695.
Kaufman, D. B., and McIntosh, R. M. (1971). *Clin. Res.* **19,** 221.
Keller, R. (1974). *Immunology* **27,** 285–298.
Keller, R. (1976). *In* "Immunobiology of the Macrophage" (D. S. Nelson ed.), pp. 487–508. Academic Press, New York.
Keller, R., Keist, R., and Ivatt, R. J. (1974). *Int. J. Cancer* **14,** 675–683.

Kleinerman, E. S., and Muchmore, A. V. (1981). *Proc. Am. Assoc. Cancer Res.* **22,** 277.
Kleinerman, E. S., Zwelling, L. A., Howser, D., Barlock, A., Young, R. C., Decker, J. M., Bull, J., and Muchmore, A. V. (1980a). *Lancet* **2,** 1102–1105.
Kleinerman, E. S., Zwelling, L. A., and Muchmore, A. V. (1980b). *Cancer Res.* **40,** 3099–3102.
Koopman, W. J., Gillis, M. H., and David, J. R. (1973). *J. Immunol.* **110,** 1609–1614.
Latta, J. S., and Gentry, R. P. (1958). *Anat. Rec.* **132,** 1.
Lauder, I., Aherne, W., Stewart, J., and Sainsbury, R. (1977). *J. Clin. Pathol.* **30,** 563–568.
Lemmel, E., Hurd, E. R., and Ziff, M. (1971). *Clin. Exp. Immunol.* **8,** 355–362.
McCarthy, P. L., Shaw, J. E., and Remold, H. G. (1979). *Cell. Immunol.* **46,** 409–415.
Makinodan, T., Santos, G. W., and Quinn, R. P. (1970). *Pharmacol. Rev.* **22,** 189–247.
Mantovani, A. (1977). *Cancer Res.* **37,** 815–820.
Mantovani, A., Tagliabue, A., Vecchi, A., and Spreafico, F. (1976a). *Eur. J. Cancer* **12,** 381–387.
Mantovani, A., Vecchi, A., Tagliabue, A., and Spreafico, F. (1976b). *Eur. J. Cancer* **12,** 371–379.
Mantovani, A., Tagliabue, A., Luini, W., Facchinetti, T., and Spreafico, F. (1977). *In* "The Macrophage and Cancer" (K. James, B. McBride, and A. Stuard, eds.), pp. 203–215. Univ. of Edinburgh Press, Edinburgh.
Mantovani, A., Luini, W., Peri, G., Vecchi, A., and Spreafico, F. (1978). *J. Natl. Cancer Inst.* **61,** 1255–1261.
Mantovani, A., Candiani, P., Luini, W., Salmona, M., Spreafico, F., and Garattini, S. (1979a). *In* "Current Trends in Tumor Immunology" (S. Ferrone, S., Gorini, R. B. Herberman, and R. A. Reisfeld eds.), pp. 139–159. Garland STPM Press, New York.
Mantovani, A., Jerrells, T. R., Dean, J. H., and Herberman, R. B. (1979b). *Int. J. Cancer* **23,** 18–27.
Mantovani, A., Polentarutti, N., Luini, W., Peri, G., and Spreafico, F. (1979c). *J. Natl. Cancer Inst.* **63,** 61–66.
Mantovani, A., Vecchi, A., Tagliabue, A., and Spreafico, F. (1979d). *In* "Tumor-Associated and their Specific Immune Response" (F. Spreafico and R. Arnon, eds.), pp. 271–286, Academic Press, New York.
Mantovani, A., Luini, W., Candiani, G. P., and Spreafico, F. (1980a). *Int. J. Immunopharmacol.* **2,** 333–339.
Mantovani, A., Peri, C., Polentarutti, N., Allavena, P., Bordignon, C., Sessa, C., and Mangioni, C. (1980b). *In* "Natural-Cell Mediated Immunity against Tumors" (R. B. Herberman, ed.), pp. 1271–1293. Academic Press, New York.
Marsland, D., Tilney, L. G., and Hirschfield, M. (1971). *J. Cell. Physiol.* **77,** 187–194.
Martin, F., Olsson, N. O., and Jeannin, J. F. (1981). *Cancer Immunol. Immunother.* **10,** 113–119.
Medgyesi, G. A., Foris, G., Dezsö, B., Gergely, J., and Bazin, H. (1980). *Immunology* **40,** 317–323.
Megirian, R. (1965). *J. Reticuloendothel. Soc.* **2,** 238–248.
Megirian, R., Warrington, D., and Laffin, R. J. (1968). *J. Reticuloendothel. Soc.* **5,** 578.
Michich, E. (1969). *Cancer Res.* **29,** 848–854.
Mizel, S. B., and Wilson, L. (1972). *Biochemistry* **11,** 2573–2578.
Moore, M., and Williams, D. E. (1973). *Int. J. Cancer* **11,** 358–368.
Nathan, C. F., Arrick, B. A., Murray, H. W., DeSantis, N. M., and Cohn, Z. A. (1980). *J. Exp. Med.* **153,** 766–782.
Nelson, D. S., ed. (1976). "Immunobiology of the Macrophage." Academic Press, New York.

Noel, G., Trouet, A., Zenebergh, A., and Tulkens, P. (1975). *In* "Adriamycin Review," pp. 99–105. (EORTC International Symposium, Brussels, May 1974). European Press, Ghent.
North, R. J. (1971). *J. Exp. Med.* **134,** 1485–1500.
Orsini, F., Epolito, C., Ehrke, M. J., and Mihich, E. (1980). *Cancer Treat. Rep.* **64,** 211–218.
Orsini, F. R., and Henderson, E. S. (1979). *Immunopharmacology* **1,** 203–210.
Orsini, F. R., and Henderson, E. S. (1980). *Immunopharmacology* **2,** 375–384.
Orsini, F. R., Pavelic, Z., and Mihich, E. (1977). *Cancer Res.* **37,** 1719–1726.
Page, A. R., Condie, R. M., and Good, R. A. (1962). *Am. J. Pathol.* **40,** 519–530.
Pekarek, J., Svejcar, J., Nouza, K., and Johanovsky, J. (1976). *Immunology* **31,** 773–779.
Pesanti, E. L., and Axline, S. G. (1975). *J. Exp. Med.* **141,** 1030–1046.
Phillips, S. M., and Zweiman, B. (1973). *J. Exp. Med.* **137,** 1494–1510.
Pick, E., and Abrahamer, H. (1973). *Int. Arch. Allergy* **44,** 215–220.
Pick, E., and Grunspan-Swirzky, A. (1977). *Cell. Immunol.* **32,** 340–349.
Poste, G., and Kirsh, R. (1979). *Cancer Res.* **39,** 2582–2589.
Purves, E. C. (1975). *Clin. Exp. Immunol.* **22,** 348–358.
Radov, L. A., Haskill, J. S., and Korn, J. H. (1976). *Int. J. Cancer* **17,** 773–779.
Ralph, P., Ito, M., Broxmeyer, H. E., and Nakoinz, I. (1978). *J. Immunol.* **121,** 300–303.
Remold-O'Donnell, E., and Alpert, H. R. (1979). *Cell. Immunol.* **45,** 221–229.
Riccardi, C., Bartocci, A., Puccetti, P., Spreafico, F., Bonmassar, E., and Goldin, A. (1979a). *Eur. J. Cancer* **16,** 23–33.
Riccardi, C., Puccetti, P., Santoni, A., Herberman, R. B., and Bonmassar, E. (1979b). *Immunopharmacology* **1,** 211–220.
Rinehart, J. J., Balcerzak, S. P., Sagone, A. L., and LoBuglio, A. F. (1974). *J. Clin. Invest.* **54,** 1337–1343.
Rinehart, J. J., Sagone, A. L., Balcerzak, S. P., Ackerman, G. A., and LoBuglio, A. F. (1975). *New Engl. J. Med.* **292,** 236–241.
Ruco, L. P., and Meltzer, M. S. (1978). *J. Immunol.* **120,** 1054–1062.
Saijo, N., Irimajiri, N., Ozaki, A., Shimizu, E., and Niitani, H. (1980). *Br. J. Cancer* **42,** 162–167.
Santoni, A., Riccardi, C., Sorci, V., and Herberman, R. B. (1980). *J. Immunol.* **124,** 2329–2335.
Schultz, R. M., Pavlidis, N. A., Chirigos, M. A., and Weiss, J. F. (1978a). *Cell. Immunol.* **38,** 302–309.
Schultz, R. M., Pavlidis, N. A., Stylos, W. A., and Chirigos, M. A. (1978b). *Cancer Treat. Rep.* **62,** 1889–1892.
Schwartz, H. S. (1976). *Biomedicine* **24,** 317–323.
Schwartz, H. S., and Grindey, G. B. (1973). *Cancer Res.* **33,** 1837–1844.
Schwartz, R. S. (1968). *Cancer Res.* **28,** 1452–1454.
Schwartz, R. S., and Andre, J. (1960). *Proc. Soc. Exp. Biol. Med.* **104,** 228–230.
Scott, M. T. (1975). *J. Natl. Cancer Inst.* **54,** 789–792.
Sharma, S. D., and Piessens, W. F. (1978a). *Cell. Immunol.* **38,** 264–275.
Sharma, S. D., and Piessens, W. F. (1978b). *Cell. Immunol.* **38,** 276–285.
Spiegelberg, H. L., and Miescher, P. A. (1963). *J. Exp. Med.* **118,** 869–890.
Spreafico, F., and Anaclerio, A. (1977). *In* "Immunopharmacology" (J. W. Hadden, R. G. Coffey, and F. Spreafico, eds.), pp. 245–278. Plenum, New York.
Spreafico, F., and Mantovani, A. (1981). *In* "Pathobiology Annual 1980" (H. L. Ioachin, ed.). Academic Press, New York.
Spreafico, F., Donelli, M. G., Bossi, A., Vecchi, A., Standen, S., and Garattini, S. (1973). *Transplantation* **16,** 269–278.

Steele, G., and Pierce, G. E. (1974). *Int. J. Cancer* **13,** 572–578.
Steele, G., Sjögren, H. O., and Ankerst, J. (1974). *Int. J. Cancer* **14,** 743–752.
Stoychkov, J. N., Schultz, R. M., Chirigos, M. A., Pavlidis, N. A., and Goldin, A. (1979). *Cancer Res.* **39,** 3014–3017.
Svennevig, J. L., Lövik, M., and Svaar, H. (1979). *Int. J. Cancer* **23,** 626–631.
Szymaniec, S., and James, K. (1976). *Br. J. Cancer* **33,** 36–50.
Tagliabue, A., Polentarutti, N., Vecchi, A., Mantovani, A., and Spreafico, F. (1977). *Eur. J. Cancer* **13,** 657–665.
Tagliabue, A., Mantovani, A., Kilgallen, M., Herberman, R. B., and McCoy, J. L. (1979). *J. Immunol.* **122,** 2363–2370.
Territo, M., and Cline, M. J. (1976). *In* "Immunobiology of the Macrophage" (D. S. Nelson, ed.), pp. 593–616. Academic Press, New York.
Terry, W. D., and Windhorst, D., eds. (1978). "Immunotherapy of Cancer: Present Status of Trials in Man," Vol. VI. Raven, New York.
Thompson, J., and Van Furth, R. (1970). *J. Exp. Med.* **131,** 429–442.
Thompson, J., and Van Furth, R. (1973). *J. Exp. Med.* **137,** 10–21.
Tomazic, V., Ehrke, M. J., and Mihich, E. (1980). *Cancer Res.* **40,** 2748–2755.
Van Furth, R., Gassmann, A. E., and Diesselhoff-Den Dulk, M. M. C. (1975). *J. Exp. Med.* **141,** 531–546.
Vassalli, J., Hamilton, J., and Reich, E. (1976). *Cell* **8,** 271–281.
Vecchi, A., Fioretti, M. C., Mantovani, A., Barzi, A., and Spreafico, F. (1976a). *Transplantation* **22,** 619–624.
Vecchi, A., Mantovani, A., Tagliabue, A., and Spreafico, F. (1976b). *Cancer Res.* **36,** 1222–1227.
Wahl, W. M., Altman, L. C., and Rosenstreich, D. L. (1975). *J. Immunol.* **115,** 476–481.
Walker, W. S. (1976). *In* "Immunobiology of the macrophage" (D. S. Nelson, ed.), pp. 91–110. Academic Press, New York.
Weissman, G., and Dingle, J. (1961). *Exp. Cell Res.* **25,** 207–211.
Werb, Z., Foley, R., and Munck, A. (1978). *J. Exp. Med.* **147,** 1684–1694.
Wessells, N. K., Spooner, B. S., Ash, J. F., Bradley, M. O., Luduena, M. A., Taylor, E. L., Wreen, J. T., and Yamada, K. M. (1971). *Science* **171,** 135–143.
Weston, W. L., Claman, H. N., and Krueger, G. G. (1973). *J. Immunol.* **110,** 880–883.
Williams, D. A., Boxer, L. A., Oliver, J. M., and Baehner, R. L. (1977). *Nature (London)* **267,** 255–257.
Wilson, L., and Bryan, L. (1974). *Adv. Cell. Mol. Biol.* **3,** 21–40.
Wilson, W. S., and Jones, R. L. (1981). *Adv. Pharmacol. Chemother.* **18,** 177–222.
Winkelstein, A., Craddock, C. G., and Lawrence, J. S. (1971). *J. Reticuloendothel. Soc.* **9,** 307–322.
Winkelstein, A., Naukin, H. R., and Mitulla, J. M. (1973). *In* "Proceedings of the Seventh Leukocyte Conference" (F. Daguillard, ed.), pp. 429–432. Academic Press, New York.
Wood, G. W., and Gollahon, K. A. (1977). *J. Natl. Cancer Inst.* **59,** 1081–10871
Yesair, D. W., Schwartzbach, E., Shuck, D., Denine, E. P., and Asbell, M. A. (1972). *Cancer Res.* **32,** 1177–1183.
Young, R. C., Ozols, R. F., and Myers, C. E. (1981). *N. Engl. J. Med.* **305,** 139–153.
Ziff, M., Hurd, E. R., Lemmel, E. M., and Jasin, H. E. (1970). *In* "Mononuclear Phagocytes" (R. Van Furth, ed.), pp. 282–297. Blackwell, Oxford.
Zschiesche, W. (1972). *J. Reticuloendothel. Soc.* **12,** 16–28.
Zweiman, B., and Phillips, S. M. (1970). *Science* **169,** 284–285.

ADVANCES IN PHARMACOLOGY AND CHEMOTHERAPY, VOL. 19

Mebendazole and Related Anthelmintics

HUGO VAN DEN BOSSCHE, FRANS ROCHETTE, AND CHRISTIAN HÖRIG

Research Laboratories
Janssen Pharmaceutica
Beerse, Belgium

I. Introduction 67
II. Chemistry and Pharmacology 69
A. Albendazole 70
B. Ciclobendazole 70
C. Fenbendazole 72
D. Flubendazole 74
E. Mebendazole 76
F. Oxfendazole 79
G. Oxibendazole 80
H. Parbendazole 81
III. Benzimidazole Carbamates in Veterinary Medicine 82
A. Introduction 82
B. Equids 83
C. Domestic Ruminants 85
D. Pig 96
E. Poultry and Birds 101
F. Dogs and Cats 102
G. Wild and Zoo Animals 106
H. Rodents 107
I. Ovicidal Activity 107
J. Resistance to Benzimidazoles 108
IV. Benzimidazole Carbamates in Human Medicine 109
A. Nematode Infections 110
B. Cestode Infections 117
V. Conclusion 118
References 119

I. Introduction

Ascaris lumbricoides has been estimated to infect one-quarter of the world's population. In a review on costs, prevalence, and approaches for control of *Ascaris* infection in Kenya, Stephenson *et al.* (1980a) collected evidence indicating that even light *Ascaris* infections may have detrimental effects on the growth of undernourished "preschool" children. These authors proved that it is simply not true that *Ascaris* infection is harmless

ISBN 0-12-032919-0

in most cases as often considered by other investigators. Ascariasis is linked not only to poor growth and protein–caloric malnutrition but also to malabsorption of macronutrients and vitamin A. In addition, the detailed study by Stephenson *et al.* (1980a) of the economic aspects of *Ascaris* infection in Kenya shows that this infection was costing Kenyans about $5 million in 1976. It is interesting that the price of a broad spectrum anthelmintic provided to all Kenyans would cost less than one-fifth of that.

Ascaris affects the growth of pigs. Spindler (1947) artificially infected pigs with *Ascaris suum* eggs and determined 126 days later the weight increase in both infected and uninfected animals. A negative correlation was found between the number of *Ascaris* and weight increase. For example, a pig with 20 worms showed a daily weight increase of 0.2 kg whereas the uninfected control gained 0.4 kg. At the end of the experiment the control had gained 49.4 kg whereas the infected pig showed a weight increase of only 27.2 kg. Stephenson *et al.* (1980b) studied the efficiency of feed utilization. In pigs infected with *Ascaris* and on a low protein diet, 6.8 kg of food was needed to gain 1 kg. In control pigs only 3.3 kg was needed.

Urquhart (1981) estimated recently that the potential loss caused by uncontrolled parasitic nematodes in ruminants would be £160 million. This was reduced to an actual loss of about £30 million by the use of anthelmintic drugs of which the cost was estimated at about £20,000.

These are just a few examples to demonstrate that treatment of parasitoses in man and animals is economic.

There is an expanding list of drugs active against a great number of parasitic helminths. The literature on broad-spectrum anthelmintic drugs has increased greatly in the last 5–10 years. The benzimidazole carbamate derivatives have especially attracted great attention. The number of publications is enormous: for mebendazole 388 in the veterinary and 349 in the human field, more than 290 for fenbendazole, 120 for albendazole, 80 for oxfendazole, and 40 for flubendazole; in short, these figures collected at the end of June 1981 indicate that it will be impossible to review all these publications.

The scope of the present overview is limited to the most promising of the benzimidazole carbamates. All the drugs to be discussed have proven highly efficacious in animals; some of them are widely used in human medicine.

It should be noted that the results presented are collected from different sources. Discrepancies between results obtained with the same anthelmintic in different countries or even the same country may be due to the use of different formulations or qualities, e.g., polymorphs, differently shaped and sized crystals, and the degree of infection.

II. Chemistry and Pharmacology

In this overview some chemical and pharmacological properties of important benzimidazole carbamates are summarized. The chemical structures of the different benzimidazole carbamate derivatives are given in Table I.

Extensive studies on the mode of action were done with mebendazole, fenbendazole, and to a lesser extent with flubendazole. Therefore only the mechanism of action of these compounds will be discussed.

TABLE I

CHEMICAL STRUCTURES OF BENZIMIDAZOLE CARBAMATE ANTHELMINTICS

General structure: R-substituted benzimidazole (N–H) with 2-position $NH-C(=O)-OCH_3$

Generic name	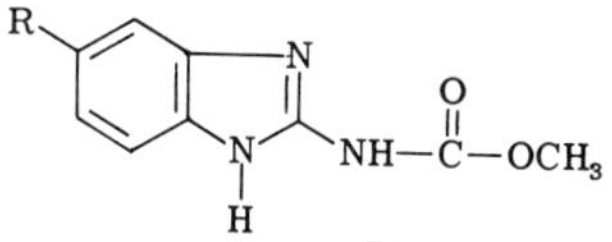 R
Albendazole	$CH_3-CH_2-CH_2-S-$
Ciclobendazole	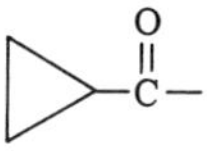 cyclopropyl$-C(=O)-$
Fenbendazole	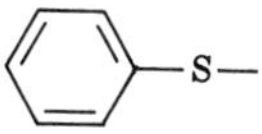 phenyl$-S-$
Flubendazole	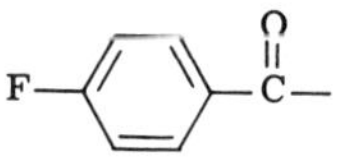 $F-$phenyl$-C(=O)-$
Mebendazole	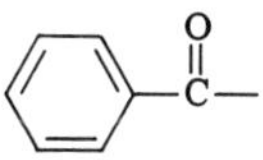 phenyl$-C(=O)-$
Oxfendazole	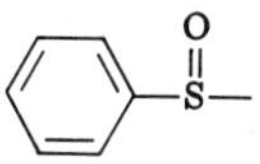 phenyl$-S(=O)-$
Oxibendazole	$CH_3-CH_2-CH_2-O-$
Parbendazole	$CH_3-CH_2-CH_2-CH_2-$

A. Albendazole

Albendazole is the generic name for methyl[5-(propylthio)-1-*H*-benzimidazol-2-yl] carbamate, a product synthesized at Smith Kline Corporation. Like the other benzimidazole carbamates it is almost insoluble in water and only slightly soluble in most organic solvents (Theodorides *et al.*, 1976a).

1. *Pharmacokinetics*

[^{14}C]Albendazole was administered to sheep (DiCuollo *et al.*, 1977) at a single oral dose of 16 mg/kg. Peak plasma levels equivalent to 3.7 μg/ml of albendazole and/or metabolites were found 15 hours posttreatment; 51% of the dose was recovered in the urine within 120 hours. Total radioactive residues in all tissues including the liver and kidney are depleted to below 0.1 ppm within a period of 10 days.

In calves peak plasma levels of 5.5 μg/ml albendazole and/or metabolites were achieved 15 hours following the administration of an oral dose of 20 mg/kg body weight; 46% of the administered dose was recovered in the urine within 72 hours. Total radioactive residues in the liver and kidney 30 days after treatment remained at 0.4 and 0.3 ppm. However, total radioactivity in muscle and fat depleted rapidly to less than 0.1 ppm within 5 days (DiCuollo *et al.*, 1977).

2. *Toxicology*

The oral LD_{50} in rats of albendazole was about 2.4 g/kg (Theodorides *et al.*, 1976b). No untoward effects were observed in sheep drenched with albendazole at dose levels of 26.5 and 37.5 mg/kg. There was a transient inappetence in the sheep drenched with 53 mg/kg. At 75 mg/kg one ram died 9 days postmedication; there was wool break in two rams and one ewe (Johns and Philip, 1977).

In a reproductive safety study no abnormalities were found in any of the lambs born to ewes dosed with 11 or 15 mg/kg on days 21, 24, and 28 after ram mounting. Three of 44 lambs born to ewes dosed with 15 mg/kg and 4 of 44 lambs born to ewes dosed with 11 mg/kg 17 days after mounting showed some skeletal abnormalities (Johns and Philip, 1977).

B. Ciclobendazole

Ciclobendazole is the generic name for methyl[5-(cyclopropylcarbonyl) 1*H*-benzimidazol-2-yl] carbamate synthesized at Janssen Pharmaceutica.

It is almost insoluble in water (0.008%) and most organic solvents (Degrémont and Stahel, 1978).

1. *Pharmacokinetics*

Pharmacokinetic studies in rats and dogs using radioactively labeled ciclobendazole are reported by Brodie *et al.* (1977). After a single oral dose of 4 mg [^{14}C]ciclobendazole per kg body weight to rats most of the dose was excreted during the first 48 hours. In the first 24 hours 52.2 and 22.4% of the administered radioactivity was excreted in the feces and urine, respectively. However, experiments with biliary cannulated rats showed that 70–80% of an oral dose of [^{14}C]ciclobendazole was eliminated in the bile. A summation of radioactivity eliminated in the urine and bile and that retained in the carcass indicated that a mean of 91.2% was absorbed.

After oral administration of [^{14}C]ciclobendazole to rats at 4, 40, or 400 mg/kg peak plasma levels occurred at 15–30 minutes representing 0.55, 3.87, and 10.53 μg/ml, respectively. Thereafter, the concentration declined with a half-life of about 20 hours.

The peak plasma concentration in the dog, after an oral dose of 4 mg [^{14}C]ciclobendazole per kg body weight, was reached at about 30 minutes and declined with a half-life of about 3 hours.

After a single oral dose of [^{14}C]ciclobendazole to dogs at a level of 4 mg/kg, most of the dose was excreted during the first 48 hours with about 80% of the dose in the feces and 10% in the urine. Anesthetised bile duct-cannulated dogs excreted between 26 and 35% of an oral dose in the bile during 24 hours, 14.5% in the urine, and 44.2% remained in the gastrointestinal tract and tissues at 24 hours.

The tissue distribution of radioactivity in rats and dogs after single or multiple doses (4 mg/kg) showed highest concentrations in the intestinal tract, liver and kidneys, organs associated with biotransformation and excretion, and also in lungs and adrenals (Brodie *et al.*, 1977).

In man treated with [^{14}C]ciclobendazole, 45 and 12% of the dose was excreted during the first 48 hours in the feces and urine, respectively.

After 5 days 72% of the dose was found in the feces and 14% in urine (Degrémont and Stahel, 1978).

2. *Toxicology*

The oral LD_{50} values found were in rats 2.46 g/kg, mice 1.03 g/kg, and rabbits 183.3 mg/kg. In dogs treated with 1.2 g/kg, besides anorexia no adverse reactions were observed (Degrémont and Stahel, 1978).

In teratological studies ciclobendazole was administered to mice, rats, and rabbits without producing teratological effects (Degrémont and Stahel, 1978).

C. Fenbendazole

Fenbendazole known chemically as methyl[5-(phenylthio)-2-benzimidazole] carbamate was synthesized by Farbwerke Hoechst in 1971. It is soluble in dimethyl sulfoxide (Düwel *et al.*, 1975; Düwel, 1979).

1. *Pharmacokinetics*

Following oral administration of [^{14}C]fenbendazole to rats, rabbits, and dogs (10 mg/kg) and to farm animals (5 mg/kg), the radioactivity was mostly excreted in the feces and only by one-tenth in the urine. An exception was the rabbit, with one-fifth in the urine. More than half of the radioactivity in the feces was unchanged fenbendazole. In the urine only a small amount ($\leq$1% of the applied dosage) of the unchanged substance was found. The principal metabolite in sheep and bovine urine results from hydroxylation at the p-place of the phenyl ring. A 2-amino derivative was also found (Düwel, 1977).

Pharmacokinetic data are summarized in Table II. Results of residue studies with nonradioactive fenbendazole in sheep, cattle, and pigs showed that in most tissues, residues after 2 days are low and approach

TABLE II

Serum and Milk Levels of Fenbendazole[a]

Species	Sample	Oral dose (mg/kg)	Time to reach maximum levels (hours)	Maximum concentration (μg/ml)	Maximum retention time (hours)	Half-live in serum (hours)
Cattle	Serum	5.0	30	0.74	96	27
		7.5	30–48	1.10	102	13
		10.0	24–30	1.60	120	14
	Milk	7.5	28	0.30	54	14
Dog	Serum	10.0	6–24	0.04–0.4		15
Pig	Serum	5.0	6–12	0.45	48	10
Rabbit	Serum	50.0	30	2.6	78	15
		100.0	48	3.6	78	21
Rat	Serum	10.0	5–7	0.19		6
Sheep	Serum	5.0	6–24	0.40	96	26

[a] Taken from Düwel (1975, 1977, 1979).

the limit of detection (0.05 mg/kg) after 5 days. However, 7 days after treatment the liver of cattle, pig, and sheep contained 0.3, 0.28, and 0.9 mg/kg, respectively. After 14 days amounts of <0.1, 0.11, and 0.2 mg/kg were found in cattle, pig, and sheep liver (Düwel, 1977).

Of interest is the study done by Prichard *et al.* (1978b). These authors compared the incorporation of radiolabel from fenbendazole in benzimidazole-susceptible with that in benzimidazole-resistant *Haemonchus contortus* and *Trichostrongylus colubriformis*. Incorporation of [^{14}C]fenbendazole and/or metabolites was significantly greater in susceptible than in resistant worms. Prichard *et al.* (1978b) also found that the rate of absorption was markedly greater if fenbendazole was administered directly into the abomasum instead of the rumen. They suggest that in sheep the rumen may act as a reservoir of fenbendazole, prolonging the period of high anthelmintic concentration in the host.

Prichard (1980) also found that sheep showing symptoms of severe infection had markedly slower absorption of fenbendazole as shown by plasma concentrations, while fenbendazole levels in the first 30 hours or more after administration were markedly reduced in the abomasum and small intestine, the sites of infection. Furthermore a significant reduction in fenbendazole uptake by *Nippostrongylus brasiliensis* in malnourished rats was found.

2. *Toxicology*

In toxicity tests involving a single administration to mice and rats it was not possible to determine the LD_{50}. For example, the oral LD_{50} is certainly >10 g/kg in rats and mice. In domestic animals the following single doses were well tolerated (apart from transient increases of individual transaminases in a few members of each group of domestic animals): cattle >2 g/kg, dog >0.5 g/kg, pig and sheep >5 g/kg.

Repeated administration of several times the therapeutic dose has also been tolerated, e.g., rat 90×1.6 g/kg, dog 90×125 mg/kg, sheep 30×45 mg/kg.

No trial has produced any evidence of teratogenic effects in rats, sheep, and cattle. At high dose some discussible effects were observed in rabbits (Delatour and Burgat-Sacaze, 1981).

3. *Mode of Action*

Investigations on the mode of action have shown that fenbendazole, like mebendazole, interferes in nematodes with the absorption of glucose and especially with the incorporation of glucose into glycogen (Düwel, 1977). In *Fasciola hepatica* fenbendazole (and mebendazole) seem to disturb the synthesis or breakdown of serotonin (thus influencing transport processes) and/or the metabolism of amino acids (Metzger and Düwel, 1974).

Within 4 to 8 hours after treatment via a stomach tube in rats infected with *Hymenolepis diminuta*, with 50 or 100 mg/kg body weight, the scolices became detached from the wall of the intestine and in 20 to 30 hours the worms were expelled from the body. The muscles of the suckers lost their tone, the scolex lost its structure, and the excretory canals dilated; 8 hours after treatment the epidermis of the tapeworm was completely destroyed. According to Düwel and Schleich (1978) these results seem to indicate that fenbendazole is neurotoxic for the worm. It should be noted that the peristalsis of the rat intestine is not increased by fenbendazole (Düwel and Schleich, 1978).

As will be discussed in the section on mebendazole, this benzimidazole carbamate interacts with cytoplasmic microtubules causing degenerative changes in the absorptive cells of parasitic nematodes and cestodes (Borgers *et al.*, 1975b). Friedman and Platzer (1978) investigated the binding and inhibitory properties of 11 benzimidazole derivatives for bovine brain tubulin. They found that fenbendazole, oxibendazole, parbendazole, and mebendazole are potent inhibitors of the initial rate of polymerization. Ireland *et al.* (1979) have described similar results with sheep brain tubulin. Friedman and Platzer (1980) also determined the inhibition constants (K_i) of mebendazole and flubendazole for bovine brain tubulin and *Ascaris suum* embryonic tubulin. The K_i of mebendazole and fenbendazole for *A. suum* embryonic tubulin were respectively 384 and 262 times smaller than the K_i of mebendazole and fenbendazole for bovine brain tubulin. These studies provide evidence that the anthelmintic activity of fenbendazole may also be based on its effects on microtubules. The consequences of such effects are discussed in the section on mebendazole.

D. Flubendazole

Flubendazole in the generic name of methyl[5-(4-fluorobenzoyl)-1*H*-benzimidazol-2-yl] carbamate, the *p*-fluoro derivative of mebendazole synthesized at Janssen Pharmaceutica. Flubendazole is insoluble in alcohol, inorganic acids, and water. It is slightly soluble in organic acids and solvents. In formic acid 34.05 g is soluble in 100 ml. The log P value, i.e., the logarithm of the partition coefficient of the substance between octanol and water, is 3.22.

1. *Pharmacokinetics*

Different studies have demonstrated that after oral treatment of rats, dogs, pig, and man, only small quantities of flubendazole are resorbed.

Plasma levels of flubendazole (radioimmunoassay) 4 hours after oral administration of 40 mg/kg were 81 ng/ml in Wistar rats and 17 ng/ml in multimammate rats. At 24 hours flubendazole levels amounted to 5.6 ng/ml. After subcutaneous injection peak flubendazole levels of 8–9 ng/ml were found 8 hours after subcutaneous administration of 40 mg flubendazole per kg to Wistar and multimammate rats. At 48 hours, plasma concentrations still represent 32% of the peak level (Michiels *et al.*, 1980a).

Plasma levels of about 0.9 and 4 ng/ml 41 days after the last treatment were found in dogs injected intramuscularly for 5 consecutive days at a dose level of 2.5 or 25 mg/kg flubendazole. Plasma levels were maximal 3–4 days after the last dose reaching peak concentrations of 2.4 and 13 ng/ml for the low and high dose levels, respectively (Michiels *et al.*, 1980b).

Pigs treated with a single dose of flubendazole at 5 mg/kg body weight were slaughtered 24, 48, and 72 hours after treatment. Plasma concentrations measured with a HPLC method were 20, 30, and less than 10 ng/ml for the various time points. Tissue levels in the liver, kidney, and muscle were approximately 10 ng/g tissue up to 72 hours after treatment. Levels in fat varied between 60 and 70 ng/g (Michiels *et al.*, 1977).

Plasma levels of flubendazole in man are extremely low. For example, after a 100-mg dose peak levels (1–4 hours after dosing) were less than 0.4 ng/ml, indicating that less than 0.2% of the administered dose was present in the whole plasma volume. All plasma levels measured, even after a 2-g dose, were lower than 1 ng/ml when flubendazole was given 2 hours before a light meal, consisting of three pieces of bread with butter and marmelade. Plasma levels were considerably higher (about 4 ng/ml) when flubendazole was given directly after a heavy breakfast, consisting of three pieces of bread with ham, eggs, and milk.

When specifically ^{14}C-labeled flubendazole was administered orally to male Wistar rats at a dose of 10 mg/kg, practically all the radioactivity was recovered in the excreta within 4 days. Seven percent was excreted with the urine and 89% with the feces. The fecal radioactivity was mainly due to unchanged flubendazole, and the urinary radioactivity almost exclusively to metabolites. The main identified metabolites resulted from a carbamate hydrolysis and reduction of the ketone; the former metabolites were found in both feces and urine, the latter was present in urine mainly as glucuronide (Meuldermans *et al.*, 1977).

2. *Toxicology* (*Thienpont et al., 1978*)

Toxicity studies were performed in various laboratory animals. The oral LD_{50} exceeded 2560 mg/kg in all species studied. Neither behavioral nor toxic effects were observed in mice, rats, and guinea pigs. In the chronic toxicity test in rats and dogs no side effects were observed, either clinically or histopathologically. No embryotoxic and teratogenic effects were seen in rats dosed from day 6 through day 15 of pregnancy with 2.5–40 mg/kg and in rabbits dosed from day 6 through day 18 of pregnancy with 10–40 mg/kg.

3. *Mode of Action*

The mode of action of flubendazole is identical to the mode of action of mebendazole and will therefore be dealt with in the next section.

E. Mebendazole

Mebendazole or methyl[5-(benzoyl)-1*H*-benzimidazol-2-yl] carbamate (Janssen Pharmaceutica) is almost insoluble in water and ethanol. In dimethyl sulfoxide its solubility is 2.4 g/100 ml. The log *P* value, i.e., the logarithm of the partition coefficient of the substance between octanol and water, is 3.10.

1. *Pharmacokinetics*

Mebendazole is poorly absorbed from the intestinal tract. The quantity of mebendazole and metabolites excreted via the urine depends on the species. As the survey in Table III shows, the excretion via the urine is only 1% in dogs, whereas in pigs almost 50% of the administered dose is found.

In rats, mebendazole is excreted almost completely unaltered via the feces. The only metabolite that is found in the feces is (2-amino-1*H*-benzimidazol-5-yl) phenylmethanone, which has no anthelmintic activity. This metabolite represents 14.8% of the total radioactivity found in the urine after treating rats with [^{14}C]mebendazole; 7% is the parent com-

TABLE III

Excretion of Mebendazole and Metabolites[a]

Species	Oral dose (mg/kg)	Time after treatment (hours)	Excretion (% of dose administered)		
			Feces	Urine	Total
Rat	2.5	24	82.7	5.1	87.8
		0–96	85.6	5.8	91.4
	10.0	0–96	92.1	12.6	104.7
Dog	10.0	0–96	90.5	0.9	91.4
Pig	1.0	0–96	45–64	32–48	93–96

[a] Source of information: Department of Drug Metabolism, Janssen Pharmaceutica.

pound and 18% methyl[5-(α-hydroxy-α-phenylmethyl-1*H*-benzimidazol-2-yl)] carbamate formed by reduction of the ketone group of mebendazole (Meuldermans *et al.*, 1977).

After Wistar rats and multimammate rats were treated with an oral dose of 40 mg/kg of mebendazole, their plasma levels (RIA method) reached 400 and 130 ng/ml, respectively, at 4 hours after drug administration. Plasma levels decreased rapidly to 37.8 ng/ml at 8 hours in the multimammate group but remained near peak levels in the Wistar rats (349 ng/ml). By 24 hours, mebendazole in the latter group had almost disappeared from the plasma. After subcutaneous administration, mebendazole was absorbed more gradually, reaching peak levels for either strain of about 60–70 ng/ml within 4–8 hours after injection. At 48 hours, plasma levels in the Wistar rat had decreased to 9.3 ng/ml (Michiels *et al.*, 1980a).

In jirds infected with *Echinococcus multilocularis* that were treated with 100 to 1000 ppm mebendazole in the food, plasma concentrations of the drug (HPLC method) varied between 118 and 1062 ng/ml. It is of interest to note that in infected animals, drug plasma levels above 73.7 ng/ml were associated with significant decrease of parasitic weights (Schantz *et al.*, 1981).

In humans, after receiving orally 200 mg/day for 3 days, plasma levels never exceeded 30 ng mebendazole per ml and 90 ng/ml of the amino derivative described above (Demoen *et al.*, 1973).

After oral administration of 1.5 g mebendazole to fasting volunteers, only plasma concentrations $\leq$5 ng/ml were found. Measurable plasma concentrations of 5–39.5 ng/ml were found if mebendazole tablets were swallowed during a meal (Münst *et al.*, 1980). In a patient with cholestasis, a plasma concentration of 112 ng/ml was found which is much higher than the plasma concentrations measured in normal subjects who received similar doses (Münst *et al.*, 1980).

The absorption of mebendazole by parasitic worms after treating the host was also studied (Van den Bossche and Janssen, 1981). When turkeys were treated with 63 ppm of mebendazole in the food for 48 hours, 6.7 ng of mebendazole and/or metabolites were found per *Syngamus trachea* worm pair. Even smaller amounts of mebendazole reached the rat pinworm, *Syphacia muris*. Twenty four hours after oral treatment of the rat host with a single therapeutic dose of 2.5 mg/kg, 60 pg of mebendazole was found.

2. *Toxicology* (*Janssen Pharmaceutica, 1972; Marsboom, 1973*)

Pharmacologically, mebendazole is almost an inert substance. It has no effect on the central nervous system and it has no analgesic, hypnotic, or anticonvulsive effects.

The acute oral toxicity of mebendazole was evaluated in various animal species. The oral LD_{50} values are higher than 1.28 g/kg in mice, rats, and guinea pigs and higher than 0.64 g/kg in rabbits, dogs, and cats. In chickens and pheasants, no side effects were noticed after treatment with 1 or 1.28 g/kg. No clinical abnormalities were shown in sheep treated with 320 mg/kg. The temperature and the cardiac and respiratory rhythm of horses treated with 40 mg/kg remained normal. The only side effects reported were transient softening of the feces and diarrhea affecting some pigs, and, in one study, horses given 400 mg/kg body weight had diarrhea.

Dogs tolerated daily doses of 40 mg/kg body weight for 104 weeks with no hematologic, clinical, or histologic changes. After daily treatment of horses with a standard dose of 5 g mebendazole for 19 to 74 days the intake of food, weight, physical appearance, and blood analysis were normal.

When mebendazole is given to dogs, sheep, pigs, and horses during organogenesis, no teratogenic or embryotoxic effects were observed; in rats when 40 mg of mebendazole per kg body weight was given, some skeleton abnormalities were seen. Mebendazole does not affect the fertility of rats when a dose of 40 mg/kg is given to male and female rats for respectively 14 and 60 days prior to mating and further throughout gestation. Also when the same dose was given to rats from the sixteenth day of gestation throughout a 3-week lactation period, no effect on mortality, pregnancy, weight, and intake of food could be shown. The number of the offspring, their weight at birth, and their weight increase were not affected either.

3. *Mode of Action*

Mebendazole affects *in vitro* and *in vivo* the glucose uptake by nematodes and cestodes (Van den Bossche, 1972, 1976; Van den Bossche and De Nollin, 1973; De Nollin and Van den Bossche, 1973). For example, 40% inhibition of the *in vitro* glucose uptake by *Ascaris* is achieved after 24 hours incubation in the presence of 8×10^{-8} *M*. This decreased glucose uptake is followed by an increased utilization of endogenous glycogen and/or decreased synthesis of this polysaccharide (Van den Bossche, 1972, 1976; Rahman and Bryant, 1977). What is the basis of the mebendazole induced impairment of glucose absorption?

In *Ascaris* most of the mebendazole is taken up by the esophagus and intestinal cells where it was mainly found in the cytoplasmic fraction partly bound to proteins with a molecular weight of about 100,000 and 50,000–60,000. Both molecular weights correspond relatively well to those of the dimer and monomer of tubulin. Tubulin is the functional subunit of microtubules which participate in several important cell functions, e.g., the transport of materials within cells.

Both mebendazole (Borgers *et al.*, 1975a,b; Verheyen *et al.*, 1976) and its fluorine analog flubendazole (Verheyen *et al.*, 1976) induce the disappearance of the cytoplasmic microtubules of the tegumental or intestinal cells of cestodes or nematodes. This is followed by a block in transport of secretory vesicles. This may lead to impaired coating of the membranes, followed by a decreased digestion and absorption of nutrients.

Mebendazole shares with other benzimidazole derivatives the ability to bind to tubulin and to inhibit the assembly of microtubules (Hoebeke *et al.*, 1976; Friedman and Platzer, 1978; Ireland *et al.*, 1979). For example, Friedman and Platzer (1980a,b) presented evidence of differential binding affinities of mebendazole for *Ascaris suum* embryonic tubulin and mammalian brain tubulin. *A. suum* embryonic tubulin was 384 times more sensitive to mebendazole than bovine brain tubulin. This observation suggests that tubulin from different phylogenetic sources may have differential binding affinities. Köhler and Bachmann (1980) described the partial purification of *Ascaris* intestinal tubulin and the interaction of mebendazole with this tubulin and that of pig brain. The results presented indicated that mebendazole could bind about two times more tightly to the parasite tubulin. Therefore it is doubtful that this small differential affinity of host and parasite tubulin could be responsible for the apparently selective interaction of the drug with the cytoplasmic microtubule of the *Ascaris* intestine (Köhler and Bachmann, 1980).

It should be investigated whether the selective toxicity could be a result of differential pharmacokinetic behavior between host and parasitic helminth.

F. Oxfendazole

Methyl-5(6)-phenylsulfinyl-2-benzimidazole carbamate (oxfendazole, Syntex Research) is another potent anthelmintic (Averkin *et al.*, 1975).

1. *Pharmacokinetics*

Prichard *et al.* (1978c) determined plasma levels of fenbendazole plus metabolites (using [^{14}C]fenbendazole and liquid scintillation counting) and of oxfendazole (using a radioimmunoassay) in previously worm-free sheep experimentally infected with 5000 benzimidazole-resistant *Haemonchus contortus* and 5000 benzimidazole resistant *Trichostrongylus colubriformis*. Sheep were treated with 5 mg/kg per os. Oxfendazole produced a higher maximum concentration in plasma (almost 3 μg/ml) than fenbendazole plus metabolites (about 0.5 μg/ml). The plasma half-decay time was 22 hours for fenbendazole and 28 hours for oxfendazole.

Prichard and Hennesy (1981) found that direct intraabomasal oxfendazole (5 mg/kg) administration, to sheep artificially infected with *T. colubriformis* and *H. contortus,* resulted in the peak plasma oxfendazole concentration (about 1.25 μg/ml) occurring sooner (time of peak plasma concentration, 6 hours) and the area under the plasma oxfendazole concentration curve being reduced when compared with intraruminal administration (plasma concentration about 1.15 μg/ml; time of peak plasma concentration, 26 hours).

2. *Toxicology*

Preliminary acute toxicity studies indicated an LD_{50} value for beagle dogs of more than 1.6 g/kg and over 6.4 g/kg in rats and mice (Averkin *et al.,* 1975).

Delatour *et al.* (1977) studied the potential embryotoxicity of oxfendazole and showed that the dose recommended for sheep must be strictly respected for the ewe at the beginning of the period of gestation. In fact a dose 4.5 times the therapeutic dose is teratogenic and embryotoxic when given on the seventeenth day of gestation.

The same authors also found oxfendazole to be embryotoxic in rats treated daily with 15.75 and 21 mg/kg from the eighth to the fifteenth day of the gestation period. It is of interest to note that fenbendazole was not embryotoxic at a dose of 119.6 mg/kg given to rats for the same period (Delatour *et al.,* 1977).

3. *Mode of Action*

The limited solubility of oxfendazole precluded accurate measurements of the concentrations of drug causing 50% inhibition of brain microtubule assembly (Ireland *et al.,* 1979). However the benzimidazole carbamates seem to have in common the property to bind to tubulin so that a similar mode of action may be proposed.

Oxfendazole inhibits the fumarate stimulated oxidation of NADH in mitochondria from susceptible *Haemonchus contortus;* 100% inhibition was achieved at 5×10^{-5} *M* (Prichard *et al.,* 1978c). Further studies are needed to determine the involvement of oxfendazole's (and other benzimidazole carbamates) interference with energy metabolism in its anthelmintic properties.

G. Oxibendazole

Oxibendazole or methyl[5-(*n*-propoxy)-1*H*-benzimidazol-2-yl] carbamate is a product synthesized at Smith Kline Corporation. It is insoluble in water and only slightly soluble in most organic solvents (Theodorides *et al.,* 1973).

1. *Pharmacokinetics*

Oral administration of ^{14}C-labeled oxibendazole at 53 mg/kg body weight to sheep resulted in a peak plasma level of 2.43 μg/ml after 6 hours. Approximately 34% of the administered dose was recovered in the urine in 24 hours, with an additional 6% recovered after 216 hours (Theodorides *et al.*, 1973).

2. *Toxicology*

A single dose of 300 mg/kg body weight was well tolerated by sheep. Oxibendazole was administered orally to mated Long Evans rats from day 6 through day 15 of gestation at dose levels of 1, 3, 10, and 30 mg/kg. There were no adverse effects upon pregnancy rate, mortality, implantation efficiency, resorptions, fetal size, ossification variations, or malformations (Theodorides *et al.*, 1973).

Delatour *et al.* (1976a) studied the possible effects of oxibendazole in rat and sheep. They found oxibendazole devoid of teratogenic activity. However at doses four times the therapeutic dose this parbendazole derivative was found to be embryotoxic in both species.

3. *Mode of Action*

Friedman and Platzer (1978), using bovine brain tubulin as experimental model, found oxibendazole like the other 2-carbamomethoxy-5-substituted benzimidazoles, to be a potent inhibitor of microtubule polymerization and five times more potent than the antimitotic agent colchicine. Further studies are needed to investigate oxibendazole's effect on the microtubular system of helminths.

H. PARBENDAZOLE

Parbendazole is the generic name of methyl-5(6)-butyl-2-benzimidazole carbamate, synthesized in 1966 at the Smith Kline and French laboratories. (Actor *et al.*, 1967).

1. *Pharmacokinetics*

Oral administration of [^{14}C]parbendazole to swine resulted in a peak plasma concentration after 6 hours. In 24 hours 11% of the radioactivity was detected in the urine, which consisted of the parent compound and two metabolites. Tissue residues were less than 0.1 ppm 21 days after oral administration of 50 mg [^{14}C]parbendazole per kg body weight (Actor *et al.*, 1967).

In sheep, tissue residues in muscle, fat, skin, liver, kidney, heart, bile, and plasma were less than 0.1 ppm 16 days after the administration of an oral dose of 45 mg [^{14}C]parbendazole/kg (Actor *et al.*, 1976).

The structures of seven metabolites isolated from sheep and cattle and from two fungi (*Cunnighamella bainieri* and *Paecilomyces* spp.) were determined by Dunn *et al.* (1973). The two major metabolites isolated from both sheep and cattle were shown to be methyl-5(6)-(3-carboxypropyl)-2-benzimidazole carbamate and methyl-*threo*-5(6)-(1,2-dihydroxybutyl)-2-benzimidazole carbamate. The first-mentioned metabolite was also produced by *C. bainieri*.

2. *Toxicology*

A single oral dose of parbendazole was well tolerated by sheep and swine. In subacute experiments in sheep, 75 mg/kg per day and 250 mg/kg per day (normal dose used is 20 mg/kg) were administered for 6 consecutive days. None of the animals died, though animals showed anorexia, weight loss, and a slight reduction in bromosulfalein clearance time. At autopsy the only significant lesions were acute irritation of the omasum and reticulum and abnormally liquid rumenal contents (O'Brien, 1970). The oral LD_{50} for rats and mice exceeds 4 g/kg body weight (Actor *et al.*, 1967).

Lapras *et al.* (1973) reported congenital abnormalities in lambs from ewes treated with parbendazole between the ninth and twenty-first day of gestation. Delatour *et al.* (1974, 1976b) found parbendazole to be embryotoxic and teratogenic in rats.

3. *Mode of Action*

Using an *in vitro* model Friedman and Platzer (1978) showed that parbendazole, like the other benzimidazole carbamates, can bind to bovine brain tubulin and prevent the polymerization process.

III. Benzimidazole Carbamates in Veterinary Medicine

A. Introduction

The purpose of this section is to provide a comprehensive review of the benzimidazole carbamates of use in veterinary medicine up to 1981. In such a review the results can only be selected and summarized. For special details the reader therefore is referred to the original publications cited in the reference list. For fenbendazole, Düwel (1980) has reviewed the scientific journals up to autumn 1978.

B. Equids

1. *Introduction*

Of the different benzimidazole carbamates, experimental and or clinical data in equine helminthiasis are available for albendazole, fenbendazole, mebendazole, oxfendazole, oxibendazole, and parbendazole. Four of them have been developed and registered for clinical use in horses. Details on dosage, formulation, and trade names are summarized in Table IV.

2. *Mebendazole*

The anthelmintic activity of mebendazole has been evaluated using autopsy data in 115 horses and 5 donkeys naturally infected with several species of worms.

Mebendazole at a standard dose of 5 to 10 mg/kg is highly effective against *Parascaris equorum,* the large strongylus *Alfortia edentata, Delafondia vulgaris, Strongylus equinus,* and *Strongylus* spp., a great number of small strongyles, e.g., *Craterostomum* spp., *Gyalocephalus capitatus, Oesophagodontus* spp., *Poteriostomum* spp., *Trichonema* spp., and *Triodontophorus* spp., and the pinworms *Oxyuris equi* and *Probstmayria vivipara.* At 20 mg/kg the cestodes *Anoplocephala* are expelled and at 20 mg/kg for 5 days an efficacy between 95 and 100% was observed in horses infected with the lungworm *Dictyocaulus arnfieldi*.

TABLE IV

Benzimidazole Carbamates in Equids

Anthelmintic	Tradename	Formulations	Company
Albendazole	Not registered in horses		Smith Kline
Fenbendazole	Panacur	10% suspension 22% powder	Hoechst
Mebendazole	Telmin	10% granulate	Janssen Pharmaceutica
	Telmin paste	20 g paste at 20%	
	Telmin + trichlorfon	40 g paste (mebendazole 4 g + 18.360 g trichlorfon)	
Oxfendazole	Synanthic	Powder/pellets	Syntex
Oxibendazole	Anthelcide-EQ.	10% suspension	Norden
	Vermikin Equiminthe	20 g paste, 2 g oxibend.	Thekan France
	Equiminthe plus	Paste 2.5 oxibendazole, 5 g dichlorvos	Virbac
Parbendazole	Not registered in horses		Smith Kline

The stomach worms *Trichostrongylus axei, Habronema* spp. and *Strongyloides westeri* also seem to be sensitive to mebendazole. However, a too small number of animals has been treated to evaluate the anthelmintic activity. A larvicidal effect on the L_4-larvae of *O. equi* and *P. vivipara* was also observed. The anthelmintic efficacy of mebendazole and other benzimidazole derivatives observed at therapeutic doses is given in Table V.

The clinical investigation of mebendazole granules and paste in horses was conducted in Belgium, the Netherlands, Great Britain, France, Germany, South Africa, and the United States (Callear and Neave, 1971; Guilhon *et al.,* 1971; Walker and Knight, 1972; Reinecke and Le Roux, 1972; Saupe and Nitz, 1972; McCurdy *et al.,* 1976; Muylle *et al.,* 1979). The younger horses received 2 g and the older 4 g of the active substance (standard dose of 5 to 10 mg/kg). The pure substance and the granules were well accepted by all animals, including thoroughbreds and Welsh ponies which in general are very refractory to oral medication. Mebendazole paste replaced the granules when deworming via the feed was difficult or impossible, i.e., to treat sick horses that eat very little or not at all, stubborn one of 2-year-old foals, unweaned foals, and especially horses which remain in the pasture and receive no additional feed.

In horses no side effects were noted following single oral doses as high as 600 mg/kg. Mebendazole is highly palatable and well tolerated even by severely infected or debilitated animals. Gravid mares had a normal pregnancy. It is compatible with other treatments and can be prescribed for horses being treated with insecticides, tranquilizers, or muscle relaxants. Since mebendazole is so well accepted, routine deworming is easy to perform (Marsboom, 1975; Bennett *et al.,* 1974).

3. *Other Benzimidazoles* (*Table V*)

Albendazole has about the same spectrum as mebendazole. However, only limited autopsy data are available to evaluate its efficacy (Colglazier *et al.,* 1977).

Fenbendazole at a dose of 5 mg/kg is sufficient to remove the greater part of the gastrointestinal worm burden. By raising the dose to 7.5 mg/kg the effect on immature forms is enhanced and even *Parascaris equorum* can be effectively attacked (Düwel, 1980). At 50 mg/kg it reduces *Strongyloides* infections in foals (Enigk *et al.,* 1974). It is efficacious against a large proportion of immature stages of the horse strongyles (Duncan and Reid, 1978).

Oxfendazole is efficacious against *Strongylus* spp., small strongyles, and mature *Oxyuris equi* at dose levels as small as 1.1 mg/kg and against *Parascaris equorum* at the dose level of 10 mg/kg. Oxfendazole did not seem to cause adverse reactions in the treated horses. However, a transient liquifying of the feces of a horse treated at the dose of 100 mg/kg has been seen (Lyons *et al.*, 1977).

Oxibendazole is effective against adult large strongyles and against adult and larval stages of the pinworm *Oxyuris equi*. It is inactive against tapeworms, lungworms, and abdominal worms (*Setaria equina*) (Kates *et al.*, 1975). When the dose is raised to 15 mg/kg, high efficacy is obtained against the small strongyles and *Probstmayria*.

Little information is available on the use of parbendazole in horse (Ostman and Scheidy, 1970; Verberne and Mirck, 1975; Drudge and Lyons, 1969). So far the product has not been registered in horses. Parbendazole proved to have a fairly narrow safety margin in horses. Verberne and Mirck (1975) reported side effects such as laxation (soft dung, diarrhea), anorexia, and listlessness with parbendazole at the therapeutic dose of 7.5 mg/kg. Half the therapeutic dose of parbendazole (2.5 to 3.75 mg/kg) administered on 2 consecutive days led, as a rule, to only slight toxic symptoms and proved highly effective.

4. *Conclusion*

Because of their safety, their easy method of administration, and their broad spectrum, most of the benzimidazole carbamates are the drug of choice to be used in routine deworming, even up to one treatment every 6 weeks.

C. Domestic Ruminants

1. *Introduction*

With tiabendazole (Brown *et al.*, 1961), the tetrahydroimidazoles tetramisole (Thienpont *et al.*, 1966) and levamisole, the benzimidazoles are now considered the most potent anthelmintics with the widest range of efficacy against the economically important helminth parasites of domestic ruminants. The story of the 2-amino substituted benzimidazole anthelmintics started with parbendazole (Actor *et al.*, 1967), and evolved over mebendazole (Brugmans *et al.*, 1971), oxibendazole (Theodorides *et al.*, 1973), fenbendazole (Baeder *et al.*, 1974), oxfendazole (Averkin *et al.*, 1975), albendazole (Theodorides *et al.*, 1976a), and flubendazole (Thienpont *et al.*, 1978). The available formulations and trade names are given in Table VI.

2. *Sheep and Goats*

a. Mebendazole. Mebendazole has been extensively tested under a wide variety of conditions in Argentina, Australia, Belgium, USSR, En-

TABLE V

ANTHELMINTIC EFFICACY OF BENZIMIDAZOLE CARBAMATES IN EQUIDS[a,b]

Worm species	Anthelmintic						References[c]
	Albendazole	Fenbendazole	Mebendazole	Oxfendazole	Oxibendazole	Parbendazole	
Lungworms							
Dictyocaulus arnfieldi		+++	+++		0		1,2,3
Stomach worms							
Trichostrongylus axei		+	(+)	(+++)			1,4,5,6,7
Habronema spp.		+++	(+)	(+)			1,5,8,9,10,11
Small intestine worms							
Parascaris equorum	+++	++–+++	+++	++	(+++)	+++	1,3,5,6,8,9,11,12,13, 14,15,16,17,18
Strongyloides westeri		+++	+	(+)?	+		1,5,9,19,20,21,22
Large intestine worms							
Large strongyles							
Delafondia (*Strongylus*) *vulgaris*	+++	+++	+++	+++	++–+++	+++	1,3,5,6,8,9,11,12,13, 15,16,17
Alfortia (*Strongylus*) *edentata*	+++	+++	+++	+++	++–+++		1,3,5,8,9,12,15,16,17

Strongylus equinus	+++	++	+++	+++	(+++)		1,3,8,9,11,12,15,16,18
Strongylus spp. (unspecified)		+++	+++				1,9,18
Small strongyles							
Triodontophorus spp.	+++	+++	+++	+++	+++		1,3,5,9,12
Oesophagodontus spp.	+++	+++	+++	+++	+++		1,3,5,10,12
Craterostomum spp.	+++	+++	+++	+++	+++		1,3,5,10,12
Trichonema spp.	+++	+++	++–+++	+++	+++		1,3,6,7,9,10,11,12
Poteriostomum spp.	+++	+++	+++	+++	+++		1,3,5,10,12
Gyalocephalus spp.	+++	+++	+++	+++	+++		1,3,5,10,12
Small strongyles (unspecified)	+++	++–+++	+++	++–+++	+++		1,3,5,8,9,11,12,15,18
Pinworms							
Oxyuris equi	+++	+++	+++	+++	+++	+++	1,3,5,6,8,9,11,12,13, 15,16,17,18
Probstmayria vivipara		+++	+++		+++		1,3,10
Cestodes							
Anoplocephala spp.		+++	+++	(+)?	0		1,3,5,8,18,23

[a] Classification efficacy: +++, 95–100%; ++, 80–100%; +, 0–100%; 0, none; ( ), insufficient or no autopsy data.

[b] Doses are given in the text.

[c] 1. Düwel (1980); 2. Clayton and Neave (1979); 3. Kates *et al.* (1975); 4. Walker and Knight (1972); 5. Lyons *et al.* (1977); 6. Duncan and Reid (1978); 7. Nawalinski and Theodorides (1976); 8. Bradley and Radhakrishnan (1973); 9. Janssen Pharmaceutica (1981); 10. Reinecke and Le Roux (1972); 11. Colglazier (1979); 12. Colglazier *et al.* (1977); 13. Ostmann and Scheidy (1970); 14. Smith Kline (1978); 15. Bennett (1973); 16. McCurdy *et al.* (1976); 17. Guerrero and Sharp (1979); 18. Lyons *et al.* (1981); 19. Stoye (1972); 20. Callear and Neave (1971); 21. Ribbeck and Kuller (1976); 22. Drudge *et al.* (1980); 23. Kelly and Bain (1975).

TABLE VI

BENZIMIDAZOLE CARBAMATES IN DOMESTIC RUMINANTS

Anthelmintic	Tradename	Formulations	Company
Albendazole	Valbazen	Suspension 1.9, 2.5, 5, 7.5, 10%,	Smith Kline
		Boli 20%;	
		Pellets 1%	
Fenbendazole	Panacur	Suspension 2.5, 10%	Hoechst
	Axilur	Granulate 22%	
		Boli 250 mg	
		Wormblock	
Mebendazole	Ovitelmin	Boli 1 g	Janssen Pharmaceutica
	Multispec	Suspension 5%	
Oxfendazole	Synanthic	Boli 568 mg	Wellcome
	Systamex	Suspension 2.265% or 9.06%	Syntex
Oxibendazole	Loditac	Suspension 5, 7.5, 10%	Smith Kline
		Premix 5, 30%	
		Powder 30%	
Parbendazole	Helmatac	Boli 1.2 g, 1.8 g	Smith Kline
		Powder 30%	
		Pellets 3.2%	
	Worm Guard	Suspension 4%	

gland, France, Germany, and South Africa (Taboa, 1972; Guilhon and Barnabe, 1973; Varga and Janisch, 1975a,b; Wallnoefer, 1977; Ribbeck and Winter, 1978; Janssen Pharmaceutica, 1981). In sheep and goats it is registered for the control of gastrointestinal nematodes, lungworms, and tapeworms. The anthelmintic efficacy of mebendazole and other benzimidazole carbamates is listed in Table VII.

Doses as low as 5 mg/kg are 100% active against *Cooperia* sp., *Strongyloides papillosus, Chabertia ovina,* and *Bunostomum* spp. In some studies 100% efficacy against *Haemonchus contortus* was found at 2.5 mg/kg. One single standard dose of 15 mg/kg controls all economically important roundworms including the lungworm *Dictyocaulus filaria* and eliminates scolices and protoglottides of the tapeworms *Moniezia* and *Avitellina*. At 3 × 15 mg/kg mebendazole is effective against the small lungworms *Protostrongylus* and *Muellerius*. At higher doses of 50 mg/kg for 3–14 days high efficacy has been proven against the cysts of *Taenia hydatigena, Taenia ovis,* and *Echinococcus granulosus*. Preliminary data reveal some activity of mebendazole against the liver fluke *Fasciola hepatica*.

Mebendazole has also been used in wild ruminants (Dollinger, 1973; Kutzer *et al.,* 1974; Pav *et al.,* 1975). It is mixed through the concentrated feed, wetted biscuits, or with pelleted feed for mouflons, deer, roe deer, fallow deer, alces, etc. at 15 mg/kg in the feed for 2 consecutive days or 3 mg/kg in the feed for 10 consecutive days. Mebendazole has a very wide margin of safety and causes no side effects. It has a safety factor up to 40 after a single oral dosage. It can be safely used at a standard dose (±15 mg/kg) in sheep and goats of all ages, sex, condition, feeding regimes, stages of pregnancy, or breeding cycle (Marsboom, 1973). Two days after treatment no traces of mebendazole were detectable in the milk. Mebendazole has no effect on cheese quality. The withholding period between treatment and slaughter is 7 days.

b. Albendazole. Theodorides *et al.* (1976a) reported that albendazole, a recent member of the benzimidazole carbamates, has a spectrum of activity covering gastrointestinal nematodes, lungworms, tapeworms, and to some extent liver fluke. At 3.8 mg/kg its efficacy against mature and immature gastrointestinal nematodes is in the high 90s as with most benzimidazoles. Efficacy against lungworms, *Nematodirus, Bunostomum, Strongyloides,* and *Trichuris* is somewhat less (Theodorides, 1977). Albendazole is also active against the adult liver fluke. However, it is not recommended for the treatment of outbreaks of acute fascioliasis caused by immature liver fluke attack.

Albendazole shows the characteristic high safety of benzimidazoles with a minimum toxic dose rate of more than 10 times the therapeutic dosage for roundworm and up to 5 times the fluke dose rate. The maximum tolerated dose is 53 mg/kg in sheep. It is teratogenic in sheep at dosages of 11 mg/kg or greater given on day 17 of pregnancy (Theodorides, 1977). It may not be used by ewes during tupping and for 1 month after removing rams. Ten days should elapse between treatment and the slaughter of sheep for human consumption.

c. Fenbendazole. Fenbendazole's efficacy is in line with benzimidazoles in general. The range of activity covers practically all important nematodes of the abomasum, and intestines, together with the large lungworms. The protostrongylids can be affected up to 100% with single doses of 15 mg/kg or more. Its activity against tapeworms in sheep is not complete at dosages recommended for nematodes and it is registered with the wording "aids in tapeworm control," but at a dose of 10 mg/kg tapeworm infection can be clinically and parasitologically cured. High doses (>100 mg/kg) are active against *Fasciola* and *Dicrocoelium*. Fenbendazole seems to be active against the hypobiotic larval stages of various strongylids in sheep. Multiple dosing gives better results. Low levels of 0.25 mg/kg/day for 14 days to 1.4 mg/kg/day for 4 days are extremely effective against a variety of gastrointestinal nematodes including inhibited *Ostertagia* larvae and *Dictyocaulus filaria* (Düwel, 1980; Kutzer *et al.*, 1974). The withholding period is 5 days.

TABLE VII

ANTHELMINTIC EFFICACY OF BENZIMIDAZOLE CARBAMATES IN SHEEP AND GOATS[a,b]

Worm species	Anthelmintic							References[c]
	Albendazole	Fenbendazole	Flubendazole	Mebendazole	Oxfendazole	Oxibendazole	Parbendazole	
Lungworms								
Dictyocaulus filaria	++–+++	+++		+++	+++		0	1,2,3,4,5,6,7
Muellerius capillaris		++		(+++)			0	3,7,8,9
Protostrongylus rufescens	++	+++		(+++)			0	3,7,8,10
Capreocaulus ocreatus		+++		(++)				3,4
Stomach worms								
Haemonchus contortus	+++	+++	+++	+++	+++	++–+++	+++	1,3,4,5,6,11, 12,13,14, 15,16,17
Ostertagia circumcincta	+++	+++	+++	++–+++	+++	++–+++	+++	2,3,4,5,6,12, 13,14,15, 17,18,19
Trichostrongylus axei	+++	+++	+++	+++	+++	++–+++	+++	4,12,13,15, 17,20,25
Small intestine worms								
Trichostrongylus spp.	+++	+++	+++	+++	+++	++–+++	+++	2,3,4,5,6,12, 14,15,16, 19,21
Nematodirus spathiger	+++	+++		+++	+++	++–+++	++–+++	1,3,4,5,6,13, 14,15,17, 18,19,20, 21,22
Cooperia sp.	+++	+++	++–+++	+++	+++	+++	+++	3,4,6,13,14, 15,17,22,23
Strongyloides papillosus	++	++–+++	+–+++	+++	+–++	+++	++–+++	3,4,5,12,13, 14,15,17,23

Bunostomum sp.	++–+++	+++	+++	+++	+++	++–+++	++–+++	3,4,12,13,14, 15,17,23
Gaigeria pachyscelis	+++	+++		+++	+++		+++	3,4,5,21,24
Capillaria sp.	+–+	+++	+++	(+++)	++–+++			3,4,12,13,23
Large intestine worms								
Chabertia ovina	+++	+++	+++	+++	+++	+++	+++	3,4,5,12,13, 14,15,21, 22,24,25,26
Oesophagostomum spp.	+++	+++		+++	+++	+++	+++	3,4,5,6,13,14, 15,21,24, 25,26
Trichuris ovis	+	++	+++	+	+		+	3,4,12,13,15, 21,23
Cestodes								
Avitellina sp.	+++			+++				4,24
Moniezia sp.	+++	++–+++		+++	+++		0	1,3,4,6,7,23, 26
Thysanosoma actinioides	+++							11
Cysts of *T. hydatigena*				+++				27,28
Cysts of *E. granulosus*				++				29
Cysts of *Taenia ovis*				++				30
Trematodes								
Fasciola hepatica	++	++		+			0	3,7,23,31,32
Dicrocoelium dendriticum	+++	+++						3,33

[a] Classification efficacy: +++, 95–100%; ++, 80–100%; +, 0–100%; 0, none; ( ), insufficient or no autopsy data.

[b] Doses are given in the text.

[c] 1. Theodorides *et al.* (1976d); 2. Ross *et al.* (1978); 3. Düwel (1980); 4. Janssen Pharmaceutica (1981); 5. Berger (1980); 6. Michael *et al.* (1979); 7. Lämmler *et al.* (1969); 8. Taboa (1972); 9. Sprink (1979); 10. Cordero-del-Campillo *et al.* (1980); 11. Craig and Shepherd (1980); 12. Thienpont (1978); 13. Kistner *et al.* (1979); 14. Theodorides *et al.* (1973); 15. Ostmann and Scheidy (1970); 16. Gibson and Parfitt (1971); 17. Ross (1968); 18. Foix (1979); 19. Thomas and Reid (1980); 20. Baker and Fisk (1977); 21. Shone *et al.* (1970); 22. Downey (1977); 23. Theodorides *et al.* (1976a); 24. Theodorides (1977); 25. Kelly and Hall (1979); 26. Daněk *et al.* (1970); 27. Oguz (1977); 28. Oguz (1976); 29. Tinar (1979); 30. Heath and Lawrence (1978); 31. Campbell and Hall (1979); 32. Chevis and Kelly (1978); 33. Himonas and Liakos (1980).

d. Flubendazole. Flubendazole is not registered as an anthelmintic for sheep or cattle. Preliminary data indicate an excellent efficacy at 10 mg/kg against the most important gastrointestinal nematodes (Thienpont *et al.*, 1978).

e. Oxfendazole. Averkin *et al.* (1975) reported that oxfendazole is effective against most important genera of nematodes in the gastrointestinal tract and lungs of sheep. Especially *Chabertia ovina* and *Oesophagostomum verulosum*, parasitic in the colon of sheep and goats, appeared highly susceptible. Exceptions are *Strongyloides papillosus* and *Capillaria* sp. *Trichuris ovis* was the most resistant parasite to oxfendazole (Kistner *et al.*, 1979). Oxfendazole has a 40- to 60-fold safety factor in sheep. It has no teratogenic effect in ewes. Combination with certain flukicides may cause toxicity (Montgomery and Montgomery, 1977). The withholding period between treatment and slaughter is 4 days.

f. Oxibendazole. Oxibendazole has been reported to be effective against a variety of gastrointestinal nematodes in sheep (Theodorides *et al.*, 1973). It is not registered for control of lungworms or tapeworms. The efficacy against *Nematodirus* is more variable with a mean efficacy of about 90% (Hopkins, 1978). A single oral dose of 300 mg/kg was well tolerated by sheep. The safety margin is greater than 60-fold. Teratogenic effects were not detected in sheep at dosages of 30 mg/kg or in cattle at dosages up to 75 mg/kg (Theodorides, 1977). The withholding period between treatment and slaughter is 7 days.

g. Parbendazole. Parbendazole at doses of 15–30 mg/kg is active against most of the important gastrointestinal nematodes in sheep (Actor *et al.*, 1967). It is not registered for lungworm or tapeworm control. Parbendazole is found to be noneffective against *Fasciola hepatica, Moniezia*, lungworms, and is less effective against *Nematodirus* and *Trichuris* (Lämmler *et al.*, 1969). The safety margin of parbendazole in sheep is of the same order as tiabendazole. It is however teratogenic in sheep and produces an embryotoxic effect at 60 mg/kg if given to ewes on day 14 to 24 of pregnancy. The withholding period is 6 days in milk and 3 weeks for meat.

3. *Cattle* (*Table VIII*)

a. Albendazole. Albendazole has in cattle about the same spectrum as in sheep. At 7.5 mg/kg it can be used for the treatment of roundworms, lungworms, and tapeworm infections, including type II ostertagiasis. It is less active against *Haemonchus* sp. *D. viviparus*, and only slightly active against *Trichuris* sp. Variable results were obtained against inhibited fourth stage larvae of *O. ostertagi* in cattle (Williams *et al.*, 1977, 1981). Albendazole at 50 mg/kg has been shown to affect the cysticerci of *Taenia saginata* in calves resulting in a decreased viability of the cysticerci and rapid resolution of the lesions (Lloyd *et al.,* 1978). For the additional treatment of adult liver-fluke infections the dose has to be doubled (15 mg/kg). However in cattle naturally infected with *F. hepatica* efficacy against the adult flukes was rather poor (57 to 63%) and no dose related trend was noticed (Bradley *et al.,* 1981). No side effects were observed at a dose up to 75 mg/kg. Albendazole has a 10-fold safety margin for nematodes and cestodes and a 5-fold safety margin for fascioliasis. The lactating animals currently producing milk for human consumption may not be dosed. Pregnant cows and heifers may not be dosed the first month of pregnancy. Fourteen days should elapse between treatment and the slaughter of cattle for human consumption (Smith Kline, 1978).

b. Fenbendazole. Fenbendazole efficacy against internal parasites is in line with the benzimidazoles in general, i.e., high efficacy against lungworms and gastrointestinal worms; somewhat less active against *Trichuris* sp. and *Strongyloides* sp. Its spectrum includes tapeworms. It does have activity against trematodes *F. hepatica* and *Paramphistomum* but not at economically practical dosages.

In Australia fenbendazole has a registered claim of 80 to 90% efficacy against inhibited fourth stage larvae of *O. ostertagi* in cattle. These larvae, previously refractory to treatment, are responsible for the outbreak of the dangerous winter ostertagiasis or type II ostertagiasis. There have been several reports of high efficacy. However, in some studies the effect was described as variable or inadequate (Düwel, 1980).

Single oral doses of 500 mg/kg are well tolerated. The minimum lethal dose for cattle is 750 mg/kg or 100 times the therapeutic dosage. Fenbendazole does not produce teratogenic effects in cattle. The withholding period between treatment and slaughter is 14 days.

c. Mebendazole. Mebendazole in cattle is only registered for tapeworm infections, at 15 mg/kg. Insufficient data are available to evaluate its anthelmintic efficacy against the important nematodes. At the dose rates tested high efficacy was obtained against most gastrointestinal nematodes (except *Ostertagia*) and against the cestode *Moniezia* sp. (Janssen Pharmaceutica, 1981).

d. Oxfendazole. Oxfendazole's spectrum includes gastrointestinal nematodes, tapeworms, and lungworms. The slightly lower efficacy of oxfendazole against *Strongyloides* sp. is similar to that of fenbendazole. Borgsteede (1977) also reported that the activity against *Strongyloides* and *Moniezia* was variable. It removes 90% of the arrested larvae of *O. ostertagia* (Armour and Duncan, 1978). Oxfendazole has at least a 10-fold safety factor in sheep and cattle but combination with certain flukicides may cause toxicity (Montgomery and Montgomery, 1977).

TABLE VIII

ANTHELMINTIC ACTIVITY OF BENZIMIDAZOLE CARBAMATES IN CATTLE[a,b]

Worm species	Anthelmintic						References[c]
	Albendazole	Fenbendazole	Mebendazole	Oxfendazole	Oxibendazole	Parbendazole	
Lungworms							
Dictyocaulus viviparus	++-+++	+++		+++			1,2,3,4,5,6
Stomach worms							
Haemonchus sp.	++-+++	+++	+++	+++	++-+++	+++	3,4,5,6,7,8,9,10,11, 12,13,14,15,16,17
Ostertagia ostertagi	+++	+++	+	+++	+++	++-+++	2,3,5,6,7,8,9,10,11, 13,14,16,17,18, 19,20
Trichostrongylus axei	+++	+++	+++	+++	+++	+++	3,5,6,7,8,9,10,11, 13,14,15,16,17,19
Small intestine worms							
Trichostrongylus sp.	+++	+++		+++	+++	+++	4,5,8,10,11,12,13,17
Cooperia sp.	+++	+++	++-+++	+++	++-+++	+++	3,4,5,6,8,9,10,11,13, 14,15,16,17,18, 19,20
Bunostomum phlebotomum	+++	+++	+++	+++	++-+++	+++	4,5,6,8,11,12,13,14, 15,17
Strongyloides papillosus	+++	+++	+++	(++)	++-+++		5,6,8,13,21
Nematodirus sp.	+++	+++		+++	++	++-+++	3,5,13,16,17

Toxocara vitulorum		+++					5
Capillaria sp.	−++	+++		+++		+++	5,21
Large intestine worms							
Chabertia ovina		+++		+++			5
Oesophagostomum radiatum	+++	+++	+++	+++	+++	+++	4,5,6,9,10,11,13,14, 16,17
Trichuris sp.	+	++−+++	+++	++	++−+++	++−+++	3,4,5,6,8,11,12, 13,17
Subcutaneous connective tissue							
Parafilaria bovicola		+++					5
Cestodes							
Moniezia sp.	+++		+++	(+++)	+		6,11,21,23
Cysts of *Taenia saginata*	++						24
Trematodes							
Fasciola hepatica	+	+					5,10,21,22,25
Fascioloides magna	++						21,24
Paramphistomum sp.		++					25

[a] Classification efficacy: +++, 95–100%; ++, 80–100%; +, 0–100%; ( ), insufficient or no autopsy data.

[b] Doses are given in the text.

[c] 1. Benz and Ernst (1978); 2. Downey (1978); 3. Downey (1976); 4. Todd and Mansfield (1979); 5. Düwel (1980); 6. Janssen Pharmaceutica (1981); 7. Williams *et al.* (1977a); 8. Theodorides *et al.* (1976d); 9. Benz (1977); 10. Herlich (1977); 11. Williams *et al.* (1977b); 12. Ogunsusi (1979); 13. Theodorides *et al.* (1976c); 14. Benz (1968); 15. Bradley (1968); 16. Rubin (1968); 17. Ostmann and Scheidy (1970); 18. Armour and Duncan (1978); 19. Rubin (1969); 20. Ross (1970); 21. Smith Kline (1978); 22. Bradley *et al.* (1981); 23. Ciordia *et al.* (1978); 24. Lloyd *et al.* (1978); 25. Theodorides and Freeman (1980).

e. Oxibendazole. Oxibendazole's spectrum includes all gastrointestinal nematodes. It is not registered for control of lungworms or tapeworms. At 5–10 mg/kg its efficacy is similar to that in sheep, i.e., the efficacy is somewhat less for *Haemonchus placei, Cooperia* spp., *Bunostomum,* and *Strongyloides.* At higher doses (15 mg/kg) the burdens of larvae from the abomasum and small intestines were reduced for 93–95% (Theodorides *et al.,* 1976c).

f. Parbendazole. In cattle parbendazole has at 30 mg/kg high efficacy against gastrointestinal nematodes. Its activity is somewhat less against *Ostertagia, Nematodirus,* and *Trichuris.* It is not registered for lungworms or tapeworms. The therapeutic index is about 1/40. A dose of 1000 mg/kg has no toxic effects. Young cattle treated with 120 mg/kg on 3 consecutive days show no toxic signs. The withholding period for milk and meat is 5 days.

D. Pig

Introduction

A permanent solution for the worm problem in pig farming should be sought in a combination of strict hygienic measures with both individual and industrial deworming. Industrial deworming is the systematic deworming of all pigs on the farm. This is achieved by treatment at tactical intervals, taking into consideration the prepatent period, with the aim of obtaining and keeping the "whole" farm worm-free.

An anthelmintic that has to serve as an industrial dewormer must satisfy a whole new area of conditions. It must be active against the most

TABLE IX

Benzimidazole Carbamates in Pigs

Anthelmintic	Trademark	Formulations	Company
Fenbendazole	Panacur 4%	Powder 4%	Hoechst
Flubendazole	Flubenol 5%	Powder 5%	Janssen Pharmaceutica
Mebendazole	Mebenvet 5 and 50%	Powder 5 and 50%	Janssen Pharmaceutica
Oxibendazole	Loditac P_5 and P_{30}	Premix 5 and 30%	Smith Kline
	Loditac sachet	Powder 5%	Smith Kline
	AM 313	Granules 4.5 g/1000 g	Smith Kline
	Bovinol 5	Suspension 5%	Labo Thersa
Oxfendazole			Syntex
Parbendazole	Helmatac 30	Premix 30%	Smith Kline
	Vermix, Pigomix 10%	Powder 10%	Proligo/Socavet

important adults, and if possible also the immature stages found in the pig. It must have a wide safety margin so that no side effects occur even after a possible overdose or a prolonged dosing period. The palatability of the medicated food must be excellent. The newer benzimidazoles meet most of these conditions (Table IX). Especially flubendazole was developed as an industrial dewormer for pigs. The anthelmintic activity of therapeutic doses of benzimidazole carbamates is given in Table X.

a. Flubendazole. The parafluor analog of mebendazole, flubendazole, is comparable to the parent compound concerning parasitological properties, but differs from it by its better tolerance in the pig. After administration, for 5 to 10 days, in very low concentrations of 30 ppm flubendazole in the feed, the substance is active against *Metastrongylus, Ascaris, Strongyloides, Oesophagostomum,* and *Trichuris. Hyostrongylus* seems to be less sensitive (91.5%) but the clinical data however reveal high activity (De Keyser, 1980). At higher dose rates (100 ppm for 10 days) flubendazole completely eliminates *Globocephalus* (Kutzer, 1978). An administration of 32 to 125 ppm flubendazole for 14 days is 100% active against *Trichinella,* even against the encysted phase (Bogan, 1980; Thienpont and Vanparijs, 1980). Flubendazole at 10 mg/kg for 10 days is active against *Cysticercus cellulosae* (Teelez-Giron *et al.,* 1980; Galdamez Toledo, 1980). A treatment of 30 ppm flubendazole for 10 days kills the migrating larvae of *Ascaris suum* (Thienpont *et al.,* 1978). Flubendazole inhibits the oviposition, even of more resistant worms such as *Macracanthorhynchus* at 30 ppm for 10 days (Fernandes, 1977).

In clinical trials in Belgium and Germany, flubendazole's activity against the nematodes of the pig was examined in field conditions and on pigs of different ages and sexes (De Keyser, 1980). For group treatment, flubendazole was mixed with a normal commercial feed; it was mixed with a small quantity of feed for individual treatment. Various treatment schedules were tried: the length of treatment was 1, 5, or 10 days. For the 10-day treatment, each sow received about 1 kg medicated feed twice a day. Before and after treatment fecal samples were taken for coprological examination. In mixed infections, *Hyostrongylus rubidus* and *Oesophagostomum dentatum* were differentiated after coproculture.

According to the data obtained from the coprological examination, flubendazole appears to have good anthelmintic activity after a single treatment of 5 mg/kg body weight as well as after a 5- or 10-day treatment with medicated feed. Flubendazole is also an effective anthelmintic against the most important wild boar nematodes (Prosl and Kutzer, 1979), especially against the lungworms (100–150 ppm for 10 days) (Kutzer, 1978).

TABLE X

ANTHELMINTIC EFFICACY OF BENZIMIDAZOLE CARBAMATES IN PIGS[a,b]

Worm species	Anthelmintic							References[c]
	Alben-dazole	Fenben-dazole	Fluben-dazole	Meben-dazole	Oxfen-dazole	Oxiben-dazole	Parben-dazole	
Lung worms								
Metastrongylus sp.		+ – +++	+++		++ – +++		0	1,2,3,4,5
Stomach worms								
Hyostrongylus rubidus		+++	++	+	+++		++	1,4,5,6,7,8
Physocephalus sexalatus		+++	(+++)					2,5
Ascarops strongylina			+++					2
Kidney worms								
Stephanurus dentatus		+++		+++				5,9
Small intestine worms								
Ascaris suum	+++	+ – +++	+++	+++	+++	+++	+++	1,3,4,5,6,10,11,12
Strongyloides ransomi		+ – +++	+++	++	+	++	+++	1,2,5,11,12,13

Large intestine worms								
Oesophagostomum sp.	+++	+++	+++	+++	+++	+++	+++	1,2,3,4,5,6,7,10, 11,12,13
Trichuris suis	+++	++	+++	+++	+-+++	+-+++	+-+++	1,2,3,4,5,6,10,11, 12,14,15
Globocephalus urosubulatus		(+-+++)	(+++)					
Cestodes								
Cysticercus cellulosae			+++					16,17
Cysticercus tenuicollis				+++				18
Echinococcus granulosus (hydatid cysts)				++				19
Trichinella spiralis			+++					20,21

[a] Classification efficacy: +++, 95–100%; ++, 80–100%; +, 0–100%; 0, none; ( ), insufficient or no autopsy data.

[b] Doses are given in the text.

[c] 1. De Keyser (1980); 2. Fernandes (1977); 3. Corwin (1979); 4. Taffs (1970); 5. Düwel (1980); 6. Janssen Pharmaceutica (1981); 7. Kingsbury *et al.* (1981); 8. Pêcheur *et al.* (1971); 9. Brandt *et al.* (1976); 10. Theodorides *et al.* (1976a); 11. Theodorides (1968); 12. Chang and Wescott (1969); 13. Enigk (1976); 14. Kutzer (1978); 15. Prosl and Kutzer (1979); 16. Tellez-Giron *et al.* (1980); 17. Galdamez Toledo (1980a); 18. Langnes (1976); 19. Pavlowski *et al.* (1976); 20. Bogan (1980); 21. Thienpont and Vanparijs (1980).

b. Albendazole. Preliminary experiments with albendazole indicate that low doses (5–10 mg/kg) are effective against *Ascaris, Oesophagostomum,* and *Trichuris* (Theodorides *et al.,* 1976).

c. Fenbendazole. A total therapeutic dose of 5 mg/kg fenbendazole or 5 ppm during 5–6, or if necessary 10 days is active against all economically important nematodes of the digestive tract, including *Trichuris.* Furthermore, the kidney worm *Stephanurus dentatus* and certain lungworms (*Metastrongylus* spp.) are highly susceptible to fenbendazole. An ovicidal effect has also been demonstrated in case of *Stephanurus.* Larvicidal activity against *A. suum, H. rubidus,* and *Oesophagostomum* sp. has been found (Düwel, 1980).

d. Mebendazole. Mebendazole has about the same parasitologic properties as flubendazole. Even at 4–8 ppm mebendazole in the feed for 5 days, or 1.25 mg/kg at one intake, it is 100% active against *Ascaris* (Janssen Pharmaceutica, 1981). At higher dose rates (100 ppm for 10 days) mebendazole completely eliminates the kidney worm *Stephanurus* (Brandt *et al.,* 1976; Hutchinson, 1981). It has a high activity at 25 mg/kg for 5 to 10 days against *Cysticercus tenuicollis* (Langnes, 1976) and the hydatid cysts of *Echinococcus granulosus* (Pavlowski *et al.,* 1976). The pig is slightly sensitive to mebendazole: at overdosage or inadequate mixing of the feed, a transient softening of the feces or sometimes diarrhea is observed.

e. Oxfendazole. Oxfendazole is effective in removing the common nematodes of pigs. This was particularly obvious in the case of *Ascaris suum, Oesophagostomum dentatum,* and mixed populations of *Metastrongylus apri* and *M. pudendotectus.* However, the effect against *Trichuris suis* was variable, with fluctuations in efficacy unrelated to the progressive increase in dose (Corwin, 1979). A dose rate of 4.5 mg provides anthelmintic activity against adult and immature *Oesophagostomum* and *Hyostrongylus* (Kingsbury *et al.,* 1981).

f. Oxibendazole. Oxibendazole is given at three dose levels: 15 mg/kg as a single dose, medicated feed at a concentration of 100 ppm for 6 days, and medicated feed at a concentration of 15 ppm for 50 days. Efficacy against *Ascaris* and *Oesophagostomum* is 100% for the three treatment schedules. Efficacies for the three dosage regimens against *Trichuris* were 74.5, 100, and 80.4%, respectively (Grisi and Lima, 1981). *Strongyloides* was eliminated by 93% with a 15 mg/kg dose (Stoye and Bürger, 1981).

g. Parbendazole. Parbendazole, given in the feed at an oral dose rate of 30 mg/kg, removes effectively *A. suum, Oesophagostomum,* and *Strongyloides.* Action against *Metastrongylus* spp. was not observed, and was variable against *Trichuris* (42 to 100%). Indirect evidence indicated that it was highly effective against *H. rubidus* (Pêcheur *et al.,* 1971). An ovicidal effect on the eggs of *Oesophagostomum* spp. and *H. rubidus* or an influence by parbendazole on subsequent larval development in fecal culture was also noticed (Chang and Wescott, 1969; Taffs, 1970).

E. Poultry and Birds

Introduction

The introduction of the benzimidazoles, with their broad spectrum of activity, their large safety margins, and their possibility to be given with the feed, has created a successful alternative for individual deworming (Table XI).

a. Mebendazole. The anthelmintic activity and safety of mebendazole in poultry was tested in 18,897 pheasants and 1006 partridges, in 1476 geese and ducks, and in 8043 chickens, turkeys, and guinea fowl (Thienpont *et al.*, 1973; Varga, 1973; Enigk *et al.*, 1973, 1975a,b,c; Kobulej, 1974; Enigk and Dey-Hazra, 1975; Beer, 1979; Schricke *et al.*, 1973). The results of some critical tests, control tests, and clinical data can be summarized as follows.

1. *Chicken, turkey, guinea fowl:* Mebendazole administered in the feed at 60 ppm for 7 days is highly active against the roundworms *Ascaridia, Heterakis,* and *Capillaria*. When administered for 10 days it is active against the tapeworm *Raillietina*.
2. *Pheasant and partridge:* A 2-week treatment of 120 ppm mebendazole in the feed eliminates not only the large and small roundworms (*Ascaridia, Heterakis*), but also the hairworms in the crop (*Capillaria*) and in the intestine (*Trichostrongylus*) and the tapeworm *Syngamus*.
3. *Goose and duck:* Geese and ducks generally live in natural surroundings. They feed on grass and other elements which they find. To be sure that domesticated geese or ducks receive a complete therapeutic dose of

TABLE XI

Benzimidazole Carbamates in Poultry and Birds

Anthelmintic	Tradename	Formulation	Company
Fenbendazole	Panacur 4%	Powder 4%	Hoechst
Mebendazole	Mebenvet 5%	Powder 5%	Janssen Pharmaceutica
Oxibendazole	Ucamix V oxibendazole	Powder 5%	Socavet France
Parbendazole	Ucamix V parbendazole	Powder 10%	Socavet France

120 ppm mebendazole (±30 mg/kg/day) the substance is administered for 7 to 14 days. At this dosage it is active against the nematode of the gizzard *Amidostomum,* the small roundworm *Heterakis,* the hairworms *Capillaria* and *Trichostrongylus,* and against different tapeworms (*Hymenolepis* spp. and *Drepanidotaenia*).

Larvicidal activity has been proven for *Ascaridia* at 30 mg/kg (Lal *et al.,* 1975), *Heterakis* and *Capillaria* at 3 × 8–10 mg/kg (Enigk *et al.,* 1975b), *Syngamus* at 40 mg/kg (Thienpont *et al.,* 1978), and against *Amidostomum* at 3 × 3 mg/kg (Enigk *et al.,* 1975c).

The recommended dose of mebendazole in poultry in general and in wild birds, in particular, was established according to the optimum anthelmintic effect. It is recommended that the therapeutic dose during the laying period not be exceeded.

b. Fenbendazole. For *fenbendazole,* poultry have been the subjects of numerous investigations with artificial infections and treatment during the prepatent period (Düwel, 1980). The results substantiate the good effects on adult *Ascaridia, Capillaria,* and *Heterakis* in chickens (Enigk *et al.,* 1975b; Tiefenbach, 1976), *Syngamus, Heterakis,* and *Capillaria* (6 × 60 ppm) in turkey, pheasant, and partridge, and on *Amidostomum, Streptocara,* and *Trichostrongylus* (6 × 60 ppm or 1 × 1.25 mg/kg) in geese. It can also be applied in zoo birds and rapacious birds (Düwel, 1980). Larvicidal effect has been proven against *Ascaridia, Capillaria,* and *Syngamus* (Enigk *et al.,* 1975b; Tiefenbach, 1976).

c. Parbendazole. At 0.05% in the diet for 24 hours or 30 mg/kg *Parbendazole* is highly active against *Ascaridia* and *Heterakis.* It is not recommended that parbendazole be given to poultry in the laying period (Actor *et al.,* 1967; Ostmann and Scheidy, 1970).

F. Dogs and Cats

Introduction

Preventing worm infection in dogs and cats is hardly feasible, due to the numerous routes of infection. A dog or cat may be infected by paratenic hosts, by fleas and lice, from the floor, via water, or just by eating fish, meat, or offal. Young dogs even harbor *Toxocara* worms before their birth, having been infected by their mother during gestation. It is clear that the use of anthelmintics is only one part of the total intestinal parasite control program. Sanitation, control of intermediate hosts or exposure to intermediate hosts, good nutrition and husbandry, isolation of new animals until checked or dewormed, decontamination of the environment, and client education are all factors that should be considered in an effective control program (Roudebush, 1980).

The first anthelmintics with a narrow spectrum such as phenothiazine, *n*-butylchloride, methylbenzene and dichlorophene combinations, piperazine, diethylcarbamazine, phthalofyne, and dithiazanine were developed from 1940 to 1957. Tiabendazole, organophosphates (dichlorvos), tetramisole and levamisole, pyrantel, and morantel were the first real broad-spectrum anthelmintics against nematodes. The newer benzimidazoles widened this spectrum to include cestodes (Table XII). Specific cesticidal agents with activity against cestodes alone are bunamidin [Scolaban (Burroughs-Wellcome)], niclosamide [Yomesan (Bayer)], and praziquantel [Droncit (Bayer)]. Like mebendazole, nitroscanate [Lopatol (Ciba Geigy)] also is said to be active against cestodes and nematodes. The anthelmintic activities of therapeutic doses of benzimidazole carbamates are given in Table XIII.

a. Mebendazole. Because of its efficacy and wide safety margin mebendazole may be given in standard doses. Standard doses of 100 mg/animal b.i.d. result in a complete elimination of the ascarids, *Toxocara canis, Toxascaris leonina,* and *Toxocara cati.* In comparison to other worm species, adult ascarids may be readily treated therapeutically. Such worms are large and dwell in the anterior part of the small intestine, and feed on the intestinal chyme of the host. An orally administered anthelmintic such as mebendazole will therefore be readily and regularly ingested by these roundworms. It is however very important to get a 100% efficacy, especially against *T. canis.* These ascarids are not only very fertile, one female produces 200,000 eggs per day, but they are very harmful to the pups and are a human health hazard (larva migrans visceralis).

Hookworms and whipworms fix themselves onto or are embedded in the intestinal epithelium. The therapeutic treatment of these worm species

TABLE XII

BENZIMIDAZOLE CARBAMATES IN DOGS AND CATS

Anthelmintic	Tradename	Formulation	Company
Mebendazole	Telmin KH	Tablets 100 mg	Janssen Pharmaceutica
Fenbendazole	Panacur	Granules	Hoechst
		Powder 4%	Hoechst
Oxibendazole	Polyverkan	Sugar tablets with 200 mg niclosamide 40 mg oxibendazole	Labo. Thekan France

TABLE XIII

ANTHELMINTIC ACTIVITY OF BENZIMIDAZOLE CARBAMATES IN DOGS AND CATS[a,b]

	Anthelmintic				
Worm species	Albendazole	Fenbendazole	Mebendazole	Parbendazole	References[c]
Lungworms					
Filaroides hirthi	++				1
Paragonimus kellicotti	+++				2
Heartworms					
Angiostrongylus vasorum			(+++)		3,4,5
Dirofilaria immitis			(+++)		6
Stomach worms					
Physaloptera rara			+	+++	4,7,8
Intestine worms					
Ascarids					
Toxocara canis	+++	+++	+++	+++	4,8,9,10,11,12
Toxocara cati		++	+++		4,12,13
Toxascaris leonina		+++	+++		4,12
Ascarids (not specified)		+++			12
Hookworms					
Uncinaria stenocephala		+++	+++	+++	4,8,12,13
Ancylostoma tubaeforme			+++		4,13
Ancylostoma caninum	+++	+++	+++	+++	4,8,10,11,12,14
Capillaria aerophila			(+++)		4
Trichuris vulpis		+++	+++	+++	2,4,12,13 7,10,13,15
Cestodes					
Taenia hydatigena		++	+++	+++	4,9,12,16,17,18
Taenia pisiformis			+++		4
Taenia sp.		++	+++		4,7,9,12
Hydatigera taeniaeformis			+−+++		4,9,12,13
Dipylidium caninum		+	+		4,12
Echinococcus granulosus			+++		4,17,18
Mesocestoides corti	+?		+		19

[a] Classification efficacy: +++, 95–100%; ++, 80–100%; +, 0–100%; (), insufficient or no autopsy data.

[b] Doses are given in the text.

[c] 1. Georgi *et al.* (1978); 2. Dubey *et al.* (1978); 3. Guiraud (1976); 4. Janssen Pharmaceutica (1981); 5. Drade and Guiraud (1977); 6. McCall and Crouthamel (1976); 7. McCurdy and Guerrero (1977); 8. Theodorides and Laderman (1968); 9. Vanparijs and Thienpont (1973); 10. Chaia *et al.* (1973); 11. Stehle (1977); 12. Düwel (1980); 13. Guerrero (1978); 14. Chandrasekharan *et al.* (1979); 15. Akusawa and Deguchi (1975); 16. Gemmell (1977); 17. Gemmell (1978); 18. Gemmell (1975); 19. Grevel and Eckert (1973).

is therefore less easy. When mebendazole is given for a sufficiently long period, i.e., a standard dose for 3 days (hookworms) and a standard dose for 3 to 5 days (whipworms) these worms are also completely expelled.

The standard dose 100 mg b.i.d. for 5 days has high efficacy against *Taenia* spp., *Hydatigera*, and *Echinococcus* (200 mg b.i.d. for 5 days). The cestodes *Dipylidium* and *Mesocestoides* are less sensitive to mebendazole. High doses (40 to 100 mg/kg) during a long period of 10 to 30 days are very effective against heartworms (Guiraud, 1976). Even the stomach worm *Physaloptera rara* seems to be sensitive to mebendazole (McCurdy and Guerrero, 1977). Under field conditions, the anthelmintic activity of mebendazole was studied in dogs and cats in Belgium, Denmark, The Netherlands, France, Germany, and the United States (Vanparijs and Thienpont, 1973; Ockens, 1974; Boncompte and Roca Torres, 1975; McCurdy and Guerrero, 1977; Guerrero, 1978; Guerrero *et al.*, 1981). Weight in dogs varied from 1.5 kg (miniature poodles) to 98 kg (St. Bernard) and in cats from 1.5 to 5 kg. After fecal examination, the anthelmintic activity of mebendazole was confirmed. Most observations referred to the clinical improvement after treatment, especially healthy fur and weight increase.

b. Albendazole. Administration of 50 mg/kg *albendazole* for 3 days was fully active against *Toxocara canis* and *Ancylostoma caninum*. It has activity against *Paragonimus kellicotti* at 50 mg/kg for 14–21 days in cats as determined by ova production, change in worm morphology, and reduction in pulmonary lesions (Dubey *et al.*, 1978). Albendazole (25 to 50 mg/kg twice daily for 5 days) is also active against the dog lungworm *Filaroides hirthi* (Georgi *et al.*, 1978).

c. Fenbendazole. Fenbendazole is effective against the important gastrointestinal helminths. Worm elimination extends over several days depending on the parasite species. A good effect, including *Taenia* spp. can be achieved by a single dose of 100 mg/kg or by dividing this dose over 5 days. Dry formulations such as granules or powder give better anthelmintic effects than liquid formulations. However, these differences in efficacy disappear if the suspension is mixed with the feed (Düwel, 1980).

Killing of *Toxocara* larvae in pregnant bitches is of special importance. In preliminary experiments, helminth-free whelps were born to bitches which had received fenbendazole 50 mg/kg each day as a long-term treatment during gestation. The results indicate that fenbendazole might be effective in preventing prenatal infections in dogs (Düwel and Strasser, 1978; Dubey, 1979).

d. Oxfendazole. Oxfendazole has a good effect on *Echinococcus* and *Taenia* (Gemmell *et al.*, 1979). But the drug is not developed for use in domestic pets.

e. Parbendazole. Critical tests in dogs have shown that *parbendazole* at 25 mg/kg/day in oral doses divided into 4 consecutive days was completely efficacious against natural infections with hookworms (*Ancylostoma, Uncinaria*), ascarids (*Toxocara*), whipworms (*Trichuris*), and the stomach worm *Physaloptera* (Theodorides and Laderman, 1968).

G. Wild and Zoo Animals

Wild animals are fairly resistant to parasitic infections, but, when confined in small areas, they may become severely affected by parasites. Newly imported zoo animals are often infected with worms. In addition, stress due to transport and adaptation decreases resistance enhancing the risk of verminosis, as well as its severity. Therefore, parasitic control and a broad-spectrum anthelmintic are imperative during the adaptation period.

Because of the large individual sensitivity and great variety in size of zoo and wild animals, and because of the large range of worm species, an anthelmintic for such animals should meet high requirements. It should have a broad spectrum of activity, i.e., against roundworms and tapeworms and a high margin of safety. It should be risk-free for any animal species. The anthelmintic has to be stable under any climatological conditions or in any feed, even when pelleted and should not have an influence on taste or smell of the feed. The benzimidazole carbamates comply with all these conditions. Mebendazole and fenbendazole are particularly well documented as anthelmintics in wild and zoo animals. A dosage generally had to be based on estimated body weight and as it is often impossible to ascertain the dose actually ingested; these dosages specified as giving a reliable anthelmintic effect must only be regarded as a guideline.

Mebendazole can be given to wild ruminants, carnivores, primates, equids, and rodents (hares, rabbits) either during a shorter period at high dosage (15 mg/kg in the feed for 2 consecutive days) or during a longer period at low dosage (3 mg/kg in the feed for 10 consecutive days). The short treatment is intended for animals in captivity and animals that show up regularly at feeding places; the long treatment is intended for animals that live in nature and are not regular visitors of feeding places (Dollinger, 1973; Hohenester, 1973; Meier, 1974; Kutzer *et al.*, 1974; Pav *et al.*, 1975; Elze *et al.*, 1976; Forstner *et al.*, 1976; Vercruysse *et al.*, 1976; Wankel and Schultze, 1976).

Fenbendazole has been tested in 65 animal species including ungulata, carnivores, primates, snakes, lizards, and reptiles. It is taken up readily and completely by such fastidious species as doucs and proboscis monkeys. Even in monitor lizards, which are prone to vomiting, fenbendazole has not been found to cause vomiting. The dosages vary from 1×5 to 1×100 mg/kg (Düwel, 1980).

H. Rodents

Rodents like the rat, mouse, rabbit, guinea pig, and hamster are the most commonly used small laboratory animals. They harbor different parasites which occur commonly in the colonies. For the eradication of these parasites and thus providing worm-free animals for experiments of all kinds, the benzimidazole carbamates, especially the well-documented mebendazole (Trane and De Carneri, 1972; Dollinger and Beglinger, 1974; Thienpont *et al.*, 1974; Kelly *et al.*, 1975; Coles and McNeillie, 1977) and fenbendazole (Düwel, 1980), are suitable. To deworm a colony 125–150 ppm mebendazole in the diet for 1 to 3 weeks can be used. A dose of 50 ppm mebendazole continuously in the feed keeps the rodents wormfree.

I. Ovicidal Activity

Inhibition of embryonation and hatching of nematode eggs by benzimidazole anthelmintics is well documented. Generally nematode eggs are sterilized in less than 24 hours after treatment of the host.

Ovicidal activity *in vitro* has been proven for all the benzimidazole carbamates against *Nematospiroides dubius* in mice (Coles and McNeillie, 1977) for fenbendazole and parbendazole against sheep nematodes (*Nematodirus, Trichostrongylus, Haemonchus,* and *Ostertagia*) (Düwel, 1980; Cooper and Nephews, 1968) and for mebendazole against *Ancylostoma* spp., *Necator* (Banerjee *et al.*, 1972), and *Ascaris lumbricoides* (Arfaa, 1978).

After treatment of the host an ovicidal effect was seen for albendazole in sheep nematodes within 8–12 hours following administration (Smith Kline, 1978). Fenbendazole sterilized worm eggs of *Parascaris* and *Strongylus* in horses and of different nematodes in sheep (Düwel, 1980).

For mebendazole, eggs incapable of further development were found in feces or horses (*Strongylus*), sheep (*Haemonchus*), dogs (*Ancylostoma, Toxocara*), and man (*Trichuris*) (Fabrello, 1973; Wagner and Chavarra, 1974; Chandrasekharan *et al.*, 1979; Janssen Pharmaceutica, 1981). Nonviable eggs were observed after treatment of sheep with oxfendazole (Ogunsusi, 1979) and after treatment of calves with parbendazole (Borgsteede, 1974).

Most benzimidazoles (albendazole, fenbendazole, mebendazole, oxibendazole, parbendazole) will kill fluke eggs in animals (Coles and Briscoe, 1978; Düwel, 1980). However, the importance of killing fluke or nematode eggs in an animal is not of practical importance, unless dosed animals are kept off pasture until nonviable eggs are passed and subsequently graze on egg- or larval-free land.

J. Resistance to Benzimidazoles

Resistance is not a recently recognized phenomenon. It has been known since the introduction of drugs for the treatment of infectious diseases of man and animals. This has applied particularly to bacteria and protozoa as well as various insects. Resistance to anthelmintics can be defined as a significant increase in the ability of individuals within a population to tolerate doses that would prove lethal to the majority of susceptible individuals in a normal population of the same species (Hall and Kelly, 1979). This ability is heritable. For anthelmintics, the first resistance was reported for phenothiazine in the United States, 15 years after the introduction of that chemical. Strains of *Haemonchus contortus* resistant to tiabendazole were first reported in 1964, just 3 years after its introduction for commercial use, and for parbendazole in 1970 and more recently against the newer benzimidazoles. Up to now resistance against benzimidazoles has been reported for nematodes in sheep, goats, and horses. It occurred mostly in limited areas where benzimidazole anthelmintics had been used intensively.

1. *Sheep*

The first report of tiabendazole resistance with *Trichostrongylus colubriformis* was that of Hotson *et al.* (1970) in Australia. Hall *et al.* (1978) reported that this strain was resistant to all benzimidazoles. However, it was susceptible to levamisole and morantel. A side resistance to a TBZ-resistant *H. contortus* strain was demonstrated for parbendazole, oxfendazole, mebendazole. This strain was fully susceptible to other anthelmintics (Campbell *et al.,* 1978). In a current survey benzimidazole resistance in *Ostertagia* spp. has been detected in sheep flocks in the Goulburn and Orange districts in Australia (Prichard *et al.,* 1980).

2. *Cattle*

Whether or not resistance occurs among cattle nematodes is unclear. Kelly and Hall (1979a) speculated that hypobiosis in *O. ostertagi* may be partially drug induced.

3. *Goat*

Benzimidazole resistance in *H. contortus* and *T. colubriformis* is present, especially where goats are reared under intensive management conditions (Prichard *et al.,* 1980).

4. *Horse*

Resistance of small strongyles of horses to benzimidazole anthelmintics has been reported in Britain (Round *et al.,* 1974), the United States (Drudge *et al.,* 1974), and Canada (Slocombe and Cote, 1977). Resistant strains of small strongyles are believed to be widespread in Australia (Barger and Lisle, 1979). The frequency of resistance appeared to be directly related to the intensity of drug use.

As Round *et al.* (1974) stated, drug tolerance must not be considered a failure of a particular drug but rather a misuse of the drug (e.g., underdosing). Tolerance can be corrected by using anthelmintics with a different mode of action. Levamisole for instance seems to select positively against benzimidazole-resistant *Ostertagia* spp. in sheep (Donald *et al.,* 1980). Even at a reduced dose of 5.3 mg/kg it controlled adult benzimidazole-resistant *H. contortus* and *T. colubriformis* (Coles *et al.,* 1979). Alternation of drugs is essential in areas where resistance is diagnosed. To reduce dependence on anthelmintics Prichard (1980) suggests integration of pasture and animal management together with the use of two chemically unrelated compounds in a slow rotation, changing at approximately yearly intervals.

IV. Benzimidazole Carbamates in Human Medicine

Mebendazole is an active drug against a huge number of nematodes and cestodes. The practical knowledge was reviewed by Janssen (1974), and a short survey of the clinical literature was prepared by Keystone and Murdock (1979). Single 100 mg-doses and a 3-day treatment with 100 mg b.i.d. are extremely well tolerated. Even very high doses (up to 200 mg/kg/day) used for a long treatment period (up to 5 years) in the treatment of, e.g., hydatid disease are usually well tolerated. Due to the fact that high doses of mebendazole affect systemically localized parasites such as larval forms of *Echinococcus* sp., anaphylatic reactions cannot be completely excluded.

Flubendazole is structurally closely related to mebendazole. Clinical trials indicated a therapeutic potential and dosage requirements that are similar to those of the predecessor substance, mebendazole. Hitherto, side effects were not reported.

Ciclobendazole is another anthelmintic with a benzimidazole carbamate structure. Clinical trials indicated in hookworm diseases a lower efficacy if compared with mebendazole (Degrémont and Stahel, 1978; Guggenmoos *et al.,* 1978). The substance is usually well-tolerated. Results of trials with long-term use of high doses are not available.

Albendazole, which is marketed as a veterinary anthelmintic, has been recently tried in man. Preliminary reports (Garin *et al.*, 1980; Pene, 1980) allow the conclusion to be drawn that a dose of 4 to 8 mg/kg may be effective in the treatment of human oxyuriasis, ascariasis, trichuriasis, and cestode and hookworm infections. At a single dose of 400 mg Pene *et al.* (1981) found a cure rate of 100, 70–90, and 29–77% in the treatment of ascariasis, ancylostomiasis (*Necator americanus*), and trichuriasis, respectively.

In the following, the indications will be described according to worm classes.

A. Nematode Infections

1. *Oxyuriasis*

Enterobius vermicularis. Mebendazole is very effective against *Enterobius vermicularis*. Several reports (Table XIV) on successful treatment with a single dose of 100 mg, which should be repeated after 2 weeks, are available (Arada *et al.*, 1978; Brugmans *et al.*, 1971; Cho *et al.*, 1977; Fierlafijn and Vanparijs, 1973; Lecomte-Ramioul, 1975; Lengyel *et al.*, 1978; Lormans *et al.*, 1975). Higher doses do not improve the efficacy in the *Enterobius* treatment (Brugmans *et al.*, 1971) and the single dose is at least as effective as a single dose of pyrvinium pamoate 5 mg/kg (Miller *et al.*, 1974).

Flubendazole is very effective against *Enterobius vermicularis,* and a single dose of 100 mg will be, in principle, sufficient (Arada *et al.*, 1978). This was confirmed by Danis *et al.* (1980) who observed a 92% cure rate. Other publications describe results obtained with 200 mg daily for 3 days (Becquet and Labarrière, 1980; Schenone *et al.*, 1977). Bourée *et al.* (1978) administered 600 mg daily for 3 days. The overall cure rates were 80 to 100%, and usually higher doses did not yield better results. Hence, the recommended dosage is one single 100-mg dose, which should be repeated after 2 weeks (Danis *et al.*, 1980).

Ciclobendazole can be used as a single 100-mg dose, with repetition after 1 week, as was shown in kindergarten children with oxyuriasis. A cure rate of 94% was obtained (Bächlin and Degrémont, 1979).

2. *Trichuriasis*

a. Trichuris trichiura. Mebendazole is the drug of choice in the treatment of infections with *Trichuris trichiura,* if 100 mg is given twice daily for 3 consecutive days (Blechman, 1975; Chanco *et al.*, 1973; Davison, 1979; De Saedeleer, 1975; Guggenmoos *et al.*, 1978; Lengyel *et al.*, 1975; Maqbool *et al.*, 1975; Miller *et al.*, 1974; Vasallo and Herrero, 1978). Some investigators recommend higher doses and a 4-day treatment period (Dalal *et al.*, 1980; Shah, 1979), a longer duration of treatment (Pereira *et al.*, 1979; Scragg and Proctor, 1978), or a combination with levamisole (Wagner and Rexinger, 1978). Usually, however, the standard treatment is used which at the same time covers the dosage schedule needed in the treatment of other infections (Table XIV), and which is superior to 1200 mg ciclobendazole daily for 3 days (Guggenmoos *et al.*, 1978).

Flubendazole yields very good results in *Trichuris* infections. A daily dose of 200 mg, given at once or split into two intakes, for 3 days, cured 80 to 100% of the patients in a single course (Becquet and Labarrière, 1980; Canese *et al.*, 1978; Danis *et al.*, 1980; Nozais, 1978; Schenone *et al.*, 1977). The administration of 300 mg daily for 3 days (Penot *et al.*, 1978), 600 mg daily for 3 days (Bourée *et al.*, 1978), or 500 mg twice daily for 1 week (Combescot and Duong, 1980) did not improve the results, whereas 300 mg daily on 2 consecutive days was less effective (Cabrera *et al.*, 1980). Thus, 100 mg twice daily for 3 days is an optimal dosage.

A daily dose of 200 mg ciclobendazole, given at once or in two intakes, for 3 days is recommended for the treatment of trichuriasis, yielding cure rates of about 80% (Degrémont and Stahel, 1978; Guggenmoos *et al.*, 1978). A dosage increase to 400 mg daily did not produce better results. Stürchler *et al.* (1980) cured 93% of their patients with a single dose of 1 g or 200 mg b.i.d. for 3 days; however, as shown above, the lower standard dose is nearly equieffective.

b. Capillaria philippinensis. The treatment of intestinal capillariasis (Pudoc disease) requires a longer duration of administration of higher daily mebendazole doses. The recommended standard schedule is 100 mg four times daily for 20 days. Some clinical reports are available which, however, do not strictly apply to this schedule. Bhaibulaya *et al.* (1977) used 200 mg b.i.d. for 2 weeks; Singson *et al.* (1975) applied daily doses of 100, 200, 300, or 400 mg for 10, 14, 20, and 30 days and observed the best results with 400 mg for at least 20 days. Tidball *et al.* (1978) treated their patients for 15 days with 400 mg daily and found mebendazole superior to tiabendazole, particularly with respect to side effects.

3. *Ascariasis*

Ascaris lumbricoides. The high efficacy of mebendazole against *Ascaris* infections has been demonstrated in patients with this particular infection (Seo *et al.*, 1978), as well as in patients who were multiply infected or belonged to a nonhomogeneously infected population (Table XIV). The preferred dosage regimen is 100 mg b.i.d. for 3 days, which is the same as

TABLE XIV

SURVEY OF STUDIES IN DIFFERENT WORM INFECTIONS

Investigators	*Entero-bius*	*Trich-uris*	*Asca-ris*	*Neca-tor*	Hook-worm	*Ancy-lostoma*	*Tricho-stron-gylus*	*Strongy-loides*	*Taenia*	*Hyme-nolepis*
Arfaa and Farahmandian (1976)		×	×	×		×	×			
Aspöck *et al.* (1977)		×	×						×	×
Banerjee *et al.* (1972)				×		×				
Banzon *et al.* (1976)		×	×		×					
Bekhti (1974)	×	×	×			×		×	×	
Biagi *et al.* (1974)	×	×	×							×
Bina *et al.* (1977)			×		×					
Borda *et al.* (1976)				×						
Cabrera and Cruz (1980)		×	×		×					
Chaia (1980)		×	×		×					
Chavarria *et al.* (1973)		×	×	×	×					
Chongsuphajaisiddhi *et al.* (1978)		×	×		×			×		
Degrémont and Baumgartner (1975)		×	×			×				
Foba-Pagou *et al.* (1980)		×	×	×					×	

Gatti *et al.* (1972)		×	×		×		×		
Goldsmid (1974)	×	×	×		×		×		×
Guggenmoos *et al.* (1978)		×	×		×				
Hutchison *et al.* (1975)		×	×		×				×
Islam and Chowdbury (1976)		×	×		×		×		
Kaba *et al.* (1978)		×	×			×			
Klein (1970)		×				×			
Lionel *et al.* (1975)		×	×	×					
Miller *et al.* (1974)	×	×							
Musgrave *et al.* (1979)		×			×		×		×
Nagalingam *et al.* (1976)		×	×		×				
Narmada *et al.* (1974)	×	×	×						
Padelt *et al.* (1979)	×	×							
Sargent *et al.* (1975)		×							
Seah (1976)		×	×		×				
Shah (1979)		×	×			×			
Sinniah *et al.* (1980)		×	×	×					
Stürchler *et al.* (1980)		×	×		×				
Vakil *et al.* (1975)		×	×		×			×	
Vandepitte *et al.* (1973)		×	×			×	×		
Wagner and Rexinger (1978)		×	×						
Wolfe and Wershing (1974)		×	×						

in the treatment of trichuriasis and ancylostomiasis, the main accompanying infections. However, mebendazole also appears to be promising given as a single 600-mg dose during mass treatment of this soil-transmitted helminthiasis (Cabrera *et al.*, 1980).

In the flubendazole treatment of *Ascaris* infections, a cure rate between 80 and 100% was found after a single course of 200 mg daily for 3 days (Becquet and Labarrière, 1980; Canese *et al.*, 1978; Danis *et al.*, 1980; Nozais, 1978; Schenone *et al.*, 1977). Higher doses did not improve the therapeutic outcome (Bourée *et al.*, 1978; Penot *et al.*, 1978).

The sensitivity of this species to ciclobendazole is also very high and cure rates between 93 and 100% were obtained after daily intake of 200 or 400 mg for 3 days (Degrémont and Stahel, 1978; Guggenmoos *et al.*, 1978), while Stürchler *et al.* (1980) observed an 88% cure rate after single 1 g doses or 200 mg b.i.d. for 3 days.

4. *Ancylostomiasis (Hookworm Disease)*

Necator americanus and Ancylostoma duodenale. Both species are very sensitive to mebendazole. The standard treatment regimen is 100 mg b.i.d. for 3 days and cure rates between 80 and 100% after a single course are obtained. There are many clinical reports on successful treatment of these infections (Table XIV).

The flubendazole sensitivity of these two species is very high and cure rates between 80 and 99% are reported, if, in a single course, 200 mg daily for 3 days (Canese *et al.*, 1978; Danis *et al.*, 1980; Nozais, 1978) or higher doses (Becquet and Labarrière, 1980; Bourée *et al.*, 1978; Combescot and Duong, 1980; Penot *et al.*, 1978) are used. Thus, the standard regimen of 200 mg daily for 3 days is sufficient.

5. *Creeping Eruption (due to Larval Forms of Ancylostoma braziliense and Ancylostoma caninum)*

Boland and Agger (1980) describe the rapid resolution of lesions from creeping eruption in one patient following a course of 100 mg mebendazole b.i.d. for 3 days, while a second patient needed further treatment with tiabendazole.

A successful flubendazole treatment of creeping eruption is reported by Jacquemin (1980). The 18-month-old patient was treated for 5 days with 100 mg twice daily. The lesions began to disappear on the fifth day. Despite the good result the investigator recommends treatment for 6 or 7 days.

6. *Trichostrongyliasis*

Trichostrongylus spp. The report of Arfaa and Farahmandian (1976) indicates the activity of mebendazole against *Trichostrongylus* spp. in man. Levamisole, however, is judged superior in view of the cure rate as well as reduction in egg count.

7. *Strongyloidiasis*

Strongyloides stercoralis. Following the single dose schedule, mebendazole is less effective against *S. stercoralis* (Table XIV) than against the above mentioned species. If, however, 100 mg b.i.d. for 3 days is used as proposed by Chongsuphajaisiddhi *et al.* (1978), a mean drop in larval counts by 82% can be obtained. Musgrave *et al.* (1979) applied a 4-day course and cured 14 of 21 children.

The therapeutic result with flubendazole in this infection obviously depends upon the total duration of treatment, because after 200 to 300 mg daily for 3 to 4 days about 50% of the patients were cured (Danis *et al.*, 1980; Penot *et al.*, 1978), and even after 600 mg daily for 3 days this number was not higher than 54% after one course, whereas 67% were cured after two courses (Bourée *et al.*, 1978).

8. *Trichinosis*

Trichinella spiralis. High doses of mebendazole for a period of about 2 weeks are mandatory in the treatment of trichinosis. The number of cases described in the literature is rather small (Ozeretskovskaja *et al.*, 1978, 1980; Sonnet and Thienpont, 1977; Thienpont, 1976). Klein *et al.* (1980) found the activity of 100 mg b.i.d. for 5 days starting not later than on day 28 after infection, superior to that of tiabendazole particularly with respcct to allergic side effects. The main difficulty in trichinosis is killing the muscle larvae. This requires effective plasma levels of the poorly absorbed drug and, hence, a dosage schedule as follows: (1) initial dosage, three times daily 200 mg; (2) then, stepwise dosage increase to 1200–1500 mg, divided into three daily portions, and the highest dose being given for 10 days. Vujošević *et al.* (1977) propose a somewhat different schedule: during the first 4 days, 100 mg is given 3 times daily, followed by a 6-day treatment with 200 mg twice daily.

Up to now, there is little experience with flubendazole in trichinosis treatment. Basically, the problems are the same as with mebendazole: once muscle larvae are present, a treatment for at least 2 weeks with a maximum dose of 1500 mg is needed in order to reach active plasma levels. As long as the worm remains in the gastrointestinal tract, 300 mg daily for 5 days is sufficient to eradicate the parasite (Bourée *et al.,* 1976).

9. *Dracontiasis*

Dracunculus medinensis. According to Shafei (1976), mebendazole is effective in the treatment of patients infected with adult guinea worms. Spontaneous expulsion of degenerated and fragmented worms was seen as well as relief of pain, tenderness, and swelling. The dosage schedule was four times daily 200 mg for 6 days. Kale (1975) had less favorable results using twice daily 200 mg for 5 or 7 days; however, the spontaneous expulsion rate and the relapse rate were in favor of the drug.

10. *Filariasis*

Experimental studies with mebendazole and flubendazole have indicated macrofilaricidal activity. Particularly, recent reports by Denham *et al.* (1978, 1979) indicated the efficacy against *Brugia pahangi.* Clinical trials are going on to evaluate the antifilarial properties of both mebendazole and flubendazole in patients infected with *Wuchereria bancrofti, Brugia malayi,* or *Onchocerca volvulus* (Van den Bossche, 1981). So far, only a few publications are available.

a. Wuchereria bancrofti. Mebendazole at a dosage of 6 mg/kg daily for 10 days following an 8-day treatment with levamisole 3 mg/kg daily prevented the recurrence of microfilarial activity otherwise seen after withdrawal of levamisole, but was unable to produce zero counts (Narasimham *et al.,* 1978). Chantin *et al.* (1975) reported an incomplete, protracted microfilaricidal activity of single doses of 200 to 400 mg mebendazole which, however, had less side effects than diethylcarbamazine.

b. Dipetalonema perstans. Goldsmid and Rogers (1976) describe two *D. perstans* infections which improved under 400 mg twice daily for 14 days. In one case the microfilariae disappeared, whereas the other patient relapsed during the follow-up period. Maertens and Wery (1975) observed disappearance of *D. perstans* microfilariae from the blood after a combination therapy of mebendazole with levamisole.

c. Onchocerca volvulus. Maertens and Wery (1975) as well as Kale (1978) were unable to demonstrate any significant improvement in microfilarial count after 200 to 300 mg daily for 1 to 4 weeks, partly in combination with levamisole. However, in both studies the authors did not evaluate the embryostatic properties of mebendazole in contrast to the recent report by Copeman (1979) for *Onchocerca gibsoni* in cattle.

Results from a recent double-blind study (Rivas-Alcala *et al.*, 1981) suggest that mebendazole may be a useful alternative to diethylcarbamazine in the treatment of onchocerciasis. Mebendazole was given orally, 1 g twice a day for 28 days. The systemic side effects observed with mebendazole were considerably fewer than those observed with diethylcarbamazine.

B. Cestode Infections

1. *Taeniasis*

Taenia saginata and T. solium. Mebendazole is active against these tapeworm species. The therapeutic outcome, however, is clearly dose-dependent. The most promising regimens are 300 mg b.i.d. for 3 days (Arambulo *et al.*, 1978; Chavarria *et al.*, 1977) and 200 mg b.i.d. for 4 days (Katz and Zicker, 1973), with cure rates between 90 and 95%. Only Vakil *et al.* (1975) had therapeutic failures using this schedule. Aspöck *et al.* (1977), Bekhti (1974), and Foba-Pagou *et al.* (1980) observed some therapeutic effect after 100 mg b.i.d. for 3 days, which was rated unsatisfactory if compared with the excellent effect of mebendazole against other helminthiases. A daily dose of 600 mg for 3 to 4 days is an effective treatment in taeniasis.

2. *Hymenolepiasis*

Hymenolepis nana. Clinical results indicate some efficacy of mebendazole against *Hymenolepis*. Several investigators used 200 mg for either 3 or 4 days, with a maximum cure rate of 40% (Goldsmid, 1974; Hutchison *et al.*, 1975), a low but detectable efficacy (Aspöck *et al.*, 1977), or without any effect (Musgrave *et al.*, 1979). Probably, a higher daily dose for a longer period can help to improve the outcome.

3. *Echinococcosis*

Larval echinococcosis can be treated either surgically or with systemically acting anthelmintics, and even in addition to surgery, systemic treatment may be desired (Gamble *et al.*, 1979; Garcia *et al.*, 1980; Tögel, 1979). Finally, mebendazole could offer an acceptable expedient for inoperable cases. Experimental and therapeutic studies with mebendazole as a systemically acting anthelmintic have been carried out and summarized (Beard *et al.*, 1978; Schantz *et al.*, 1981; Editorial, 1979). Long-term administration of high daily doses results in detectable plasma levels, and even here the drug tolerance was good. Recently, Murray-Lyon and

Reynolds (1979) report on unspecific febrile reactions in two patients, while Miskovitz and Javitt (1980) observed a not clearly drug-related leukopenia with relative neutropenia in one patient. Alopecia which subsides after the end of the therapy has been described (Beard *et al.*, 1978; Kern *et al.*, 1979).

Echinococcus granulosus and E. multilocularis. The treatment of human echinococcosis requires doses of 30 to 60 mg/kg/day, subdivided into three intakes. Treatment takes at least 1, usually several months (Ammann *et al.*, 1978, 1979; Bekhti *et al.*, 1977, 1980; Kern *et al.*, 1979; Müller *et al.*, 1980; Starke, 1979; Werczberger *et al.*, 1979) but reports on drug administration for 1 (Brandimarte *et al.*, 1980; Kayser, 1980), 3 (Wilson *et al.*, 1978), and even 5 years (Wilson and Rausch, 1980) are available. If mebendazole treatment is used as an adjuvant therapy to surgical intervention, lower doses for a shorter period might be sufficient (Lüdin *et al.*, 1977; Nolla *et al.*, 1979). Although mebendazole is far from being an ideal chemotherapeutic agent in the treatment of human echinococcosis, as can be understood from the extremely high doses and long treatment periods, it can be helpful in the treatment of otherwise infaust cases.

The experience with flubendazole in the treatment of echinococcosis is preliminary. Three patients with *E. granulosus* were treated by Bourée *et al.* (1977) for 5 to 12 months using 2 g daily. The results are encouraging. At the XII International Congress of Hydatidology Bourée *et al.* (1981) reported on 20 patients who were treated for 2 months to 3 years. About one-half of the patients benefited from the treatment. Petigny *et al.* (1980) describe the treatment of one patient using 2 g daily after extirpation of multiple hydatid cysts. The drug is well tolerated and results are similar to those which might be expected under mebendazole therapy. However, this is not conclusive and more studies are needed.

V. Conclusion

The studies discussed here just gave an idea of the anthelmintic properties of the benzimidazole carbamates. Tools are available to provide better health for the populations in developing countries and to reduce the wastage of livestock products due to helminthiasis.

ACKNOWLEDGMENTS

The authors wish to thank H. Vanhove, R. Jacobs, C. Maes, G. Heylen, and D. Verkuringen for their assistance in the preparation of this manuscript. The authors gratefully acknowledge P. A. J. Janssen, R. Marsboom, M. Rogiers, and D. Thienpont for a number of fruitful discussions.

References

Actor, P., Anderson, E. L., DiCuollo, C. J., Ferlanto, R. J., Hoover, J. R. E., Pagano, J. F., Ravin, L. R., Scheidy, S. F., Stedman, R. J., and Theodorides, V. J. (1967). *Nature (London)* **215,** 321–322.

Akusawa, M., and Deguchi, N. (1975). *Jpn. J. Parasitol.* **24,** 357–361.

Ammann, R., Akovbiantz, A., and Eckert, J. (1978). *Abstr. Jahresversamml. Schweiz. Ges. Gastroenterol., Montreux 1978* p. 44.

Ammann, R., Akovbiantz, A., and Eckert, J. (1979). *Schweiz. Med. Wochenschr.* **109,** 148–151.

Arada, E. V., Agustin, E. C., Bagasao, M. G., Chung, E. O., Diadula, H. M., Ibarra, A. N., Libarnes, R. L., Lim, A. C., Padilla, E. P., and Tan, E. S. (1978). *J. Manila Med. Soc.* **16,** 39–46.

Arambulo, P. V., Cabrera, B. D., and Cabrera, M. G. (1978). *Acta Trop.* **35,** 281–286.

Arfaa, F. (1978). *Iran. J. Public Health* **7,** 186–195.

Arfaa, F., and Farahmandian, I. (1976). *In* "Chemotherapy" (J. D. Williams and A. M. Geddes, eds.), Vol. 6, pp. 11–22. Plenum, New York.

Armour, J., and Duncan, J. L. (1978). *Vet. Rec.* **102,** 263–264.

Aspöck, H., Flamm, H., Picher, O., and Wiedermann, G. (1977). *Wien. Med. Wochenschr.* **127,** 88–91.

Averkin, E. A., Beard, C. C., Dvorak, C. A., Edwards, J. A., Fried, J. H., Kilian, J. C., Schiltz, R. A., Kistner, T. P., Drudge, J. H., Lyons, E. T., Sharp, M. L., and Corwin, R. M. (1975). *J. Med. Chem.* **18,** 1164–1166.

Bächlin, A., and Degrémont, A. (1979). *Praxis* **68,** 1183–1185.

Baeder, C., Bähr, H., Christ, O., Düwel, D., Kellner, H. M., Kirsch, R., Loewe, H., Schultes, E., Schütz, E., and Westen, H. (1974). *Experientia* **30,** 753–754.

Baker, N. F., and Fisk, R. A. (1977). *Am. J. Vet. Res.* **38,** 1315–1316.

Banerjee, D., Prakash, O., and Kaliyugaperumal, V. (1972). *Indian J. Med. Res.* **60,** 562–566.

Banzon, T. C., Singson, C. N., and Cross, J. H. (1976). *J. Philipp. Med. Assoc.* **52,** No. 7–8.

Barger, I. A., and Lisle, K. A. (1979). *Aust. Vet. J.* **55,** 594–595.

Beard, T. C., Rickard, M. D., and Goodman, H. T. (1978). *Med. J. Aust.* **2,** 633–635.

Becquet, R., and Labarrière, F. (1980). *Med. Actuelle* **7** (10).

Beer, J. (1979). *World Pheasant Assoc. J.* **5,** 98–104.

Bekhti, A. (1974). *Acta Gastro-Enterol. Belg.* **37,** 302–306.

Bekhti, A., Schaaps, J.-P., Capron, M., Dessaint, J.-P., Santoro, F., and Capron, A. (1977). *Br. Med. J.* **2,** 1047–1051.

Bekhti, A., Nizet, M., Capron, M., Dessaint, J. P., Santoro, F., and Capron, A. (1980). *Acta Gastro-Enterol. Belg.* **43,** 48–65.

Bennett, D. G. (1973). *Vet. Med. Small Anim. Clin.* **68,** 604–609.

Bennett, D. G., Bickford, A. A., and Lund, J. E. (1974). *Am. J. Vet. Res.* **35,** 1003–1004.

Benz, G. W. (1968). *J. Am. Vet. Med. Assoc.* **153,** 1185–1188.

Benz, G. W. (1977). *Am. J. Vet. Res.* **38,** 1425–1426.

Benz, G. W., and Ernst, J. V. (1978). *Am. J. Vet. Res.* **39,** 1107–1108.

Berger, J. (1980). *J. S. Afr. Vet. Assoc.* **51,** 51–58.

Bhaibulaya, M., Benjapong, W., and Noeypatimanond, S. (1977). *J. Med. Assoc. Thailand* **60,** 507–509.

Biagi, F., Smyth, J., and Gonzalez, C. (1974). *Prensa Med. Mex.* **49,** 3–5.

Bina, J. C., Figueiredo, J. F. M., Barreto Ailho, A., and Carvalho, F. (1977). *Rev. Inst. Med. Trop. São Paulo* **19,** 47–51.

Blechman, M. G. (1975). *Curr. Ther. Res.* **18,** 800–803.
Bogan, J. A. (1980). *Drugs Today* **16,** 306–310.
Boland, T. W., and Agger, W. A. (1980). *Wis. Med. J.* **79,** 32–34.
Boncompte Antonijuan, P., and Roca Torres, J. (1975). *Panorama Vet.* 443–452.
Borda, C. E., Rea, M. J., and Borda, R. W. (1976). *Prensa Med. Argent.* **63,** 55–58.
Borgers, M., De Nollin, S., Verheyen, A., Vanparijs, O., and Thienpont, D. (1975a). *J. Parasitol.* **61,** 830–843.
Borgers, M., De Nollin, S., Verheyen, A., De Brabander, M., and Thienpont, D. (1975b). *In* "Microtubules and Microtubular Inhibitors" (M. Borgers and M. De Brabander, eds.), pp. 497–508. Elsevier, Amsterdam.
Borgsteede, F. H. M. (1974). *Tijdschr. Diergeneeskd.* **99,** 991–995.
Borgsteede, F. H. M. (1977). *Tijdschr. Diergeneeskd.* **102,** 801.
Bourée, P., Kouchner, G., and Gascon, A. (1976). *Bull. Soc. Pathol. Exot.* **69,** 177–181.
Bourée, P., Cazin, A., Gascon, A., Kouchner, G., and Molimard, R. (1977). *Bull. Soc. Pathol. Exot.* **70,** 365–371.
Bourée, P., Cazin, A., and Kouchner, G. (1978). *Abstr. Int. Congr. Parasitol., 4th, Warsaw* p. 26.
Bourée, P., Jerray, M., Thulliez, P., and Djenayah, F. (1981). *Abstr. Int. Hydatidol. Congr., 12th, Algiers* p. 49.
Bradley, R. E. (1968). *Am. J. Vet. Res.* **29,** 1979–1982.
Bradley, R. E., and Radhakrishnan, C. V. (1973). *Am. J. Vet. Res.* **34,** 475–477.
Bradley, R. E., Randell, W. F., and Armstrong, D. A. (1981). *Am. J. Vet. Res.* **42,** 1062–1064.
Brandimarte, C., Ribotta, G., Frediani, T., Lalloni, L., and Giunchi, G. (1980). *Ital. J. Gastroenterol.* **12,** 306–308.
Brandt, J., Aguilera, R., and Rodriguez, J. (1976). *Rev. CENIC (Cent. Nac. Invest. Cient.), Cienc. Biol.* **7,** 91–101.
Brodie, R. R., Mayo, B. C., Chasseaud, L. F., and Hawkins, D. R. (1977). *Arzneimittelforschung* **27,** 593–598.
Brown, H. D., Matsuk, A. H., Ilves, I. R., Peterson, L. J., Harris, S. A., Sarett, L. H., Egerton, J. R., Yakstis, J. J., Campbell, W. C., and Cuckler, A. C. (1961). *J. Am. Chem. Soc.* **83,** 1764–1765.
Brugmans, J. P., Thienpont, D. C., Van Wijngaarden, I., Vanparijs, O. F., Schuermans, V. L., and Lauwers, H. L. (1971). *J. Am. Med. Assoc.* **217,** 313–316.
Cabrera, B. D., and Cruz, A. C. (1980). *Acta Med. Philipp.* **16,** 55–57.
Cabrera, B. D., Valdez, E. V., and Go, T. G. (1980). *S.E. Asian J. Trop. Med. Public Health* **11,** 502–506.
Callear, J. F. F., and Neave, R. M. S. (1971). *Br. Vet. J.* **127,** 41–43.
Campbell, N. J., and Hall, C. A. (1979). *Res. Vet. Sci.* **26,** 90–93.
Campbell, N. J., Hall, C. A., Kelly, J. D., and Martin, I. C. A. (1978). *Aust. Vet. J.* **54,** 23.
Canese, A., Canese, J., de De Vargas, H., Galeano, A., Moleon, A., and Alsina, P. (1978). *Rev. Paraguaya Microbiol.* **8,** 31–33.
Chaia, G. (1980). *In* "Health Policies in Developing Countries" (C. Wood and Y. Rue, eds.), Int. Congr. Symposium Ser. No. 24, pp. 103–108. Royal Society of Medicine, London.
Chaia, G., Chiari, L., Martins, C. A., Moura Aranjo, S., Barbosa de Abreu, I., Filho, A. A., and Fuchigami, K. S. (1973). *Rev. Inst. Med. Trop. São Paulo* **15,** 239–247.
Chanco, P. P., Tulane, M. P. H., and Atienza, M. R. (1973). *Philipp. J. Microbiol. Infect. Dis.* **2,** 27–38.
Chandrasekharan, K., Ramadas, K., Cheeran, J. V., and Paily, E. P. (1979). *Kerala J. Vet. Sci.* **10,** 159–162.
Chang, J., and Wescott, R. B. (1969). *Am. J. Vet. Res.* **30,** 77–80.

Chantin, L., Merlin, M., and Laigret, J. (1975). *Bull. Soc. Pathol. Exot.* **68,** 198–204.
Chavarria, A. P., Swartzwelder, J. C., Villarejos, V. M., and Zeledon, R. (1973). *Am. J. Trop. Med. Hyg.* **22,** 592–595.
Chavarria, A. P., Swartzwelder, J. C., Villarejos, V. M., and Zeledon, R. (1977). *Am. J. Trop. Med. Hyg.* **26,** 118–120.
Chevis, R. A. F., and Kelly, J. D. (1978). *N. Z. Vet. J.* **26,** 218–220.
Cho, S.-Y., Ahn, Y.-R., Ryang, Y.-S., and Seo, B.-S. (1977). *Korean J. Parasitol.* **15,** 100–108.
Chongsuphajaisiddhi, T., Sabcharoen, A., Attanath, P., Panasoponkul, C., and Radomyos, P. (1978). *Ann. Trop. Med. Parasitol.* **72,** 59–63.
Ciordia, H., Campbell, H. C., and Stuedemann, J. A. (1978). *Am. J. Vet. Res.* **39,** 517–518.
Clayton, H. M., and Neave, R. M. S. (1979). *Vet. Rec.* **104,** 571–572.
Coles, G. C., and Briscoe, M. G. (1978). *Vet. Rec.* **103,** 360–361.
Coles, G. C., and McNeillie, R. M. (1977). *J. Helminthol.* **51,** 323–326.
Coles, G. C., Briscoe, M. G., and Simpkin, K. G. (1979). *Vet. Rec.* **105,** 470.
Colglazier, M. L. (1979). *Am. J. Vet. Res.* **40,** 384–386.
Colglazier, M. L., Enzie, F. D., and Kates, K. C. (1977). *J. Parasitol.* **63,** 724–727.
Combescot, C., and Duong, T. H. (1980). *Med. Malad. Infect.* **10,** 735–738.
Cooper and Nephews, Ltd. (1968). "Parbendazole. A New Broad Spectrum Anthelmintic for Sheep and Goats." Technical Services Department, Johannesburg.
Copeman, D. B. (1979). *In* "Report of the 3rd Meeting of the Scientific Working Group on Filariasis": WHO/TDR/FIL-SWG (3)/79.3.
Cordero-del-Campillo, M., Rojo-Vazquez, F. A., and Diez-Banos, P. (1980). *Vet. Rec.* **106,** 458.
Corwin, R. M. (1979). *Am. J. Vet. Res.* **40,** 297–298.
Cotteleer, C., and Joossens, G. (1974). *Ann. Med. Vet.* **118,** 239–242.
Craig, T. M., and Shepherd, E. (1980). *Am. J. Vet. Res.* **41,** 425–426.
Dalal, N. J., Vakil, B. J., and Shah, P. N. (1980). *Indian Pediatr.* **17,** 689–692.
Daněk, J., Pavliček, J., and Zajiček, D. (1970). *Helminthologia* **11,** 243–246.
Danis, M., Datry, A., Meunier, Y., and Gentilini, M. (1980). *Gaz. Med. Fr.* **87,** 5444–5446.
Davison, R. P. (1979). *Med. J. Aust.* **2,** 401–402.
Degrémont, A., and Baumgartner, M. W. (1975). *Schweiz, Med. Wochenschr.* **105,** 1830–1832.
Degrémont, A., and Stahel, E. (1978). *Schweiz. Med. Wochenschr.* **108,** 1430–1433.
De Keyser, H. (1980). *Tieraerztl. Prax.* **8,** 163–170.
Delatour, P., and Burgat-Sacaze, V. (1981). *Recl. Med. Vet.* **157,** 213–218.
Delatour, P., Lorgue, G., Lapras, M., and Deschanel, J.-P. (1974). *Bull. Soc. Sci. Vet. Med. Comparee* **76,** 147–154.
Delatour, P., Lorgue, G., Courtot, D., and Lapras, M. (1976a). *Recl. Med. Vet.* **152,** 467–470.
Delatour, P., Lorgue, G., Lapras, M., and Richard, Y. (1976b). *C. R. Acad. Sci. Ser. D* **282,** 517–518.
Delatour, P., Debroye, J., Lorgue, G., and Courtot, D. (1977). *Recl. Med. Vet.* **153,** 639–645.
Demoen, P., Van Aelst, C., Loomans, J., Verhaegen, H., De Cree, J., Verbruggen, F., and Ringoir, S. (1973). *Janssen Pharm., Clin. Res. Rep.* R 17 635/36.
Denham, D. A., Suswillo, R. R., and Rogers, R. (1978). *Trans. R. Soc. Trop. Med. Hyg.* **72,** 546–547.
Denham, D. A., Samad, R., Cho, S. Y., Suswillo, R. R., and Skippins, S. C. (1979). *Trans. R. Soc. Trop. Med. Hyg.* **73,** 673–676.

De Nollin, S., and Van den Bossche, H. (1973). *J. Parasitol.* **59,** 970–976.
De Saedeleer, G. (1975). *Louvain Med.* **94,** 41–48.
DiCuollo, C. J., Miller, J. A., Colman, W. F., Kraeer, P. M., and Wong, M. Y. (1977). *Proc. Int. Conf. WAAVP, 8th, Sydney.*
Dollinger, P. (1973). *Verhandlungsber. Int. Symp. Erkrankung. Zootiere, 15th, Kolmarden.*
Dollinger, P., and Beglinger, R. (1974). Unpublished report, Universität Zürich.
Donald, A. D., Waller, P. J., Dobson, R. J., and Axelsen, A. (1980). *Int. J. Parasitol.* **10,** 381.
Downey, N. E. (1976). *Vet. Rec.* **99,** 267–270.
Downey, N. E. (1977). *Vet. Rec.* **101,** 260–263.
Downey, N. E. (1978). *Vet. Rec.* **103,** 427–428.
Drade, T., and Guiraud, C. (1977). *Proc. World Congr. WSAVA, 6th, Amsterdam* pp. 141–142.
Drudge, J. H., and Lyons, E. T. (1969). *Proc. Int. Conf. Equine Infect. Dis., 2nd, Paris* p. 310.
Drudge, J. H., Lyons, E. T., and Tolliver, S. C. (1974). *Am. J. Vet. Res.* **35,** 1409–1412.
Drudge, J. H., Lyons, E. T., Tolliver, S. C., and Kubis, J. E. (1980). *Equine Pract.* **2,** 23–34.
Dubey, J. P. (1979). *Am. J. Vet. Res.* **40,** 698–699.
Dubey, J. P., Hoover, E. A., Stromberg, P. C., and Toussant, M. J. (1978). *Am. J. Vet. Res.* **39,** 1027–1031.
Duncan, J. L., and Reid, J. F. S. (1978). *Vet. Rec.* **103,** 332–334.
Dunn, G. L., Gallagher, G., Davis, L. D., Hoover, J. R. E., and Stedman, R. J. (1973). *J. Med. Chem.* **16,** 996–1002.
Durez, J., and Pécheur, M. (1972). *Ann. Med. Vet.* **116,** 669–675.
Düwel, D. (1975). *Berl. Muench. Tieraerztl. Wochenschr.* **88,** 418–419.
Düwel, D. (1977). *Pestic. Sci.* **8,** 550–555.
Düwel, D. (1979). Panacur. Information brochure, Hoechst A. G., Frankfurt (Main).
Düwel, D. (1980). Panacur, Axilur. Summary and Evaluation of the Worldwide Published Investigations, Hoechst A. G., Frankfurt (Main).
Düwel, D., and Schleich, H. (1978). *Zentralbl. Veterinaermed. Reihe B* **25,** 800–805.
Düwel, D., and Strasser, H. (1978). *Dtsch. Tieraerztl. Wochenschr.* **85,** 189–241.
Düwel, D., Hajdu, P., and Damm, D. (1975). *Berl. Muench. Tieraerztl. Wochenschr.* **88,** 131–134.
Editorial (1979). *Br. Med. J.* **2,** 563.
Elze, K., Danner, G., and Tamin, E. (1976). *Verhandlungsber. Int. Symp. Erkrankung. Zootiere, 18th, Innsbruck* pp. 219–224.
Enigk, K. (1976). *Tieraerztl. Umsch.* **31,** 360–362.
Enigk, K., and Dey-Hazra, A. (1975). *Wild Hund* **78,** 236–239.
Enigk, K., Dey-Hazra, A., and Batke, J. (1973). *Avian Pathol.* **2,** 67–74.
Enigk, K., Dey-Hazra, A., and Batke, J. (1974). *Dtsch. Tieraerztl. Wochenschr.* **81,** 605–628.
Enigk, K., Dey-Hazra, A., and Batke, J. (1975a). *Dtsch. Gefluegelwirtsch. Schweineprod.* **27,** 131–132.
Enigk, K., Dey-Hazra, A., and Batke, J. (1975b). *Tieraerztl. Umsch.* **30,** 324–329.
Enigk, K., Dey-Hazra, A., and Batke, J. (1975c). *Acta Parasitol. Pol.* **23,** 367–372.
Fabrello, N. R. (1973). *Gac. Vet.* **35,** 586–591.
Fernandes, B. F. (1977). Unpublished report, Universidade Federal do Paraná, Brazil.
Fierlafijn, E., and Vanparijs, O. F. (1973). *Trop. Geogr. Med.* **25,** 242–244.
Foba-Pagou, R., Kegoum, E., Same-Ekobo, A., Eben-Moussi, E., Faucher, P., Carrie, J., and Ripert, C. (1980). *Bull. Soc. Pathol. Exot.* **73,** 171–178.
Foix, J. (1979). *Rev. Med. Vet. (Toulouse)* **130,** 1511–1522.
Forstner, M. J., Wiesner, H., Jonas, D., and Kraneburg, W. (1976). *Zool. Garten* **46,** 401–416.
Friedman, P. A., and Platzer, E. G. (1978). *Biochim. Biophys. Acta* **544,** 605–614.

Friedman, P. A., and Platzer, E. G. (1980a). *In* "The Host-Invader Interplay" (H. Van den Bossche, ed.), pp. 595–604. Elsevier, Amsterdam.
Friedman, P. A., and Platzer, E. G. (1980b). *Biochim. Biophys. Acta* **630,** 271–278.
Galdamez Toledo, O. E. (1980). Thesis, Universidad Nacional Autonoma de Mexico.
Gamble, W. G., Segal, M., Schantz, P. M., and Rausch, R. L. (1979). *J. Am. Med. Assoc.* **241,** 904–907.
Garcia, M. L. L., Montes, J. A. R., Herreros, A. T., Fernandez, J. S., Prianes, L. A., and de Lis, S. F. (1980). *Rev. Clin. Esp.* **159,** 133–136.
Garin, J. P., Mojon, M., Piens, M. A., and Rossignol, J. F. (1980). *Abstr. Int. Congr. Trop. Med. Malaria, 10th, Manila* p. 148.
Gatti, F., Krubwa, F., Lonti, M., Vandepitte, J., and Thienpont, D. (1972). *In* "Advances in Antimicrobial and Antineoplastic Chemotherapy" (M. Hejzlar, M. Semonsky, and S. Masak, eds.), pp. 453–455. Urban & Schwarzenberg, Munich.
Gemmell, M. A., Johnstone, P. D., and Oudemans, G. (1975). *Res. Vet. Sci.* **19,** 229–230.
Gemmell, M. A., Johnstone, P. D., and Oudemans, G. (1977). *Res. Vet. Sci.* **23,** 115–116.
Gemmell, M. A., Johnstone, P. D., and Oudemans, G. (1978). *Res. Vet. Sci.* **25,** 107–108.
Gemmell, M. A., Johnstone, P. D., and Oudemans, G. (1979). *Res. Vet. Sci.* **26,** 389–390.
Georgi, J. R., Slauson, D. O., and Theodorides, V. J. (1978). *Am. J. Vet. Res.* **39,** 803–806.
Gibson, T. E., and Parfitt, J. W. (1971). *Br. Vet. J.* **127,** 201–206.
Goldsmid, J. M. (1974). *S. Afr. Med. J.* **48,** 2265–2266.
Goldsmid, J. M., and Rogers, S. (1976). *S. Afr. Med. J.* **50,** 1129–1132.
Grevel, V., and Eckert, J. (1973). *Schweiz. Arch. Tierheilkd.* **115,** 559–578.
Grisi, L., and Lima, M. M. (1981). *Int. Conf. Vet. Parasitol., 9th, Budapest* p. 153.
Guerrero, J. (1978). *Prac. Vet.* **49,** 15–17.
Guerrero, J., and Sharp, M. L. (1979). *Equine Pract.* **1,** 53–55.
Guerrero, J., Pancari, G., and Michael, B. (1981). *Am. J. Vet. Res.* **42,** 425–427.
Guggenmoos, R., Akhtaruzzaman, K. M., Rosenkaimer, F., Gaus, W., Bienzle, U., and Dietrich, M. (1978). *Tropenmed. Parasitol.* **29,** 423–426.
Guilhon, J., and Barnabé, R. (1973). *Bull. Acad. Vet. Fr.* **46,** 299–303.
Guilhon, J., Couradeau, G., and Barnabé, R. (1971). *Bull. Acad. Vet. Fr.* **44,** 311–315.
Guiraud, C. (1976). *Anim. Compagnie* **1,** 65–73.
Hall, C. A., and Kelly, J. D. (1979). *New S. Wales Vet. Proc.* **15,** 32–36.
Hall, C. A., Kelly, J. D., Campbell, N. J., Withlock, H. V., and Martin, I. C. A. (1978). *Res. Vet. Sci.* **25,** 364.
Heath, D. D., and Lawrence, S. B. (1978). *N. Z. Vet. J.* **26,** 11–15.
Herlich, H. (1977). *Am. J. Vet. Res.* **38,** 1247–1248.
Himonas, C. A., and Liakos, V. (1980). *Vet. Rec.* **107,** 288–289.
Hoebeke, J., Van Nijen, G., and De Brabander, M. (1976). *Biochem. Biophys. Res. Commun.* **69,** 319–324.
Hohenester, H. (1973). Unpublished report, Zoologisch-Parasitologisches Institut der Tieraerztlichen Fakultaet der Universitaet Muenchen.
Hopkins, T. (1978). *Refresh. Course Vet.* **2,** 615–629.
Hotson, I. K., Campbell, N. J., and Smeal, M. G. (1970). *Aust. Vet. J.* **46,** 356.
Hutchison, G. W. (1981). *Res. Vet. Sci.* **30,** 175–180.
Hutchison, J. G. P., Johnston, N. M., Plevey, M. V. P., Thangkhiew, I., and Aidney, C. (1975). *Br. Med. J.* **2,** 309–310.
Ireland, C. M., Gull, K., Gutteridge, W. E., and Pogson, C. I. (1979). *Biochem. Pharmacol.* **28,** 2680–2682.
Islam, N., and Chowdbury, N. A. (1976). *S.E. Asian J. Trop. Med. Public Health* **7,** 81–84.
Jacobs, D. E. (1977). *Symp. Assoc. Vet. Ind., 3rd, London* pp. 45–52.
Jacquemin, J. L. (1980). *Nouv. Presse Med.* **9,** 1779.
Janssen, P. A. J. (1974). *In* "Progress in Drug Research" (E. Jucker, ed.), Vol. 18, pp. 191–203. Birkhaeuser, Basel.

Janssen Pharmaceutica (1972). Mebendazole Synopsis.
Janssen Pharmaceutica (1981). Research Data.
Johns, D. J., and Philip, J. R. (1977). *Proc. Int. Conf. WAAVP, 8th, Sydney.*
Kaba, A. S., Luvwezo, M., Nzuzi, K., and Thienpont, D. (1978). *Ann. Soc. Belge Med. Trop.* **58,** 241–249.
Kale, O. O. (1975). *Am. J. Trop. Med. Hyg.* **24,** 600–605.
Kale, O. (1978). *Tropenmed. Parasitol.* **29,** 163–167.
Kates, K. C., Colglazier, M. L., and Enzie, F. D. (1975). *Vet. Rec.* **97,** 442–444.
Katz, N., and Zicker, F. (1973). *Rev. Soc. Bras. Med. Trop.* **7,** 225–229.
Kayser, H. J. S. (1980). *S. Afr. Med. J.* **58,** 560–563.
Kelly, J. D., and Bain, S. A. (1975). *N. Z. Vet. J.* **23,** 229–232.
Kelly, J. D., and Hall, C. A. (1979a). *New S. Wales Vet. Proc.* **15,** 19–31.
Kelly, J. D., and Hall, C. A. (1979b). *Adv. Pharmacol. Chemother.* **16,** 89–128.
Kelly, J. D., Chevis, R. A. F., and Goodman, H. T. (1975). *Int. J. Parasitol.* **5,** 275–280.
Kern, P., Dietrich, M., and Volkmer, K.-J. (1979). *Tropenmed. Parasitol.* **30,** 65–72.
Keystone, J. S., and Murdoch, J. K. (1979). *Ann. Intern. Med.* **91,** 582–586.
Kingsbury, P. A., Rowlands, T., and Reid, J. F. S. (1981). *Vet. Rec.* **108,** 10–11.
Kistner, T. P., Wyse, D., Schiltz, R. A., Averkin, E., and Cary, A. (1979). *Vet. Parasitol.* **5,** 195–204.
Klein, E. (1970). *Dtsch. Med. Wochenschr.* **97,** 1215–1216.
Klein, J. S., Zakharenko, D. F., Dolgina, L. E., Braginets, V. P., and Linkov, I. A. (1980). *Abstr. Int. Conf. Trichinellosis, 5th, Noordwijk* p. 118.
Kobulej, T. (1974). *Proc. Int. Congr. Parasitol., 3rd, Munich* **II,** 763–764.
Köhler, P., and Bachmann, R. (1980). *In* "The Host-Invader Interplay" (H. Van den Bossche, ed.), pp. 727–730. Elsevier, Amsterdam.
Kutzer, E. (1978). *Tieraerztl. Prax.* **6,** 325–334.
Kutzer, E., Prosl, H., and Frey, H. (1974). *Dtsch. Tieraerztl. Wochenschr.* **81,** 112–119.
Lal, J., Subramanian, G., and Sabir, M. (1975). *Indian J. Anim. Sci.* **45,** 807–808.
Lämmler, G., Sahai, B. N., and Zahner, H. (1969). *Br. Vet. J.* **125,** 205–211.
Langnes, A. (1976). Thesis, Freie Universität of Berlin.
Lapras, M., Deschanel, J. P., Delatour, P., Gastellu, J., and Lombard, M. (1973). *Bull. Soc. Sci. Vet. Med. Comparee* **75,** 53–61.
Lecomte-Ramioul, S. (1975). *Rev. Med. Liege* **30,** 733–736.
Lengyel, A., Levai, J., and Rovo, J. T. (1975). *Ther. Hung.* **23,** 64–67.
Lengyel, A., Albi, I., and Rovo, J. T. (1978). *Ther. Hung.* **26,** 64–66.
Lionel, N. D. W., Rajapakse, L., Soysa, P., and Aiyathurai, J. E. J. (1975). *J. Trop. Med. Hyg.* **78,** 75–77.
Lloyd, S., Soulsby, E. J. L., and Theodorides, V. J. (1978). *Experientia* **34,** 723–724.
London, C. E., Roberson, E. L., McCall, J. W., Guerrero, J., Pancari, G., Michael, B., and Newcomb, K. (1981). *Am. J. Vet. Res.* **42,** 1263–1265.
Lormans, J. A. G., Wesel, A. J. T., and Vanparijs, O. F. (1975). *Chemotherapy (Basel)* **21,** 255–260.
Lüdin, C. E., Gyr, K., and Karoussos, K. (1977). *J. Intern. Med. Res.* **5,** 367–368.
Lyons, E. T., Drudge, J. H., and Tolliver, S. C. (1977). *Am. J. Vet. Res.* **38,** 2049–2053.
Lyons, E. T., Drudge, J. H., and Tolliver, S. C. (1981). *Am. J. Vet. Res.* **42,** 685–686.
McCall, J. W., and Crouthamel, H. H. (1976). *J. Parasitol.* **62,** 844–845.
McCurdy, H. D., and Guerrero, J. (1977). *Vet. Med. Small Anim. Clin.* **72,** 1731–1733.
McCurdy, H. D., Sharp, M. L., and Sweeny, W. T. (1976). *Vet. Med. Small Anim. Clin.* **71,** 97–100.
Maertens, K., and Wery, M. (1975). *Trans. R. Soc. Trop. Med. Hyg.* **69,** 359–360.
Maqbool, S., Lawrence, D., and Katz, M. (1975). *J. Pediatr.* **86,** 463–465.

Marsboom, R. (1973). *Toxicol. Appl. Pharmacol.* **24,** 371–377.
Marsboom, R. (1975). *Equine Section, 12th Annu. Convention, Anaheim.*
Meier, H. W. (1974). *Prakt. Tierarzt* **55,** 630–638.
Metzger, H., and Düwel, D. (1974). *Proc. Int. Congr. Parasitol., 3rd, Munich* **3,** 1444–1445.
Meuldermans, W., Hurkmans, R., Swijsen, E., and Heykants, J. (1977). *Janssen Pharm. Preclin. Res. Rep.* R 17 889/5.
Michael, S. A., El Refaii, A. H., Mansour, W. H., Selim, M. K., and Higgins, A. J. (1979). *Vet. Rec.* **104,** 338–340.
Michiels, M., Heykants, J., Sneyers, R., Wignants, J., and Marsboom, R. (1977). *Janssen Pharm. Preclin. Res. Rep.* R 17 889/6.
Michiels, M., Heykants, J., Van den Bossche, H., and Verhoeven, H. (1980a). *Janssen Pharm. Preclin. Res. Rep.* R 17 635/13, 889/12, R 34 803/5.
Michiels, M., Prinsen, P., Heykants, J., and Van den Bossche, H. (1980b). *Janssen Pharm. Preclin. Res. Rep.* R 17 889/14.
Miller, M. J., Krupp, I. M., Little, M. D., and Santos, C. (1974). *J. Am. Med. Assoc.* **230,** 1412–1414.
Miskovitz, P. F., and Javitt, N. B. (1980). *Am. J. Trop. Med. Hyg.* **29,** 1356–1358.
Montgomery, I. W., and Montgomery, J. D. (1977). *Abstr. Int. Conf. WAAVP, 8th, Sydney* p. 68.
Müller, E., Akovbiantz, A., Bircher, J., Eckert, J., Wissler, K., and Ammann, R. W. (1980). *Joint Meet. R. Soc. Trop. Med. Hyg. Schweiz. Ges. Tropenmed. Parasitol., Basel.*
Münst, G. J., Kalaganis, G., and Bircher, J. (1980). *Eur. J. Clin. Pharmacol.* **17,** 375–378.
Murray-Lyon, I. M., and Reynolds, K. W. (1979). *Br. Med. J.* **2,** 1111–1112.
Musgrave, I. A., Hawes, R. B., Jameson, J. L., Sloane, R. A., and Quayle, P. A. (1979). *Med. J. Aust.* **2,** 403–405.
Muylle, E., Oyaert, W., and Rogiers, M. (1979). *Vlaams Diergeneeskd. Tijdschr.* **48,** 279–282.
Nagalingam, I., Lam, L. E., Robinson, M. J., and Dissanaike, A. S. (1976). *Am. J. Trop. Med. Hyg.* **25,** 568–572.
Narasimham, M. V. V. L., Roychowdhury, S. P., Das, M., and Rao, C. K. (1978). *S.E. Asian J. Trop. Med. Public Health* **9,** 571–575.
Narmada, R., Jagadeeswara Rao, M., Adinaraynan, P., and Balagopal, Raju, V. (1974). *Indian Pediatr.* **11,** 417–419.
Nawalinski, T., and Theodorides, V. J. (1976). *Am. J. Vet. Res.* **37,** 469–471.
Neave, R. M. S., and Callear, J. F. F. (1973). *Br. Vet. J.* **129,** 79–82.
Nolla Salas, M., Alvarez Lerma, F., Torres Rodriguez, J. M., and Nolla Panades, R. (1979). *Ann. Med.* **65,** 1339–1360.
Nozais, J. P. (1978). *Med. Afr. Noire* **25,** 473–475.
O'Brien, J. J. (1970). *Aust. Vet. J.* **46,** 297–300.
Ockens, N. (1974). *Danske Dyrlaegeforening Meblemsblad* **57,** 923–925.
Ogunsusi, R. A. (1979). *Res. Vet. Sci.* **27,** 246–247.
Oguz, T. (1976). *Vet. Fakult. Dergisi* **23,** 383–395.
Oguz, T. (1977). *Abstr. Mediterr. Conf. Parasitol., 1st, Izmir* pp. 122–123.
Ostmann, O. W., and Scheidy, S. F. (1970). *Proc. Int. Congr. Chemother., 6th, Baltimore* **I,** 159–163.
Ozeretskovskaya, N. N., Pereverzeva, E. V., Tumolskaya, N. I., Bronstein, A. M., Morenez, T. M., and Imamkuliev, K. D. (1978). *In* "Trichinellosis" (Ch. W. Kim and Z. S. Pawlowski, eds.), pp. 381–393. Univ. Press of New England, Hanover, N. Hampshire.
Ozeretskovskaya, N. N., Morenetz, T. M., Pereverzeva, E. V., Bronstein, A. M., Veretennikova, N. L., Poverenny, A. M., Podgorodnichenko, V. K., and Karogodin, D. A. (1980). *Abstr. Int. Conf. Trichinellosis, 5th, Noordwijk* p. 116.
Padelt, H., Hölzer, E., and Steinbrück, M. (1979). *Ther. Hung.* **27,** 167–169.

Pav, J., Zajicek, D., and Zahradnikova, W. (1975). *Lesnictvi* **21,** 51–62.
Pavlowski, Z., Kozakiewicz, B., and Zatonski, J. (1976). *Vet. Parasitol.* **2,** 299–302.
Pêcheur, M., Dewaele, A., Brassine, M., and Pandey, V. S. (1971). *Ann. Med. Vet.* **115,** 175–180.
Pene, P. (1980). *Abstr. Int. Congr. Trop. Med. Malaria, 10th, Manila* p. 149.
Pene, P., Vincentelli, J.-M., Soula, G., Bourderioux, Ch., and Rossignol, J.-F. (1981). *Med. Afr. Noire* **28,** 483–485.
Penot, C., Picot, H., and Lavarde, V. (1978). *Bull. Soc. Pathol. Exot.* **71,** 370–375.
Pereira, J. F. V., Ghosh, H. K., Conklin, S., and Ryan, S. (1979). *Med. J. Aust.* **1,** 134–135.
Petigny, A., Savoye, B., Vilain, C., Boulez, J., Girard, M., and Prud'hon, M. C. (1980). *Sem. Hop.* **56,** 685–687.
Prichard, R. K. (1980). *In* "The Host-Invader Interplay" (H. Van den Bossche, ed.), pp. 731–734. Elsevier, Amsterdam.
Prichard, R. K., and Hennessy, D. R. (1981). *Res. Vet. Sci.* **30,** 22–27.
Prichard, R. K., Donald, A. D., and Hennessy, D. R. (1978a). *Vet. Rec.* **102,** 382.
Prichard, R. K., Kelly, J. D., and Thompson, H. G. (1978b). *Vet. Parasitol.* **4,** 243–255.
Prichard, R. K., Hennessy, D. R., and Steel, J. W. (1978c). *Vet. Parasitol.* **4,** 309–315.
Prichard, R. K., Hall, C. A., Kelly, J. D., Martin, I. C. A., and Donald, A. D. (1980). *Aust. Vet. J.* **56,** 239–251.
Prosl, H., and Kutzer, E. (1979). Unpublished report, Inst. for Parasitology and General Zoology, Vienna.
Rahman, M. S., and Bryant, C. (1977). *Int. J. Parasitol.* **7,** 403–409.
Reinecke, R. K., and Le Roux, D. J. (1972). *J. S. Afr. Vet. Med. Assoc.* **43,** 287–294.
Ribbeck, R., and Kuller, H. J. (1976). *Medicamentum (Berlin)* **17,** 352–356.
Ribbeck, R., and Winter, J. (1978). *Monatsh. Veterinaermed.* **33,** 706–707.
Rivas-Alcalá, A. R., Taylor, H. R., Ruvalcaba-Macías, A. M., Mackenzie, C. D., Green, B. M., Domíguez-Vázquez, A., Lugo-Pfeiffer, C., and Beltran, H. F. (1981). *Lancet* **ii,** 485–490.
Ross, D. B. (1968). *Vet. Rec.* **82,** 731–735.
Ross, D. B. (1970). *Vet. Rec.* **86,** 60–61.
Ross, D. B., Eichler, D. A., and Cameron, D. (1978). *Vet. Rec.* **102,** 556–557.
Roudebusch, P. (1980). *Canine Pract.* **7,** 67–80.
Round, M. C., Simpson, D. J., Haselden, C. S., Glendinning, E. S. A., and Baskerville, R. E. (1974). *Vet. Rec.* **95,** 517–518.
Rubin, R. (1968). *Am. J. Vet. Res.* **29,** 1385–1389.
Rubin, R. (1969). *J. Am. Vet. Med. Assoc.* **154,** 177–180.
Santiago, M. A. M., Da Costa, V. C., Benevenga, S., and Da Silva, V. P. (1973). *Veterinaria* **8,** 121–123.
Sargent, R. G., Dotterer, T. D., Savory, A. M., and Lee, P. R. (1975). *South. Med. J.* **68,** 38–40.
Saupe, E., and Nitz, K. J. (1972). *Berl. Muench. Tieraerztl. Wochenschr.* **85,** 21–24.
Schantz, P. M., Van den Bossche, H., and Eckert, J. (1982). *Z. Parasitenkd.* **67,** 5–26.
Schenone, H., Galdames, M., Inzunza, E., Jimenez, M. Romero, E., and Bloomfield, R. (1977). *Bol. Chil. Parasitol.* **32,** 85–86.
Schricke, E., Goupille, F., and Heude, B. (1973). *Recl. Med. Vet.* **149,** 1327–1338.
Scragg, J. N., and Proctor, E. M. (1978). *Am. J. Trop. Med. Hyg.* **27,** 255–257.
Seah, S. K. K. (1976). *CMA J.* **115,** 777–779.
Seo, B.-S., Cho, S.-Y., and Chai, J.-Y. (1978). *Korean J. Parasitol.* **16,** 21–25.
Shafei, A. Z. (1976). *J. Trop. Med. Hyg.* **79,** 197–200.
Shah, M. (1979). *Indian Pediatr.* **16,** 267–270.

Shivakumar, A. M., Chandra, S., and Sabir, M. (1975). *Indian Vet. J.* **52,** 136–142.
Shone, D. K., Saayman, D., Erasmus, F., and Philip, J. R. (1970). *J. S. Afr. Vet. Med. Assoc.* **41,** 61–67.
Singson, C. N., Banzon, T. C., and Cross, J. H. (1975). *Am. J. Trop. Med. Hyg.* **24,** 932–934.
Sinniah, B., Sinniah, D., and Dissanaike, A. S. (1980). *Ann. Trop. Med. Parasitol.* **74,** 619–623.
Slocombe, J. O. D., and Cote, J. F. (1977). *Can. Vet. J.* **18,** 212–217.
Smith Kline Corp. (1978). "Albendazole Scientific Publications." Philadelphia, Pennsylvania.
Smith Kline Corp. (1978). "Valbazen, Albendazole Technical Manual." Philadelphia, Pennsylvania.
Sonnet, J., and Thienpont, D. (1977). *Acta Clin. Belg.* **32,** 297–302.
Spindler, L. A. (1947). *Proc. Helminthol. Soc. Wash.* **14,** 58–63.
Sprink, H. M. (1979). *Rep. Stichting Gezondheidsdienst Dieren Gelderland, Utrecht.*
Starke, J. (1979). *Dtsch. Med. Wochenschr.* **104,** 1132–1135.
Stehle, S. (1977). *Kleintier-Prax.* **22,** 261–266.
Stephenson, L. S., Latham, M. C., and Oduori, M. L. (1980a). *J. Trop. Pediatr.* **26,** 246–263.
Stephenson, L. S., Pond, W. G., Nesheim, M. C., Krook, L. P., and Crompton, D. W. T. (1980b). *Exp. Parasitol.* **49,** 15–25.
Stoye, M. (1972). *Schweiz. Arch. Tierheilkd.* **114,** 601–613.
Stoye, M., and Bürger, H. J. (1981). *Abstr. Int. Conf. Vet. Parasitol., 9th, Budapest* p. 152.
Stürchler, D., Stahel, E., Saladin, K., and Saladin, B. (1980). *Tropenmed. Parasitol.* **31,** 87–93.
Taboa, M. (1972). Thesis, Tierärztliche Hochschule, Hannover.
Taffs, L. F. (1970). *Res. Vet. Sci.* **11,** 515–522.
Tellez-Giron, E., Ramos, M. C., and Montante, M. (1980). *Am. J. Trop. Med. Hyg.* **30,** 135–138.
Theodorides, V. J. (1977). *Proc. Symp. Assoc. Vet. Ind., 3rd, London* pp. 37–44.
Theodorides, V. J., and Freeman, J. F. (1980). *Vet. Rec.* **106,** 78–79.
Theodorides, V. J., and Laderman, M. (1968). *Vet. Med. Small Anim. Clin.* **63,** 985.
Theodorides, V. J., Laderman, M., and Pagano, J. F. (1968). *Vet. Med. Small Anim. Clin.* **63,** 370–371.
Theodorides, V. J., Chang, J., DiCuollo, C. J., Grass, G. M., Parish, R. C., and Scott, G. C. (1973). *Br. Vet. J.* **129,** 97–98.
Theodorides, V. J., Gyurik, R. J., Kingsbury, W. D., and Parish, R. C. (1976a). *Experientia* **32,** 702–703.
Theodorides, V. J., Gyurik, R. J., Kingsbury, W. D., and Parish, R. C. (1976b). *Experientia* **32,** 706.
Theodorides, V. J., Nawalinski, T., Freeman, J. F., and Murphy, J. R. (1976c). *Am. J. Vet. Res.* **37,** 1207–1209.
Theodorides, V. J., Nawalinski, T., and Chang, J. (1976d). *Am. J. Vet. Res.* **37,** 1515–1516.
Theodorides, V. J., Nawalinski, T., Murphy, J., and Freeman, J. (1976e). *Am. J. Vet. Res.* **37,** 1517–1518.
Thienpont, D. (1976). *Nouv. Presse Med.* **5,** 1759–1760.
Thienpont, D., and Vanparijs, O. (1980). *Abstr. Int. Conf. Trichinellosis, 5th, Noordwijk* p. 125.
Thienpont, D., Vanparijs, O. F. J., Raeymaekers, A. H. M., Vandenberk, J., De Moen, P. J. A., Allewijn, F. N., Marsboom, R. P. H., Niemegeers, C. J. E., Schellekens, K. H. L., and Janssen, P. A. J. (1966). *Nature (London)* **209,** 1084–1086.

Thienpont, D. C., Vanparijs, O. F. J., and Hermans, L. C. (1973). *Poult. Sci.* **52,** 1712–1714.
Thienpont, D., Vanparijs, O., Niemegeers, C., and Marsboom, R. (1978). *Arzneimittelforschung* **28,** 605–612.
Thomas, R. J., and Reid, J. F. S. (1980). *Res. Vet. Sci.* **28,** 134–136.
Tidball, J. S., Aguas, J. P., and Aldis, J. W. (1978). *S.E. Asian J. Trop. Med. Public Health* **8,** 33–40.
Tiefenbach, B. (1976). *Blau. Hefte* **55,** 204–218.
Tinar, R. (1979). *Vet. Fakultesi Dergisi* **26,** 145–168.
Todd, K. S., and Mansfield, M. E. (1979). *Am. J. Vet. Res.* **40,** 423–424.
Tögel, H. (1979). *Med. Welt* **30,** 1042–1046.
Trane, F., and De Carneri, I. (1972). *Rev. Parasitol.* **33,** 137–140.
Urquhart, G. M. (1981). Cited in *Vet. Rec.* **106,** 27.
Vakil, B. J., Dalal, N. J., and Enjetti, E. (1975). *J. Trop. Med. Hyg.* **78,** 154–158.
Van den Bossche, H., ed. (1972). "Comparative Biochemistry of Parasites," pp. 139–157. Academic Press, New York.
Van den Bossche, H., ed. (1976). "Biochemistry of Parasites and Host-Parasite Relationship," pp. 553–572. Elsevier, Amsterdam.
Van den Bossche, H. (1981). *Ann. Soc. Belge Med. Trop.* **61,** 287–296.
Van den Bossche, H., and De Nollin, S. (1973). *Int. J. Parasitol.* **3,** 401–407.
Van den Bossche, H., and Janssen, P. A. J. (1982). *Proc. Symp. Chemother. Immunol. Control Malaria, Filaria Leishmaniasis, Lucknow* (in press).
Vandepitte, J., Gatti, F., Lontie, M., Krubwa, F., Nguete, M., and Thienpont, D. (1973). *Bull. Soc. Pathol. Exot.* **66,** 165–178.
Vanparijs, O., and Thienpont, D. (1973). *Dtsch. Tieraerztl. Wochenschr.* **80,** 317–340.
Varga, I. (1973). *Magy. Allatorv. Lapja* **28,** 320–323.
Varga, I., and Janisch, M. (1975a). *Magy. Allatorv. Lapja* **30,** 336–343.
Varga, I., and Janisch, M. (1975b). *Acta Vet. Acad. Sci. Hung.* **25,** 105–111.
Vasallo, M. F., and Herrero, A. C. (1978). *Med. Klin.* (*Span. ed.*) (197), 42–46.
Verberne, L. R. M., and Mirck, M. H. (1975). *Tijdschr. Diergeneeskd.* **100,** 1143–1153.
Vercruysse, J., Kumar, V., Ceulemans, F., and Mortelmans, J. (1976). *Acta Zool. Pathol. Antverp.* **64,** 115–119.
Verheyen, A., Borgers, M., Vanparijs, O., and Thienpont, D. (1976). *In* "Biochemistry of Parasites and Host-Parasite Relationships" (H. Van den Bossche, ed.), pp. 605–618. Elsevier, Amsterdam.
Vujošević, M., Kostić, A., Ilié, L., and Žerjav, S. (1977). *Yugosl. Ital. Meet. Infect. Dis., 4th, Perugia.*
Wagner, E. D., and Chavarra, A. P. (1974). *Am. J. Trop. Med. Hyg.* **23,** 154–157.
Wagner, E. D., and Rexinger, D. D. (1978). *Am. J. Trop. Med. Hyg.* **27,** 203–205.
Walker, D., and Knight, D. (1972). *Vet. Rec.* **90,** 58–65.
Wallnoefer, E. (1977). *Wien. Tieraerztl. Wochenschr.* **64,** 129–131.
Wankel, B., and Schultze, H. (1976). *Dtsch. Tieraerztl. Wochenschr.* **83,** 463–466.
Werczberger, A., Golhman, J., Wertheim, G., Gunders, A. E., and Chowers, I. (1979). *Chest* **76,** 482–484.
Wiesner, H. (1973). *Tieraerztl. Umsch.* **28,** 135–138.
Williams, J. C., Sheenan, D., and Fuselier, R. H. (1977). *Am. J. Vet. Res.* **38,** 2037–2038.
Williams, J. C., Knox, J. W., Baumann, B. A., Snider, T. G., and Hoerner, T. J. (1981). *Am. J. Vet. Res.* **42,** 318–321.
Wilson, J. F., and Rausch, R. L. (1980). *Am. J. Trop. Med. Hyg.* **29,** 1340–1355.
Wilson, J. F., Davidson, M., and Rausch, R. L. (1978). *Am. Rev. Respir. Dis.* **118,** 747–757.
Wolfe, M. S., and Wershing, J. M. (1974). *J. Am. Med. Assoc.* **230,** 1408–1411.

ADVANCES IN PHARMACOLOGY AND CHEMOTHERAPY, VOL. 19

Chemotherapy of Human Intestinal Helminthiases: A Review, with Particular Reference to Community Treatment

D. STÜRCHLER

Swiss Tropical Institute
Medical Department
Basel, Switzerland

I. Summary . . . 129
II. Introduction . . . 130
III. The Parasites . . . 131
  A. Helminths of the Human Intestinal Tract . . . 131
  B. The Impact of Intestinal Helminths on Human Health . . . 132
IV. The Human Host . . . 136
  A. Symptoms of Intestinal Helminthiases . . . 136
  B. Indications for Anthelminthics . . . 136
  C. Reinfection . . . 137
V. The Drugs . . . 138
  A. A List of Essential Drugs . . . 138
  B. Anthelminthic Activity . . . 140
  C. Administration of Anthelminthics . . . 141
  D. Which Anthelminthic? . . . 144
  E. Drug Resistance and Drug Combinations . . . 146
  F. Supportive Treatment . . . 147
VI. Therapeutic Intervention . . . 147
  A. For Individuals . . . 147
  B. Anthelminthic Treatment in Childhood and during Pregnancy . . . 147
  C. For Communities . . . 148
  References . . . 151

I. Summary

Human intestinal helminthiases are common in many countries. Depending on their number and location intestinal helminths may cause important symptoms such as anemia and diarrhea. Even in lightly infected individuals they may impair the nutritional state, the growth rate, and resistance to infection. The latter effects are not yet well understood and are sometimes underestimated.

Efficient and well tolerable anthelminthic drugs are currently available. A list of drugs of choice for the treatment of single helminth species in

ISBN 0-12-032919-0

individual patients is given. The modern anthelminthic drugs available have brought an extension of the indications for treatment: not only of the individual symptomatic patient but also, if economically feasible, of the carrier or even a whole community.

By scoring the efficacy, the duration of treatment, the side effects, and the costs, the following five anthelminthic drugs have been identified as most suitable for mass application (in alphabetical order): levamisole, mebendazole, niclosamide, praziquantel, and pyrantel. Some principles of mass treatment are discussed and the following procedure is proposed for achieving an optimal effect: (1) obtain the agreement of the population, (2) motivate and train auxiliary personnel, (3) investigate and treat a random sample in a pilot study, (4) take a census and instruct the population, and (5) deliver the anthelminthic drug, if necessary repeatedly with appropriate spacing.

II. Introduction

Intestinal helminths of man are widely prevalent. In many instances they are "ideal" parasites, i.e., they do not lead to the death of their host. However, by their frequency and number, they are responsible for considerable morbidity and economic losses of individual persons and of whole communities. This is particularly true for nonindustrialized countries where the well being of people is vulnerable.

Treatment with anthelminthic drugs occupies an important part of the control of human intestinal helminthiases and may contribute to the improvment of individual health and to the alleviation of parasite-related suffering. This article deals principally with the chemotherapy of communities and of intestinal polyparasitism, rather than with that of individual patients or individual helminth species. Since an understanding of the principles of the epidemiology and pathophysiology of intestinal human helminthiases is essential for proper application of anthelminthics, these subjects will be part of this article.

Quite a broad variety of anthelminthics is currently available. Therefore, the clinician and epidemiologist will have to make his choice among several drugs on the basis of their efficacy, spectrum of action, tolerance, and costs. This article inevitably expresses the author's personal views on this subject.

It is hoped that the following will be useful to physicians working in this field and help them to decide whom to treat with which anthelminthic and how often.

III. The Parasites

A. Helminths of the Human Intestinal Tract

A number of helminths may inhabit the human intestinal tract (Table I). They reside in the small or large bowel, as larvae and as adults, moving freely within the bowel lumen or being attached to the intestinal wall. On reproduction, their eggs, larvae, or proglottids appear in the feces. On occasion, adults creep to the anal region or are expelled by peristalsis.

The larvae of *Anisakis* spp. and *Oesophagostomum* spp. live completely within the intestinal wall (Pinkus *et al.,* 1975; Barrowclough and Crome, 1979). The adults of *Schistosoma* spp. even live in the veins of the mesenterium or pelvis, but their eggs have to penetrate the intestinal wall. As part of their life cycle the larvae of *Ascaris lumbricoides,* of the hookworms, and of *Strongyloides sterocoralis* enter the circulation, pass to the trachea, and reenter the intestinal tract. During their tissue phase these larvae are much less sensitive to anthelminthics (Katz, 1977). The same may be true for schistosomulae and for growing larvae in the intestinal lumen. The length of prepatency (Table III) is therefore of considerable importance for determining the interval in which anthelminthic mass chemotherapy has to be administered and in which stools must be examined parasitologically after treatment (see also Section VI,C).

In this article only those intestinal helminths will be considered that have their principal location in or close to the intestinal tract, that live in it

TABLE I

HELMINTHS OCCURRING IN THE HUMAN INTESTINAL TRACT AND THEIR DEMONSTRATION IN THE FECES[a]

Location	Nematode genera	Trematode genera	Cestode genera
Small bowel	*Ascaris:* E	*Fasciolopsis:* E	*Taenia:* P E
	Necator: E (L)	*Heterophyes:* E	*Diphyllobothrium:* E (P)
	Ancylostoma: E (L)	*Metagonimus:* E	*Hymenolepis:* E
	Strongyloides: L	*Echinostoma:* E	
	Trichostrongylus: E		
	Capillaria: E		
	Anisakis: O		
Large bowel	*Trichuris:* E	*Schistosoma:* E	
	Oxyuris: (A) (E)	*Gastrodiscoides:* E	
	Oesophagostomum: O		

[a] A, adults; E, eggs; L, larvae; P, proglottids; O, not appearing in the feces.

for a protracted period of time, and the eggs, larvae, or proglottids of which appear in the stool. We therefore exclude *Anisakis* spp., *Oesophagostoma* spp., *Trichinella spiralis*, and the hepatic and lung flukes from this article.

B. The Impact of Intestinal Helminths on Human Health

The prevalence, the geographical distribution, and the helminth-related morbidity are presented in Table II.

A. lumbricoides is the most prevalent human intestinal helminth. High prevalences are reached by most of the intestinal worms using the feco-oral route of transmission. They are followed in frequency by those which are transmitted percutaneously. In some populations of tropical countries nearly all community members may be infected and the prevalence of intestinal parasitism may attain 100%. In many communities intestinal polyparasitism is frequent (Buck *et al.*, 1978).

TABLE II

The Importance of Human Intestinal Helminths[a]

Principal mode of transmission	Helminth genera	Number of infected persons in millions	Geographical distribution	Degree of morbidity
By contaminated foods and hands	*Ascaris*	About 1000	Global	Low to moderate
	Trichuris	About 500	Global	Low
	Oxyuris	500?	Global	Low
	Hymenolepis	About 50	Restricted	Low
	Trichostrongylus	About 5–10	Restricted	Low
	Oesophagostomum	?	Focal	Moderate to severe
By uncooked, infected food	*Taenia*	About 60	Restricted	Low to moderate
	Diphyllobothrium	About 2–9	Focal	Low
	Fasciolopsis	About 2–10	Focal	Low to moderate
	Capillaria	Below 0.01	Focal	Moderate to severe
	Anisakis	Below 0.01	Focal	Moderate to severe
	Heterophyes	?	Focal	Low
	Metagonimus	?	Focal	Low
	Gastrodiscoides	?	Focal	Moderate
Percutaneously	Hookworms	400–800	Global	Moderate to heavy
	Strongyloides	About 80	Restricted	Low to heavy
	Schistosoma	About 100	Restricted to focal	Moderate

[a] Data in part from Janssen (1974) and Stürchler (1981).

A. lumbricoides, T. trichiura, and the hookworms occur in most southern countries (Stürchler, 1981). *O. vermicularis* occurs worldwide. *O. vermicularis* and *Diphyllobothrium* spp. have been found among the aboriginal population as far north as the Labrador peninsula in Canada (Sole and Croll, 1980). Because of their focal occurrence and their probably low prevalence *Metagonimus yokogawai, Heterophyes heterophyes,* and *S. intercalatum* will not be discussed further.

Helminth infections may interfere with human health by several mechanisms (Grove, 1979): (1) by their location they may occupy space or lead to obstruction; (2) by their number; and (3) by the reactions of the host which they may induce.

Helminths of the human intestinal tract lead to morbidity mainly by their number. Infections of low intensity are unlikely to produce symptoms, and a carrier state is common. High worm burden on the other hand may cause significant morbidity (Tables II and IV). Intestinal helminths, unlike bacteria or protozoa, do not multiply within the host (with the few exceptions of autoinfection taking place with strongyloidiasis and oxyuriasis). Therefore, the worm load is proportional to the number of larvae entering the host and to the duration of exposure. A good measure

TABLE III

PREPATENCY PERIOD OF SOME HUMAN INTESTINAL HELMINTHS[a]

Helminth	Time
Nematodes	
Ancylostoma duodenale	35–42 days
Ascaris lumbricoides	50–80 days
Necator americanus	35–42 days
Oxyuris vermicularis	30–37 days
Stronglyloides stercoralis	17–28 days
Trichostrongylus orientalis	25 days
Trichuris trichiura	1–3 months
Cestodes	
Diphyllobothrium latum	3 weeks
Hymenolepis nana	4 weeks
Taenia saginata	10–12 weeks
Taenia solium	5–12 weeks
Trematodes	
Fasciolopsis buskii	About 3 months
Schistosoma mansoni	5–7 weeks
Schistosoma japonicum	3–10 weeks

[a] Data from Piekarski (1975).

TABLE IV

MORBIDITY FROM INTESTINAL HELMINTHS IN RELATION TO SITE OF INFECTION, NUMBER OF WORMS, AND HOST RESPONSE

	Location of worms	Number of worms	Host reaction
Intestinal	Duodenitis Anal pruritus Anal prolapse Intestinal obstruction Appendicitis Obstructive jaundice Pancreatitis	Diarrhea Bleeding: occult Bleeding: dysentery Steatorrhea	Local immune response
Extra-intestinal	Urticarial rash (creeping eruption) Löffler's syndrome	Hypochromic anemia Iron deficiency Malabsorption Hypovitaminoses Megaloblastic anemia Growth retardation	Pruritus Blood eosinophilia Humoral immune response Immunodepression? Hemolytic anaemia? Löffler's syndrome

of the previous exposure and the intensity of infection is the number of eggs excreted in the feces (Coumbaras *et al.*, 1976). Eggs can be counted by various techniques (Garcia and Ash, 1979). Egg counts indicating heavy worm infestations are shown in Table V. Likewise, the number of

TABLE V

EGG PRODUCTION BY FEMALE WORMS AND ESTIMATED NUMBER OF EGGS INDICATING HEAVY WORM LOAD[a,b]

	Number of eggs produced by one female per gram feces	Number of eggs per gram feces indicating high worm load
Ascaris	1,000–2,000	>10,000
Necator	10–40	>5,000–20,000
Ancylostoma	50–80	>10,000
Trichuris	50–100	>5,000–10,000
Trichostrongylus	?	?
Hymenolepis	?	?
Diphyllobothrium	50,000–500,000	>1–10 million
Schistosoma mansoni	1–10	>200
Schistosoma japonicum	100–200	>500
Fasciolopsis	100–300	>10,000

[a] Data in part from Muller (1975).

[b] With *Strongyloides stercoralis*, *Oxyuris vermicularis*, and *Taenia* species eggs are not usually found in the feces.

worms expelled after chemotherapy may be counted as a measure for the worm burden.

In the last few years several investigators (Blumenthal and Schultz, 1976; Mahalanabis *et al.*, 1976; Chandra, 1979; Brown *et al.*, 1980; Stephenson, 1980; Stephenson *et al.*, 1980a) have provided evidence that even light infections in asymptomatic persons may be detrimental to the state of health of the host, particularly regarding absorption of nutrients, growth, and resistance to infections. On the other hand it has been recently questioned whether a significant influence of ascaridiasis on the nutritional state of the host is clearly established (Gupta, 1981). Taken together these studies bring into doubt the concept of a healthy carrier state and give rise to the question of whether any intestinal helminthiasis should be treated, be it light or heavy and with symptoms or not (see also Section IV,B and Table VI).

TABLE VI

INDICATIONS FOR ANTHELMINTHICS

I. For individual application
  A. When symptoms and helminths are present ("classical indication")
    Diarrhea, dysentery caused by *Trichuris, Strongyloides, Schistosoma, Capillaria*
    Abdominal pain, duodenitis caused by hookworms, *Strongyloides*
    Malabsorption caused by *Strongyloides, Capillaria, Fasciolopsis, Diphyllobothrium*
    Itching, skin eruptions caused by *Oxyuris, Strongyloides,* hookworms
    Anemia caused by hookworms, *Trichuris, Schistosoma*
  B. When symptoms are present but no helminths demonstrable ("trial indication")
    1. Symptoms as under I,A suggesting intestinal helminths
    2. Blood eosinophilia considered to be caused by intestinal helminths
    3. Previous exposure to contaminated food or soil
  C. When symptoms are absent but helminths present: treatment of carriers
  D. When neither symptoms nor helminths are present ("preventive indication")
    1. Close contacts of persons infected with *Oxyuris* or *Hymenolepis*
    2. Persons with a travel history and a depressed immune system (treatment with corticosteroids, cytostatic drugs, etc.)

II. For mass application
  A. Treatment of all members of a population without parasitological screening ("eradication indication")
  B. Treatment of all members of a population found to be infected by parasitological screening ("control indication")
  C. Treatment of persons at high risk ("target indication")
    1. Without parasitological screening
      Infants
      Children
      Pregnant women
    2. After parasitological screening
      Persons with egg outputs indicating high worm load (see Table V)

IV. The Human Host

A. Symptoms of Intestinal Helminthiases

The problem of carriers and of disease caused by intestinal helminths has been discussed in Section III,B. Important symptoms of intestinal helminthiases are shown in Table IV. Of the intestinal symptoms, diarrhea, blood loss, and malabsorption are of particular importance. According to a W.H.O. scientific working group (1980) the following intestinal helminths may cause a true parasitic diarrhea: *T. trichiura, S. stercoralis, S. mansoni,* and *Capillaria philippensis*. For ascaridiasis, ancylostomiasis, and taeniasis diarrhea is not regarded as a characteristic feature. In addition to diarrhea, *S. stercoralis, C. philippensis* and probably also *Fasciolopsis buski* and *D. latum* may cause a malabsorption syndrome (Tomkins, 1979; Brasitus, 1979). Bleeding occurs when intestinal helminths damage the mucosa with their suckers or when penetrating it for migration or anchorage (Chapell, 1980). Bleeding is of particular importance with ancylostomiasis. Blood loss due to one adult worm may be 0.03 ml/day for *N. americanus* and 0.1 ml/day for *A. duodenale* (Rep, 1980).

Important extraintestinal features of intestinal helminthiases are skin lesions, anemia, and immunological disturbances. Parasitic anemia may be a result not only of blood loss and iron deficiency, but also of malabsorption of folates and vitamin B_{12}. It is not yet clear to what extent and how intestinal helminths evoke a host immune response (Wakelin, 1978). An intact immune system of the host seems necessary for controlling overwhelming or generalized infection. This is indicated by reports of disseminated, lethal strongyloidiasis in immunocompromised patients (Barr, 1978; Bradley *et al.*, 1978; Briner *et al.*, 1978). On the other hand, intestinal helminths may depress the host's immune system, either by direct influence on cells of the immune system, or indirectly by impairing the nutritional state of the host (Chandra, 1979; Glazebrook and Davis, 1979). Local pulmonary as well as systemic immune mechanisms may contribute to the appearance of Löffler's syndrome (Stürchler *et al.*, 1978). Although as yet ill understood, the effects of intestinal helminths on the immune system and on the nutritional state of the host may be important clinically and epidemiologically. This has been shown by Murray *et al.* in 1978. After deworming malnourished children heavily infected with *Ascaris,* they observed the appearance of malaria attacks in the treated but not in the control group.

B. Indications for Anthelminthics

A list of indications for anthelminthics is given in Table VI, separately for individual and for mass application. In the past, anthelminthics were mostly for deworming single, symptomatic patients ("classical indication"). However, since efficient and well tolerated broad spectrum anthelminthics have appeared on the market in the last few years (Miller, 1976; Katz, 1977; Botero, 1978; The Medical Letter, 1979; Kean and Hoskins, 1980), the indications for anthelminthics can be extended to include the treatment of patients with symptoms but without demonstrable infection ("trial indication") and of asymptomatic but exposed persons ("preventive indication"). In addition, mass application of anthelminthics has been made possible by these new drugs (Krubwa *et al.*, 1974; Arfaa *et al.*, 1977; Gupta *et al.*, 1977; Ripert *et al.*, 1978; Jancloes *et al.*, 1979; Stürchler *et al.*, 1980). Mass application can be done by treating all members of a community ("eradication indication"), or by treating only the infected population ("control indication") or a population segment which is at high risk ("target indication"). This subject is discussed further in Section VI,C.

C. Reinfection

Reinfection may abolish the effects of anthelminthic treatments in a short period of time. It is favored by (1) environmental factors such as humidity or inappropriate sanitation; (2) the parasite itself, which may multiply within the soil or an intermediate host or resist an unfavorable environment; and (3) the host by his behavior.

Human activities that favor reinfection are shown in Table VII. They have been best investigated in schistosomiasis by observing people at water sites (Dalton, 1976). In schistosomiasis, occupational, domestic, recreational, ritual, and other outdoor activities may lead to reinfection.

Much less is known about other intestinal helminthiases. Oxyuriasis is easily spread from person to person by means of contaminated fingers (Kalbermatten *et al.*, 1980; Stürchler and Peter, 1981). Anthelminthic treatment of oxyuriasis should be accompanied by health instruction. Ancylostomiasis is transmitted by contact of the unprotected skin with contaminated soil. One would expect the provision of toilets and the treatment of excreta before bringing them to the field to be the best supportive measurements for the control of the soil-transmitted intestinal nematodes, in addition to chemotherapy (Mara and Teachem, 1980; Kalbermatten *et al.*, 1980). However, it has been suggested that in the surroundings of ill maintained toilets there may be a high density of infective hookworm larvae which may enhance the transmission of ancylostomiasis (Arfaa *et al.*, 1977; Udonsi *et al.*, 1980; Stürchler *et al.*, 1980). It would be valuable to know how reinfection occurs in intestinal helminthiases.

When a substantial part of a community does not receive anthelminthic chemotherapy it may act as a human reservoir and be a source of reinfec-

TABLE VII

HUMAN BEHAVIOR AND REINFECTION WITH INTESTINAL HELMINTHS

Human behavior	Type of helminth transmitted
Poor personal hygiene (fingers, fingernails, anal region, etc.)	*O. vermicularis, H. nana,* occasionally *S. stercoralis*
Unhygienic excreta disposal (in woods, at rivers, in technically defective toilets)	The soil-transmitted helminths *A. lumbricoides* *T. trichiura* The hookworms *S. stercoralis* The helminths with intermediate host The schistosomes *F. buskii* The taenias *D. latum*
Skin to ground contact (barefoot walking, sitting on the ground)	The hookworms, *S. stercoralis*
Skin to water contact (washing, fishing, bathing)	The schistosomes
Eating of improperly prepared or stored food	*A. lumbricoides, T. trichiura, H. nana,* The taenias, *D. latum*

tion. Short course therapy does not eliminate tissue larvae, which are a source of early "reinfection."

V. The Drugs

A. A List of Essential Drugs

In 1977 a W.H.O. expert committee regarded the following anthelminthics as essential: bephenium, mebendazole, niclosamide, piperazine, tetrachloroethylene, and thiabendazole. Action Medeor, a non-profit-making organization, offers in its 1979 catalogue bephenium, niclosamide, piperazine, and stibophene as anthelminthics of low costs. In 1981 Mission Pharma, another such organization, listed the following anthelminthics: bephenium, levamisol, mebendazole, niclosamide, piperazine, and thiabendazole. The clinician and epidemiologist can probably manage most of the therapeutic problems of intestinal helminthiases with a list of a few, reliable drugs (Stürchler, 1980). Such a tentative list is presented in Table VIII. It is an extract of review articles (Janssen, 1974; Miller, 1976; Katz, 1977; Botero, 1978; The Medical Letter, 1979; Coulaud, 1980; Kean and Hoskins, 1980) and of my personal experience. In addition to the review articles mentioned, the data in Tables VIII and IX–XI have been

TABLE VIII

SPECTRUM OF ACTIVITY OF SELECTED ANTHELMINTHICS

	Nematodes							Cestodes			Trematodes		
	A. lumbricoides	*N. americanus*	*A. duodenale*	*T. trichiura*	*S. stercoralis*	*Trichostrongylus* sp.	*O. vermicularis*	*H. nana*	*Taenia* sp.	*D. latum*	*S. japonicum*	*S. mansoni*	*F. buskii*
Bephenium	—	—	—			—							
Levamisole	—[a]	—	—		—	—[a]							
Mebendazole	—[a]	—	—	—	—	—	—[a]	—	—	—			
Niclosamide								—[a]	—[a]	—[a]			
Oxamniquine												—[a]	
Piperazine	—						—						
Praziquantel								—[a]	—[a]	—	—	—[a]	?
Pyrantel	—[a]	—	—	—		—[a]	—						
Tetrachloroethylene		—	—										—
Thiabendazole	—	—	—	—	—[a]	—	—						

[a] High cure rates (over 90%).

derived from reports on individual drugs of which only some are cited here: (1) mebendazole (Partono *et al.*, 1974; Degrémont and Baumgartner, 1975; Aspöck *et al.*, 1977; Chavarria *et al.*, 1977; Seo *et al.*, 1978; Scragg and Proctor, 1978; Pereira *et al.*, 1979; Foba-Pagou *et al.*, 1980; Muttalib *et al.*, 1981); (2) pyrantel (Ripert *et al.*, 1978); (3) levamisole (Miller, 1980); (4) praziquantel (Davis *et al.*, 1979; Wegner and Thomas, 1980; Biltricide Symposium, 1981; Rim *et al.*, 1978; Groll, 1980); (5) oxamniquine (Saif *et al.*, 1978; Simposio sobre Oxamniquine, 1980; Sleigh *et al.*, 1981); and (6) niclosamide (Seftel and Heinz, 1964; Van den Bossche, 1980).

This list of drugs covers the whole spectrum of intestinal nematodes, cestodes, and trematodes considered here (Table VIII). It does not contain newly developed drugs on which clinical experience is limited, such as flubendazole (Penot *et al.*, 1978; Danis *et al.*, 1980; Bunnag *et al.*, 1980), ciclobendazole (Degrémont and Stahle, 1978; Guggenmoos *et al.*, 1978; Stürchler *et al.*, 1980), and oxantel (Lim, 1978; Margono *et al.*, 1980). Metrifonate is also excluded because it is not used for the treatment of intestinal schistosomiasis (Webbe, 1981).

B. Anthelminthic Activity

The spectrum of activity is shown in Table VIII. The majority of anthelminthics is effective against a single class of helminths. Antinematodes are bephenium, levamisole, piperazine, pyrantel, and thiabendazole. Niclosamide is an anticestode drug while oxamniquine is an antischistosome drug. Tetrachloroethylene, mebendazole, and praziquantel are active against more than one class of helminths. Tetrachloroethylene is used for the treatment of ancylostomiasis and fasciolopsiasis (Idris *et al.*, 1980). Mebendazole shows antinematode and anticestode activity. Praziquantel acts on cestodes and trematodes; its possible effects on nematodes are not established.

High cure rates (over 90%) are obtained with levamisole, mebendazole, pyrantel, and thiabendazole against some nematodes, with niclosamide and with praziquantel against some cestodes, and with praziquantel and with oxamniquine against intestinal schistosomes. The hookworms, *S. stercoralis* and *T. trichiura* are more difficult to treat than *A. lumbricoides* and *E. vermicularis*. Broad spectrum anthelminthics are preferable for the treatment of polyparasitism.

Traditional anthelminthics were purgative. Piperazine and pyrantel paralyze intestinal nematodes which are expelled by peristalsis. This mode of action might be termed "helminthostatic" (Stürchler, 1980). Other anthelminthics interfere with physiological activities of intestinal helminths such as feeding, energy production, and reproduction by blocking enzymes (Van den Bossche, 1976, 1978; Mansour, 1979; Von Brand, 1979; Chappell, 1980). Structural or ultrastructural lesions may ensue, and embryogenesis may be impaired. This mode of action might be termed "helminthocidal" or "helmintholytic." With helminthostatic drugs aberrant migration following treatment does not seem to occur. These drugs lead to expulsion of intact worms that can be identified and counted (Section III,B) and used for demonstrating prompt deworming. With helminthocidal drugs the embryogenesis of residual females may be clearly impaired, and worm expulsion seems inconstant. After single dose mebendazole treatment the time required for the expulsion of *Ascaris* with feces was 3.6 days on average (Muttalib *et al.,* 1981).

Mebendazole, pyrantel, and niclosamide are poorly absorbed from the gut and hence will reach the colon in higher concentrations than well-absorbed drugs such as thiabendazole and levamisole. The latter have a systemic effect and are therefore used for the treatment of tissue helminthiases. They may exert some anthelminthic effect on migratory larvae of intestinal nematodes (see also Section III,A).

C. Administration of Anthelminthics

Dosages and usual length of treatment are given in Table IX. In general, single dose application is used with levamisole, niclosamide (for the treatment of taeniasis), oxamniquine, praziquantel, pyrantel, and tetrachloroethylene. A multidose schedule is preferred for mebendazole, piperazine, and thiabendazole and for the treatment of hymenolepiasis with niclosamide. For mass treatment a single dose schedule is preferable. The total dose needed for optimal efficacy may vary geographically. For mass treatment it is advisable to determine the optimal dosage schedule by an initial pilot trial. A second treatment may be needed after some weeks in cases of high parasite load or when the prepatency (Table III) is assumed to be in progress.

Side effects of anthelminthics are shown in Table X. In general, anthelminthics are well tolerated, and in most instances side effects are minor and reversible. Rarely severe side effects may occur that necessitate withdrawal of treatment and hospitalization. Such side effects are neurological (with oxamniquine, piperazine, tetrachloroethylene, and thiabendazole), dermatological (with thiabendazole), and hematological (also with thiabendazole). A high degree of drug safety is demanded for mass treatment because the medical surveillance is less good than with individual patients and because many of the treated persons may be asymptomatic or even free of parasites.

Some anthelminthics may have additional effects such as antiinflam-

TABLE IX

THE ADMINISTRATION OF ANTHELMINTHICS

Drug	Helminths	Dose and length of treatment[a]
Bephenium, 5 g powder	*A. duodenale*	A and older C: 1 × 5 g/day × 1 to 3 days, C <20 kg: 1 × 2.5 g/day × 1 to 3 days
Levamisole, 30 and 150 mg tablet	*A. lumbricoides*	1 × 2.5–3 mg/kg
	Hookworms	3–6 mg/kg/day × 3 to 1 days
Mebendazole, 100 mg tablet	*A. lumbricoides* and *O. vermicularis*	A and C >2 years: 1 × 200 mg
	Hookworms	A and C >2 years: 2 × 100 mg/day × 3 days
	S. stercoralis and *Taenia* sp.	A and C >2 years: 2 × 300 mg/day × 4 days
Niclosamide, 500 mg tablet	*Taenia* sp.	A: 2 g/day, C 10–35 kg: 1 g/day 1 ×
	H. nana	First day: full dose; next 6 days: half dose
Oxamniquine, 250 mg tablet	*S. mansoni*	1 to 2 × 15 mg/kg/day × 1 to 3 days
Piperazine, 300 mg tablet of salt	*A. lumbricoides*	75 mg/kg/day × 3 days: maximal daily dose for A 4 g, for C 3 g
Praziquantel, 600 mg tablet	*S. mansoni*	40 mg/kg/day × 1 to 2 days
	S. japonicum	60 mg/kg/day × 2 days
	Taenia sp.	1 × 10 mg/kg
	H. nana	1 × 15 mg/kg
	D. latum	1 × 25 mg/kg
Pyrantel (base) 250 mg tablet 50 mg/ml suppository	*A. lumbricoides*	1 × 10 mg/kg
	Hookworms	20–10 mg/kg/day × 1 to 3 days Maximal daily dose for A 1 g
Tetrachloroethylene, 1 ml gelatine capsules	Hookworms	0.1 ml/kg/day × 1 to 3 days: maximal daily dose for A 5 ml, for C 4 ml
Thiabendazole, 500 mg tablet	*S. stercoralis*	25 to 50 mg/kg/day × 3 to 5 days: maximal daily dose for A 3 g

[a] A, adults; C, children.

matory property or immunomodulation. According to dose, timing, and the genetic background of the host, levamisole may act either as an immunostimulant or as an immunosuppressive (Renoux, 1980).

There is only limited information available on the pharmacokinetics and the side effects of anthelminthics in sick, anemic, or malnourished patients. Diarrhea may either accelerate or decrease the absorption of anthelminthics (Pritchard, 1980). Antidiarrheals such as loperamid may enhance the anthelminthic effect of anthelminthics administered to children

TABLE X

TOLERANCE OF ANTHELMINTHICS AND THEIR SIDE EFFECTS[a]

	Bephen-ium	Levami-sole	Meben-dazole	Niclosa-mide	Oxamni-quine	Piper-azine	Prazi-quantel	Pyrantel	Tetra-chloro-ethylene	Thiaben-dazole
Gastrointestinal										
Nausea, vomiting	2	0	0	1	1	1	1	1	1	2
Abdominal discomfort	2	1	1	1	0	1	2	1	1	1
Diarrhea	2	0	1	0	1	1	0	1	1	1
Other	0	0	0	0	1[b]	0	0	0	0	1[b]
Neurological										
Headache	1	1	0	0	1	1	1	1	0	2
Dizziness	1	1	0	0	1	1	1	1	2	2
Other	0	0	0	0	1[c]	3[d]	2[c]	0	3[d]	0
Cardiovascular										
Hypotension	1	0	0	0	0	2	0	0	0	1
Other	0	0	0	0	1[e]	0	0	0	0	0
Dermatological										
Rash	0	0	0	0	1	1	0	1	0	1
Other	0	0	0	0	0	0	0	0	0	3[f]
Other	0	0	0	0	0	0	0	0	0	3[g]

[a] 0, Side effects rare and reversible; 1, side effects occasional and reversible; 2, side effects frequent and reversible; 3, side effects severe, requiring hospitalization and treatment.

[b] Disturbed liver function tests.

[c] Somnolence, lethargy.

[d] Convulsion, ataxia.

[e] Alterations of electrocardiogram.

[f] Severe toxic dermatosis (Lyell syndrome).

[g] Leucopenia, agranulocytosis.

with diarrhea (Scragg and Proctor, 1978). After giving mebendazole to patients with anemia or severe malnutrition, Chavarria *et al.* (1973) did not observe significant side effects.

D. WHICH ANTHELMINTHIC?

This choice is different for individual patient therapy and for mass application.

1. *Treatment of the Individual Patient*

The physician can adjust the treatment to the individual patient's needs. Polyparasitism can be treated with the appropriate broad spectrum anthelminthic or with several anthelminthics combined or administered subsequently. The most important criteria for selecting the appropriate anthelminthic will be effectiveness and tolerance. Table XI presents a list of drugs of choice which has been computed from the references cited in Section V,A. Suggested drugs of choice for ascaridiasis are pyrantel or levamisole, for ancylostomiasis mebendazole, for trichuriasis again

TABLE XI

ANTHELMINTHIC DRUGS OF CHOICE FOR THE TREATMENT OF INDIVIDUAL PATIENTS

Helminth	First line drugs	Second line drugs
A. lumbricoides	Pyrantel × 1 dose or levamisole × 1 dose	Mebendazole × 3 days
N. americanus	Mebendazole × 3 days	Pyrantel × 3 days or thiabendazole × 2 days or tetrachloroethylene × 1–3 days
A. duodenale	Mebendazole × 3 days or pyrantel × 1 dose	Bephenium × 1–3 days
T. trichiura	Mebendazole × 3 days	Thiabendazole × 3 days
S. stercoralis	Thiabendazole × 3 days	Mebendazole × 4 days
Trichostrongylus sp.	Pyrantel × 1 dose or levamisole × 1 dose	Mebendazole × 3 days
O. vermicularis	Mebendazole × 1 dose or pyrantel × 1 dose	Piperazine × 3–7 days
H. nana	Praziquantel × 1 dose	Niclosamide × 7 days
Taenia sp.	Niclosamide × 1 dose	Praziquantel × 1 dose
D. latum	Niclosamide × 1 dose	Praziquantel × 1 dose
S. mansoni	Oxamniquine × 1 dose	Praziquantel × 1 dose
S. japonicum	Praziquantel × 1–3 days	
F. buskii	Tetrachloroethylene × 3 days or praziquantel × 1 dose?	

mebendazole, for strongyloidiasis thiabendazole, for trichostrongyliasis pyrantel or levamisole, for oxyuriasis mebendazole or pyrantel, for the cestodoses niclosamide or praziquantel, for intestinal schistosomiasis oxamniquine or praziquantel, for oriental schistosomiasis praziquantel, and for fasciolopsiasis in the near future may also be praziquantel.

2. *Mass Application*

In most instances a rigid schedule is applied for mass treatment. Here effectiveness and spectrum of the anthelminthic, length of treatment, side effects, and costs are of equal importance. Therefore, a score system is developed as follows which may facilitate the choice of the appropriate anthelminthic.

a. Effectiveness. The effectiveness and the spectrum of activity have been scored from Table VIII by attributing one point to each horizontal bar of each drug (spectrum) and an additional point for high effectiveness (>90%). The scores thus obtained are indicated in Table XII.

b. Length of Treatment. For each drug and helminth 3 points will be given when a good drug effect is achieved with one dose only, 2 points when a 2 day treatment is necessary, 1 point when 3 days are required, and 0 when the length of treatment extends above 3 days (Table IX). For example, mebendazole will score 3 for treatment of *O. vermicularis,* 0 for *S. stercoralis,* and 1 for each of the eight remaining helminthiases. The result of the calculations is again shown in Table XII.

TABLE XII

EVALUATION OF ANTHELMINTHICS FOR MASS APPLICATION[a]

Drug	Effec-tiveness	Length of treatment	Side effects	Costs	Total
Bephenium	4	8	−6	0	6
Levamisole	7	11	0	0	18
Mebendazole	12	11	0	0	23
Niclosamide	6	6	0	0	12
Oxamniquine	2	3	0	−5	0
Piperazine	2	1	−5	0	−2
Praziquantel	8	14	−4	−5	13
Pyrantel	8	14	0	−2	20
Tetrachloroethylene	3	6	−5	0	4
Thiabendazole	8	12	−12	−2	6

[a] For explanation of the score see text.

c. Side Effects. Only frequent (Table X: number 2) or severe (Table X: number 3) side effects were included. These numbers were added up for each drug and entered with a minus into Table XII.

d. Costs. When available the prices for drugs were taken from the drug indices of Medeor and of Mission Pharma which deliver drugs at low costs. For other drugs the commercial prices were taken. From these prices the costs for the treatment of an adult were calculated. The following approximate values in sFr. were obtained (2 sFr. is approximately $1 US): levamisole 0.2, niclosamide 0.2, mebendazole 0.3, piperazine 0.4, bephenium 0.5, tetrachloroethylene 0.9, thiabendazole 1.6, pyrantel 10.0, oxamniquine 15.0, and praziquantel 18.0. Cheap drugs, i.e., with costs up to 1.0 sFr. were scored 0, those between 1 and 10 were scored −2, and those with higher costs −5 (see Table XII).

In summary, Table XII identifies five effective, safe, and economically reasonable anthelminthics which are most useful for mass treatment: levamisole, mebendazole, niclosamide, praziquantel, and pyrantel. With these, all classes and all common species of human intestinal helminths can be treated successfully.

This article on drugs is concluded by summarizing the results of some recent comparative drug studies. Islam and Chowdhury (1976) compared the efficacy of a 3 day mebendazole treatment with pyrantel treatment of the same length. Cure rates for ascariasis, ancylostomiasis, trichuriasis, and strongyloidiasis were 96, 82, 71, and 67% with mebendazole, respectively, and 93, 86, 19, and 0% with pyrantel. Farid *et al.* (1977) compared single dose treatments of ancylostomiasis and ascaridiasis with levamisole, pyrantel, or bephenium and they found the following cure rates: with levamisole 100 and 93%, with pyrantel 90 and 78%, and with bephenium 73 and 81%, respectively. In a comparative study in Venezuela oxamniquine (single dose of 15 mg/kg) and praziquantel (single dose of 30 or 40 mg/kg) achieved similar cure rates and egg output reduction after 120 days (Berti *et al.,* 1979).

E. Drug Resistance and Drug Combinations

Unlike the case with bacteria and protozoa the appearance of drug resistance in intestinal helminths has, to my knowledge, not been reported so far. Therefore, the rationale for drug combinations is to increase the spectrum of activity, mainly for mass treatment and for polyparasitism. Drug combinations tested hitherto are oxantel plus pyrantel (Lim, 1978; Cabrera *et al.,* 1980), mebendazole plus pyrantel (Purnomo *et al.,* 1980), and oxantel plus pyrantel plus mebendazole (Sinniah *et al.,* 1980). Interesting combinations might be (1) a poorly absorbed antinematode drug (e.g., mebendazole) with a well absorbed (e.g., levamisole); (2) a predominantly antinematode drug (e.g., pyrantel) with a predominantly anticestode or antitrematode drug (e.g., praziquantel); and (3) an anthelminthic with an antidiarreic (see Section V,B).

F. Supportive Treatment

In addition to anthelminthics anemia may need correction with iron and folate, duodenitis and mucosal irritation may be soothed by antacids, and allergic skin manifestations of intestinal helminthiases may be treated with antihistaminics.

VI. Therapeutic Intervention

A. For Individuals

Indications for treatment have been shown in Table VI. Classically a correct parasitological diagnosis should be attempted before treatment. This is done by stool analysis (repeatedly and including concentration techniques, if necessary), then by investigations of an anal tape, of the rectal mucosa, and of the duodenal juice. Differential white blood count (for demonstrating blood eosinophilia), total immunoglobulin E concentration, and serological tests may be helpful but are not conclusive. Under optimal conditions and when economically feasible every proven infection should be treated, whether it is light or not, symptomatic or not, or whether reinfection is likely or not. Drugs of choice for individual helminths are shown in Table XI, and their administration in Table IX.

In many instances anthelminthic treatment should be supported by advice on proper behavior (Table VII), and additional medication may be indicated (Section V,F).

The effect of treatment should be followed if possible by appropriate parasitological examinations. These posttherapeutic controls should not be done too early, i.e., not before about 2 to 4 weeks, since eggs may continue to be excreted for some time even when all adult worms are dead. This is the case with schistosomiasis where the eggs within the tissue act as a reservoir. Also, the prepatency period may last up to 3 months (Table III). By that time growing larvae will have completed their development and will start with the production of eggs.

B. Anthelminthic Treatment in Childhood and during Pregnancy

In general, all drugs discussed in this article can be used with adults and with children as well (Coulaud, 1980). However, for children less than 1 year of age, the safety of the drugs is not well established. In that age group treatment should be avoided if possible. In many instances pediatric drug preparations are unnecessary—tablets may be crushed and given with some fluid.

Anthelminthic treatment during pregnancy should be avoided, particularly during the first trimester. However, when there is heavy and symptomatic infection threatening the outcome of pregnancy, e.g., severe hookworm anemia, treatment may be indicated. In that case the poorly absorbable drugs mebendazole, pyrantel, or niclosamide are preferable. However, it should be noted that mebendazole seems to be teratogenic in some experimental animals. The treatment of schistosomiasis during pregnancy should be avoided, if possible.

C. For Communities

Anthelminthic mass chemotherapy has been carried out for several reasons (see also Table VI): (1) for the eradication or the control of a particular intestinal helminthiasis or of intestinal polyparasitism (Gatti *et al.*, 1972; Krubwa *et al.*, 1974; Banzon *et al.*, 1976; Arfaa *et al.*, 1977; Arfaa and Ghadirian, 1978; Jancloes *et al.*, 1979; Stürchler *et al.*, 1980; Poldermann and Manshande, 1981; Sleigh *et al.*, 1981), and (2) for improvement of the health state of a community or of a particular population segment (Gupta *et al.*, 1977; Willett and Kilama, 1978; Stephenson *et al.*, 1980b). The advantages and disadvantages of each of these approaches will be briefly discussed here.

In populations with high prevalences of intestinal helminthiases it may be a waste of time, material, and resources to do parasitological investigations before mass chemotherapy. In addition, light infections are likely to be missed with simple and single stool analyses. Particularly costly and time consuming is to identify heavily infected population segments by counting egg outputs (Coumbaras *et al.*, 1976; Webbe, 1981). On the other hand, a substantial fraction of the population may be free of parasites and receive unnecessary treatment. This increases the costs for drugs (Stephenson *et al.*, 1980a) and poses a critical ethical problem: can healthy persons be treated for the benefit of a whole community?

A target population has to be defined first by means of epidemiological and parasitological investigations. The health care delivery system is likely to be more complex in the case of target treatment than of community treatment. Existing primary care systems such as centers for antenatal care or under fives clinics may greatly facilitate a target treatment programme. The long-term effect of target interventions may be limited by leaving some people untreated who will act as a reservoir and a source of reinfection. In fact it is sometimes a custom to regularly deworm some population segments such as children attending outpatient departments with gastrointestinal complaints. This habit of deworming children may persist in industrialized countries, though it is quite unnecessary (Stürchler and Peter, 1981).

For a successful anthelminthic mass chemotherapy I suggest the following sequence of events:

1. Community participation. The community must have identified intestinal helminthiases as one of their major health problems and want anthelminthic chemotherapy. The agreement of the community to participate may decide the successful outcome of the treatment campaign.

2. Motivation and training of auxiliary personnel. Participating health personnel and village volunteers have to be motivated, equipped, and trained. This may well take place within the villages, visible to the whole community.

3. Pilot investigation. A randomized, representative population sample is investigated clinically and parasitologically. This pilot investigation should answer the following questions: Which are the most important intestinal helminth species within this community? (In this pilot study the distinction between *N. americanus* and *A. duodenale* should be part of the investigations.) How intense are these infections? Which population segments are touched most? What is the impact of these intestinal helminths on the health state of the community (diarrhea, anemia, concomitant infections, malnutrition)?

Then this sample should receive a comparative anthelminthic treatment in order to determine which anthelminthic drug is optimal for the local needs (Stürchler *et al.*, 1980).

4. Census and information of the general population. A census seems indispensable for achieving high attendance rates. The census is best taken in the evening hours outside the harvest times by going from house to house. It should include all members of a household, as well as those working in the field or migrating, the sick, and the uncooperative. While counting the household members, information can be given on the intended campaign: where to come, what to bring, who will receive treatment, etc. It should be remembered that while sick persons are motivated to get treatment ("pressure of pain"), asymptomatic carriers or healthy persons may not be.

Jancloes *et al.* (1978) suggest that a population participation of 60 to 90% may be adequate for control of ascaridiasis with spaced single dose administration of levamisole.

5. Drug delivery and spacing. Whenever possible drugs should be dis-

tributed by the same persons that carried out the pilot investigation and the census, as this will strengthen their authority within the community.

In mass treatment a single dose administration is optimal. We found in Liberia that the participation of the village population rapidly declined from day to day with a 3 day drug schedule (Stürchler *et al.*, 1981).

Care should be taken to exclude severely sick persons, pregnant women, and children below 1 year of age from treatment, if necessary. On the other hand, reach as many persons as possible. Population movements are a major obstacle to this goal. By the arrival of untreated persons and by the departure of treated persons the fraction of the treated population is decreasing.

Migration and reinfection call for drug administration at regular intervals. Little information is available on the problem of spacing: at what interval should certain drugs be reapplied for a particular intestinal helminth? A theoretical answer is given by the length of the prepatent period (Table III). In practice, however, a 3 monthly interval is used in many cases, though there is not always a rational basis for it. After three trimestrial applications of levamisole to primary school children in the Congo the prevalence of ascaridiasis remained low for 6 months (Gatti *et al.*, 1972). In Iran, after three trimestrial doses of levamisole the prevalence of ascaridiasis remained at reduced level 1 year after treatment. It increased to its original level after 2 years, while the prevalence of trichostrongyliasis was still low at that time (Arfaa and Ghadirian, 1978). Interestingly, single dose administration had a similar effect to trimestrial application. Chaia and Da Cunha (1970) performed monthly stool analyses following the treatment of 330 school children with either thiabendazole or tetramizole for ascaridiasis, ancylostomiasis, trichuriasis, and strongyloidiasis. They observed a steady monthly increase of infection rates and of the number of excreted eggs until about 5 to 6 months after treatment, when the treated children reached the infection rates and the parasite loads of untreated controls. In 1981 Sleigh *et al.* reported the long-term effects of oxamniquine on *S. mansoni* in an endemic area of Brazil. Thirty-three months after the two-dose treatment the prevalence was still lowered by 35% and the mean egg number by 40%. Clearly, the optimal time interval for anthelminthic mass treatment is ill defined so far.

It is probable that intestinal helminthiases will neither be eradicated nor controlled even by extensive anthelminthic mass treatment programs in the near future. Even intestinal parasites might learn to survive in an ever more unfavorable environment. However, individual and community anthelminthic treatment definitely brings relief from suffering to some, and improvement of a critical health state to more.

References

Action Medeor (1979). D-4154 Toenisvorst 2, West Germany

Arfaa, F., and Ghadirian, E. (1978). *Iran. J. Public Health* **7,** 100–111.

Arfaa, F., Sahba, G. H., Farahmandian, I., and Jalali, H. (1977). *Am. J. Trop. Med. Hyg.* **26,** 230–233.

Aspöck, H., Flamm, H., Picher, O., and Wiedermann, G. (1977). *Wien. Med. Wochenschr.* **127,** 88–91.

Banzon, T. C., Singson, C. N., and Cross, J. H. (1976). *J. Philipp. Med. Assoc.* **52,** 7–8.

Barr, J. R. (1978). *Can. Med. Assoc. J.* **118,** 933–935.

Barrowclough, H., and Crome, L. (1979). *Trop. Geogr. Med.* **31,** 133–138.

Berti, J., Paez de Molina, B., and Schmidt, D. (1979). *Trib. Med. (Santiago)* **50,** 47–48.

Biltricide Symposium on African Schistosomiasis, Nairobi, 1980. (1981). *Arzneimittelforsch. Drug Res.* **30,** 535–616.

Blumenthal, D. S., and Schultz, M. G. (1976). *Am. J. Trop. Med. Hyg.* **25,** 682–90.

Botero, D. R. (1978). *Annu. Rev. Pharmacol. Toxicol.* **18,** 1–15.

Bradley, S. L., Dines, D. E., and Brewer, N. S. (1978). *Mayo Clin. Proc.* **53,** 332–335.

Brasitus, T. A. (1979). *Am. J. Med.* **67,** 1058–1065.

Briner, J., Eckert, J., Frei, D., Largiader, F., Binswanger, U., and Blumberg, A. (1978). *Schweiz. Med. Wochenschr.* **108,** 1632–1637.

Brown, K. H., Gilman, R. H., Makhduma, K., and Giashuddin, A. (1980). *Am. J. Clin. Nutr.* **33,** 1975–1982.

Buck, A. A., Anderson, R. I., Mac Rae, A. A., and Tain, A. (1978). *Tropenmed. Parasitol.* **29,** 61–70.

Bunnag, D., Harinasuta, T., Viravan, C., Jarupakorn, D., Chindanond, D., and Desakorn, V. (1980). *Asian J. Trop. Med. Public Health* **11,** 363–366.

Cabrera, B. D., Valdez, E. V., and Go, T. G. (1980). Clinical trials of broad spectrum anthelminthics against soil-transmitted helminthiasis. *S.E. Asian J. Trop. Med. Public Health* **11,** 502–506.

Chaia, G., and Da Cunha, A. S. (1970). *Rev. Inst. Med. Trop. S. Paulo* **12,** 152–160.

Chandra, R. K. (1979). *Bull. WHO* **57,** 167–177.

Chappell, L. H. (1980). "Physiology of Parasites," p. 230. Blackie, Glasgow.

Chavarria, A. P., Swartzwelder, J. C., Villarejos, V. M., and Zeledon, R. (1973). *Am. J. Trop. Med. Hyg.* **22,** 592–595.

Chavarria, A. P., Villarejos, V. M., and Zeledon, R. (1977). *Am. J. Trop. Med. Hyg.* **26,** 118–120.

Coulaud, P. (1980). *Généraliste* **291** (Suppl. 3), 3–14.

Coumbaras, A., Larivière, M., Beauvais, B., Languillat, G., and Turquet, M. (1976). *Bull. Soc. Pathol. Exot.* **69,** 95–99.

Dalton, P. R. (1976). *Bull. WHO* **54,** 587–595.

Danis, M., Datry, A., Meunier, Y., and Gentilini, M. (1980). *Gaz. Méd. France* **87,** 5444–5446.

Davis, A., Biles, J. E., Ulrich, A. M., and Wegner, D. H. G. (1979). *Bull. WHO* **57,** 767–779.

Degrémont, A., and Baumgartner, M. W. (1975). *Schweiz. Med. Wochenschr.* **105,** 1830–1832.

Degrémont, A., and Stahel, E. (1978). *Schweiz. Med. Wochenschr.* **108,** 1430–1433.

Farid, Z., Bassily, S., Miner, W. F., Hassan, A., and Laughlin, L. W. (1977). *J. Trop. Med. Hyg.* **80,** 107–108.

Foba-Pagou, R., Kegoum, E., Same-Ekobo, A., Eben-Moussi, E., Faucher, P., Carrie, J., and Ripert, C. (1980). *Bull. Soc. Pathol. Exot.* **73,** 171–178.

Garcia, L. S., and Ash, L. R. (1979). "Clinical Laboratory Manual," p. 174. Mosby, St. Louis, Missouri.

Gatti, F., Krubwa, F., Vandepitte, J., and Thienpont, D. (1972). *Ann. Soc. Belge Méd. Trop.* **52,** 19–32.

Glazebrook, P. W., and Davis, G. H. G. (1979). *Asian J. Infect. Dis.* **3,** 93–117.

Groll, E. (1980). *Acta Trop.* **37,** 293–296.

Grove, D. I. (1979). *Med. J. Aust.* **66,** 641–642.

Guggenmoos, R., Akhtarazzaman, K. M., Rosenkaimer, F., Gaus, W., Bienzle, U., and Dietrich, M. (1978). *Tropenmed. Parasitol.* **29,** 423–426.

Gupta, M. C. (1981). *Am. J. Clin. Nutr.* **34,** 2327–2328.

Gupta, M. C., Mithal, S., Arora, K. L., and Tandon, B. N. (1977). *Lancet* **16,** 108–110.

Idris, Md., Kazi Masihur, R., Muttalib, M. A., and Khan, A. K. (1980). *J. Trop. Med. Hyg.* **83,** 71–74.

Islam, N., and Chowdhury, N. A. (1976). *S.E. Asian J. Trop. Med. Public Health* **7,** 81–84.

Jancloes, M. F., Cornet, P., and Thienpont, D. (1979). *Trop. Georgr. Med.* **31,** 111–122.

Janssen, P. A. J. (1974). *In* "Progress in Drug Research" (E. Jucker, ed.), pp. 191–203. Birkhäuser-Verlag, Basel.

Kalbermatten, J. M., Julius, D. S., Mara, D. D., and Gunnerson, C. G. (1980). "Appropriate Technology for Water Supply and Sanitation," Washington, D.C. pp. 7–20. The World Bank.

Katz, M. (1977). *Drugs* **13,** 124–136.

Kean, B. H., and Hoskins, D. W. (1980). *In* "Drugs of Choice 1980–1981" (W. Modell, ed.), pp. 357–371. Mosby, St. Louis.

Krubwa, F., Gatti, F., Lontie, M., Nguete, K., Vandepitte, J., and Thienpont, D. (1974). *Méd. Trop.* **34,** 679–687.

Lim, J. K. (1978). *Drugs* **15** (Suppl. 1), 99–103.

Loria-Cortes, R., and Lobo-Sanahuja, J. F. (1980). *Am. J. Trop. Med. Hyg.* **29,** 538–544.

Mahalanabis, D., Jalan, K. N., Maitra, T. K., and Agarwal, S. K. (1976). *Am. J. Clin. Nutr.* **29,** 1372–1375.

Mansour, T. E. (1979). *Science* **205,** 462–469.

Mara, D., and Teachem, R. (1980). *J. Trop. Med. Hyg.* **83,** 229–240.

Margono, Sri S., Mahfudin, H., Rasidi, R., and Rasad, R. (1980). Oxantelpyrantel pamoate for the treatment of soil-transmitted helminths. *S.E. Asian J. Trop. Med. Public* **11,** 384–386.

Miller, M. J. (1976). *Fortschr. Arzneimittelforsch.* **20,** 433–464.

Miller, M. J. (1980). *Drugs* **19,** 122–130.

Mission Pharma (1981). ApS, Box 54, DK-3450 Alleroed, Denmark.

Muller, R. (1975). "A Manual of Medical Helminthology," p. 161. Heinemann, London.

Murray, J., Murray, A., Murray, M., and Murray, C. (1978). *Am. J. Clin. Nutr.* **31,** 1363–1366.

Muttalib, M. A., Khan, M. U., and Haq, J. A. (1981). *J. Trop. Med. Hyg.* **84,** 159–160.

Partono, F., Purnomo, F., and Tangkilisan, A. (1974). *S.E. Asian J. Trop. Med. Public Health* **5,** 258–263.

Penot, C., Picot, H., and Lavarde, V. (1978). Essai thérapeutique d'un nouvel antihelminthique en Amazonie colombienne: le flubendazole. *Bull. Soc. Pathol. Exot.* **71,** 370–375.

Pereira, J. F. V., Ghosh, H. K., Conklin, S., and Ryan, S. (1979). *Med. J. Aust.* 134–135.

Piekraski, G. (1975). *Bundesgesundheitsblatt* **18,** 413–418.

Pinkus, G. S., Coolidge, C., and Little, M. D. (1975). *Am. J. Med.* **59,** 114–120.
Poldermann, A. M., and Manshande, J. P. (1981). *Lancet* 27–28.
Pritchard, R. K. (1980). *In* "The Host Invader Interplay" (H. Van den Bossche, ed.), pp. 731–734. Elsevier, Amsterdam.
Purhomo, Partono, F., and Soewarta, A. (1980). *S.E. Asian J. Trop. Med. Public Health* **11,** 324–327.
Renoux, G. (1980). *Drugs* **19,** 89–99.
Rep. B. H. (1980). *Trop. Geogr. Med.* **32,** 251–255.
Rim, H-J., Park, Ch-Y., Lee, J-S., Joo, K.-H., and Lyu, K. S. (1978). *Kor. J. Parasitol.* **15,** 82–87.
Ripert, Ch., Durand, B., Carris, J., Riedel, D., and Bray-Zoua, D. (1978). *Bull. Soc. Pathol. Exot.* **71,** 361–369.
Saif, M., Gaber, A., Hassanein, Y. S., and Khameis, S. (1978). *J. Egypt. Med. Assoc.* **61,** 427–431.
Scragg, J. N., and Proctor, E. M. (1978). *Am J. Trop. Med. Hyg.* **27,** 255–257.
Seftel, H. C., and Heinz, H. J. (1964). *S. Afr. Med. J.* **38,** 263.
Seo, B. S., Cho, S. Y., and Chai, I. Y. (1978). *Kor. J. Parasitol.* **16,** 21–25.
Simposio sobre Oxamniquine (1980). *Rev. Inst. Med. Trop. S. Paulo* **22,** (Suppl. 4), 1–237.
Sinniah, B., Sinniah, D., and Dissanaike, A. S. (1980). *Ann. Trop. Med. Parasitol.* **74,** 619–623.
Sleigh, A. C., Mott, K. E., Franca Silva, J. T., Muniz, T. M., Mota, E. A., Barreto, M. L., Hoff, R., Maguire, J. H., Lehmann, J. S., and Sherlock, I. (1981). *Trans. R. Soc. Trop. Med. Hyg.* **75,** 234–238.
Sole, T. D., and Croll, N. A. (1980). *Am. J. Trop. Med. Hyg.* **29,** 364–368.
Stephenson, L. S. (1980). *Parasitology* **81,** 221–233.
Stephenson, L. S., Latham, M. C., and Oduori, M. L. (1980a). *J. Trop. Pediatr.* **26,** 246–263.
Stephenson, L. S., Crompton, D. W. T., Latham, M. C., Schulpen, T. W. J., Nesheim, M. C., and Jonsen, A. A. J. (1980b). *Am. J. Clin. Nutr.* **33,** 1165–1172.
Stürchler, D. (1980). *In* "Importierte Infektionskrankheiten. Epidemiologie und Therapie" (O. Gsell, ed.), pp. 121–125. Thieme, Stuttgart.
Stürchler, D. (1981). "Endemiegebiete tropischer Infektionskrankheiten," pp. 1–246. Huber, Bern.
Stürchler, D., and Peter, R. (1981). *Sozial- Präventivmed.* **26,** 317–319.
Stürchler, D., Imbach, P., Gartmann, J., and Degrémont, A. (1978). *Schweiz. Med. Wochenschr.* **108,** 1461–1464.
Stürchler, D., Stahel, E., Saladin, K., and Saladin, B. (1980). *Tropenmed. Parasitol.* **31,** 87–93.
The Medical Letter (1979). *Med. Lett.* **21,** 105–112.
Tomkins, A. M. (1979). *Trop. Doctor* **9,** 21–24.
Udonsi, J. K., Nwosu, A. B. C., and Anya, A. O. (1980). *Z. Parasitenkd.* **63,** 251–259.
Van den Bossche, H. (1976). "Biochemistry of Parasites and Host-Parasite Relationships," p. 664. Amst North-Holland Publ., Amsterdam.
Van den Bossche, H. (1978). *Nature* (*London*) **273,** 626–630.
Van den Bossche, H. (1980). *In* "Biology of the Tapeworm Hymenolepis Diminuta" (H. P. Arai, ed.), pp. 639–693. Academic Press, New York.
Von Brand, T. (1979). "Biochemistry and Physiology of Endoparasites," p. 447. Elsevier, Amsterdam.
Wakelin, D. (1978). *Nature* (*London*) **273,** 617–620.

Webbe, G. (1981). *Br. Med. J.* **283,** 1104–1106.
Wegner, D. H. G., and Thomas, H. (1980). *In* "Importierte Infektionskrankheiten, Epidemiologie u. Therapie" (O. Gsell, ed.), pp. 101–112. Thieme, Stuttgart.
Willett, W., and Kilama, W. (1978). *Clin. Res.* **26,** 282 A.
WHO (1977). *Tech. Rep. Ser. No. 615, Geneva* pp. 1–36.
WHO (1980). "Diarrhoeal Diseases Control Programme Parasite-Related Diarrhoeas." WHO unpublished document, WHO/CDD/Par/801.

Development of Radiosensitizers: A Medicinal Chemistry Perspective

V. L. NARAYANAN* AND WILLIAM W. LEE†

** Division of Cancer Treatment*
National Cancer Institute
Bethesda, Maryland
and
† SRI International
Menlo Park, California

I. Introduction 155
II. General Background 156
A. Ways to Overcome Hypoxia 156
B. Search for Radiosensitizers 158
C. Evaluation of Radiosensitizers 160
D. Mechanism of Action of Radiosensitizers 162
E. Criteria for Radiosensitizers 163
III. Structure Activity/Toxicity Determinants 163
A. Electron Affinity (Redox Potential) 163
B. Lipophilicity and Aqueous Solubility 168
C. Toxicity 169
D. Metabolism 171
E. Strategy for Designing Novel Radiosensitizers 172
IV. Medicinal Chemistry of Electron-Affinic Radiosensitizers 173
A. Early Studies 173
B. Nitrobenzenes 174
C. Nitrofurans 175
D. Nitroimidazoles, General 176
E. N-Substituted 2-Nitroimidazoles 177
F. N- and C-Substituted Nitroimidazoles 180
G. Nitroimidazoles, *in Vivo* Studies 184
H. Nitroimidazoles, Synthesis 190
I. Other Nitroheterocyclic Compounds 194
J. Other Classes of Compounds 197
V. Summary and Perspectus for the Future 198
References 200

I. Introduction

Radiosensitizers are chemicals that sensitize hypoxic tumor cells to radiation. Electron affinic radiosensitizers are the most promising of the several classes of radiosensitizers summarized in the Division of Cancer

ISBN 0-12-032919-0

Treatment (DCT), National Cancer Institute (NCI), Linear Array, Radiosensitizers, February 1978. The objective of this article is to critically review electron affinic radiosensitizers from the medicinal chemist's perspective with the goal of discovering new clinically useful radiosensitizers. As such the article will integrate the concepts and research results available on this subject from the physicochemical, radiobiological, structure–activity, synthesis, pharmacological, and clinical points of view. We hope that this integrated view will contribute to a better understanding of the relationship between molecular structure, radiobiological activity, and mode of action, thus providing a basis for the rational design and synthesis of novel radiosensitizers.

Several excellent reviews on aspects of radiosensitization, radiobiology, and clinical implications are available [see Adams (1977, 1979, 1981), Chapman (1979), Dische (1978), Fowler (1980), Fowler and Denekamp (1979), Wardman (1977, 1979), Phillips (1981), and Durand and Olive (1981)].

Beginning in 1977 the National Cancer Institute (NCI) has sponsored a program to discover and develop clinically effective radiosensitizers. To date about 400 compounds have been evaluated as potential radiosensitizers. This work was made possible primarily through two NCI contracts: one with the Institute of Cancer Research, Sutton (Adams and colleagues), and the other with SRI International, Menlo Park and Stanford University (Lee and Brown). These investigations sponsored by the NCI have permitted a systematic study of radiosensitizers, specifically of nitroimidazoles, on a large scale. The highlights of these results will be incorporated into the discussion in later sections.

II. General Background

A. Ways to Overcome Hypoxia

The presence of radioresistant hypoxic cells in the tumor is believed to be a major cause of the failure of radiation therapy. Hypoxic cells lack oxygen either chronically (Adams, 1979) or acutely (Brown, 1979; Sutherland and Franko, 1980), and this fact affords them protection against radiation. Cells are chronically hypoxic because the oxygen, supplied by capillaries, has been depleted by the metabolism of intervening cells. Experiments with many types of cells have shown that cells irradiated in air are killed about three times more readily (one-third the radiation dose) than similar cells under nitrogen; that is, the oxygen enhancement ratio (OER) is about three for many types of cells (see Fig. 1).

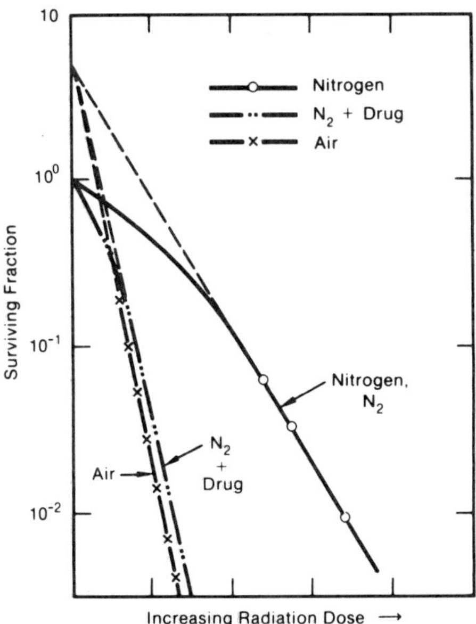

FIG. 1. Effect of radiosensitizing drug on cell survival. Drugs are usually compared *in vitro* by their enhancement ratio (ER). Sometimes the term sensitizer enhancement ratio (SER) is used. The ER is the ratio of the slope of the cell radiation survival curve for the organism under hypoxic conditions to the slope under fully oxygenated conditions. The ER for a cell culture experiment is demonstrated. This figure shows hypothetical curves much like the experimentally determined cell-survival curves for mammalian cells irradiated in air (fully oxygenated cells) and in nitrogen (hypoxic cells) in the presence and in the absence of an effective radiosensitizing drug at its most effective concentration. The curve for cell survival in nitrogen with drug is identical to that of fully oxygenated cells, indicating that the drug has the same effect on hypoxic cells as oxygen and an ER of 2.8. The oxygen enhancement ratio (OER) is 2.8, and an ER of 2.8 is about the maximum obtainable in this system. The term dose modification factor (DMF) is the ratio of the dose without drug to the dose with drug to produce the same effect. The DMF is not equal to the slope ratios (Fowler and Denekamp, 1979). The DMF is applicable to all drugs that modify radiation, be it radioprotection or radiosensitization (Phillips, 1977).

The resistance of hypoxic cells to radiation has been demonstrated in several experimental systems: cell cultures, animal tumors, and human hypoxic skin. Investigators in this field strongly believe that both animal and human tumors contain hypoxic tumor cells. For a summary see the review of Denekamp *et al.* (1977). That adequate oxygen levels can influence the clinical results of radiation is shown by the work of Bush and his colleagues (1978). Their analysis of the radiation treatment of 2803 patients with carcinoma of the cervix showed that patients who were not anemic experienced a significantly greater cure rate than those who were anemic.

A number of ways have been investigated to overcome the resistance of hypoxic tumor cells to radiation. The principal ways are summarized below.

1. Fractionation therapy. When radiation is administered in fractions at periodic intervals, the more sensitive oxygenated cells are killed initially. The hypoxic cells become reoxygenated and then are killed more readily by the next fraction of radiation (see Kallman and Rockwell, 1977). Thus, a given total dose of radiation can be more effective when administered as several fractions than as a single dose. Fractionation therapy can be used in conjunction with the other three ways discussed below.

2. Hyperbaric oxygen. This technique has been of limited use clinically. The use of high-pressure oxygen requires cumbersome and expensive pressure chambers and may cause some unwanted side effects.

3. Heavy particle radiation. There is much current interest in techniques using neutron, pi-meson, and other high linear energy transfer (LET) radiation. With heavy particles, the presence or lack of oxygen makes little difference. However, such radiation requires expensive and complex equipment.

4. Radiosensitizers. Like oxygen, these chemicals sensitize hypoxic tumor cells to radiation. The advantages of hypoxic cell radiosensitizers are that they are selective for hypoxic cells and that, unlike oxygen, they will not be consumed during cellular metabolism. In comparison to hyperbaric oxygen and heavy particle radiation, this approach is the least expensive and the most promising, and is the subject of this article.

B. Search for Radiosensitizers

The search for compounds that mimic the effects of oxygen in sensitizing hypoxic tumor cells began over two decades ago (see the review by Adams, 1977). These compounds share the properties of oxygen in that they can undergo either free radical or oxidation reactions.

1. *Radical Sensitizers*

The free radical type of sensitizers include compounds such as the stable free radical triacetoneamine-*N*-oxyl (*1*, TAN; Parker *et al.*, 1969), norpseudopelletierine-*N*-oxyl (*2*, NPPN; Sapora *et al.*, 1977), and biradical *3* (Ro-03-6061; Millar *et al.*, 1978). While compounds of this type have been effective radiosensitizers in bacterial cell culture systems, their utility has been severely restricted because of their toxicity to mammalian cells. This type of radiosensitizer will not be discussed further.

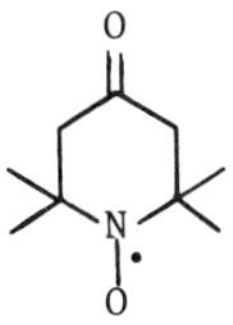

1, TAN 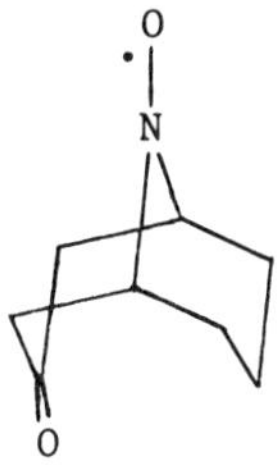   2, NPPN 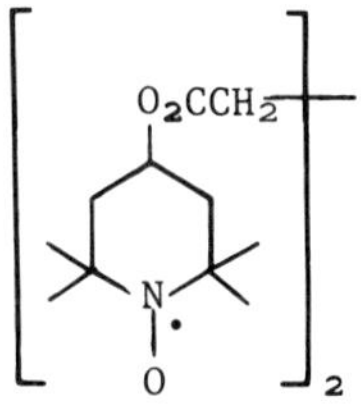   3, Ro-03-6061

2. *Electron-Affinic Sensitizers*

The major impetus for the development of electron-affinic radiosensitizers resulted from the work of Adams and Dewey (1963), who suggested that the electron affinity of compounds can be correlated with radiosensitizing effectiveness. This hypothesis led to the systematic study of a variety of compounds starting from quinones and conjugated carbonyl compounds and leading to nitrobenzenes, nitrofurans, and finally to nitroimidazoles. Two of the nitroimidazoles, metronidazole (Flagyl, *4*) and misonidazole (*5a*), are currently in clinical trials. A search for improved analogs and new types of radiosensitizers is now under way.

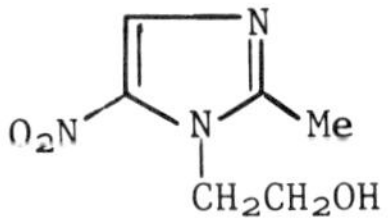

4

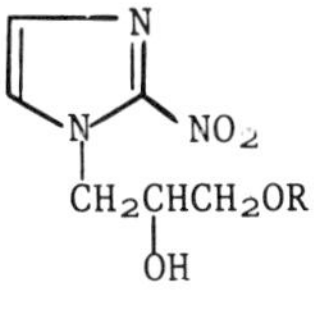

5a, R = Me
5b, R = H

3. *Other Types of Sensitizers*

Other types of radiosensitizers include compounds that bind sulfhydryl groups [*6*,*N*-ethylmaleimide (NEM), Kimler *et al.*, 1977], compounds that exhibit radiation-induced cytotoxicity (*7*, iodoacetamide, Mullenger *et al.*, 1967), and compounds that increase the fragility of the DNA to radiation (*8*, BUdR, Bagshaw *et al.*, 1967). These will not be discussed here.

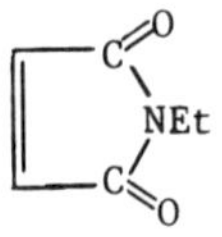

6, NEM

ICH_2CONH_2

7

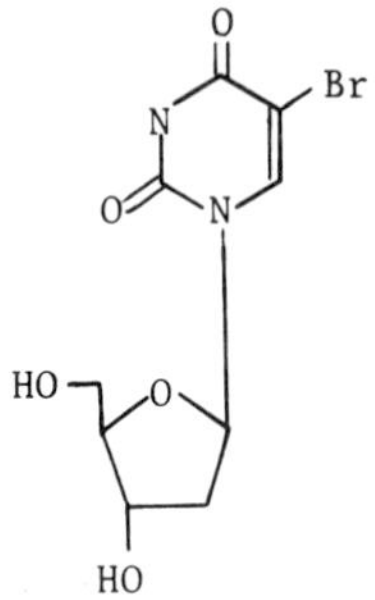

8, BUdR

4. *Other Uses for Sensitizers*

In the search for new sensitizers, some new applications of radiosensitizers have been developed and have aroused considerable interest. The first application makes use of the selective cytotoxic effect of some radiosensitizers on hypoxic cells. This subject has been discussed at a conference sponsored by the Radiosensitizer/Radioprotector Working Group, DCT, NCI, in 1979. See also Brown (1979) and Mahood and Willson (1981) for additional discussion and references on the subject.

The second application is for "chemosensitization" in which radiosensitizers enhance the effect of anticancer agents such as cyclophosphamide (Law *et al.*, 1981; Martin *et al.*, 1981; Twentyman, 1981), BCNU (Mulcahy *et al.*, 1981), and several other agents including melphalan (Roizin-Towle and Hall, 1981; Fu *et al.*, 1981; Clement *et al.*, 1980). Many of the above authors, and others as well, have reported further studies at a Conference on Chemical Modification: Radiation and Cytotoxic Drugs held at Key Biscayne, Florida, Sept. 17–20, 1981. The proceedings will appear as a special issue of the *International Journal of Radiation Oncology Biology, Physics*. A phase I clinical study of misonidazole and cyclophosphamide in solid tumors was reported at this conference (Klein *et al.*, 1981). As can be seen from the above selected references, there is intense interest in this growing area.

C. Evaluation of Radiosensitizers

1. *In Vitro Assays*

The discovery and development of radiosensitizers have been made possible by the concurrent development of multiple methods of evaluation using both *in vitro* and *in vivo* systems (see DCT Linear Array, 1978). *In vitro* systems include bacterial and mammalian cell culture systems using monolayers, single cell suspensions, or spheroids. The *in vitro* assays using both bacterial and mammalian cell culture techniques are very useful for providing rapid feedback for the development of radiosensitizers as well as for studying the mechanism of radiosensitization (Fowler and Denekamp, 1979). For example, these techniques have been helpful in developing the free radical sensitizers (TAN, *1*, Parker *et al.*, 1969), the SH-binding agents (NEM, *6*, Kimler *et al.*, 1977), and the nitrofurans (Chapman *et al.*, 1972).

2. *In Vivo Assays*

For the development of clinically useful radiosensitizers it is essential that *in vitro* assays be supplemented by *in vivo* assays. Some of the *in vivo* assays are summarized below [for details, see Fowler and Denekamp (1979), Fowler *et al.* (1976), and DCT Linear Array (1978)].

a. In Vivo–in Vitro Cell Survival. Mice bearing tumors are treated with the radiosensitizer and then irradiated. The tumors are excised, disaggregated, and single cells are plated and allowed to form colonies. The ratio of the fraction of surviving cells (counted as those able to form colonies) as compared with the control is an index of the activity of the compound. This is the most rapid of all the *in vivo* assays.

b. Tumor Growth Delay. This assay is based on the comparison of the time required for a tumor to regrow to a given size between drug treated and control mice.

c. Tumor Cure (or Survival). This assay compares the proportion of tumors locally controlled—those not recurring within a given time, say 150 days—between drug treated and control mice.

d. Epidermal Cell Survival in Vivo. Historically, this was the first *in vivo* assay that was developed. This assay is based on the regrowth of epidermal cells (Denekamp *et al.*, 1974).

e. Correlation between in Vitro and in Vivo Assays. The studies of McNally *et al.* (1978) showed that a good correlation exists between radiosensitization effectiveness *in vitro* and *in vivo* provided equal drug concentration can be achieved in both the *in vitro* and the *in vivo* systems. The above study also indicates that the intratumor concentration is a good index of the drug concentration in the hypoxic cells. However, recent work by Brown and Lee (1980), Brown and Workman (1980), and Brown and Yu (1980) has shown that this assumption is not always valid and that the transport characteristics of the particular drug determines the relative concentrations. Thus *in vitro* assays are by no means a substitute for *in vivo* assays. In fact, in the development of radiosensitizers, one should depend on multiple assays with multiple endpoints (see DCT Linear Array, 1978).

D. Mechanism of Action of Radiosensitizers

Various models for the mechanism of action of radiosensitizers have been proposed. The direct action model of Adams and Cooke (1969) is shown in Fig. 2.

The energy deposited by radiation directly on the target DNA molecule induces its polarization. The trapped electron and the positive ion can recombine or the electron can be thermalized and migrate along the DNA molecule, according to Adams and Jameson (1980). If a sensitizer with high electron affinity is available, the electron can be transferred to the sensitizer while the target cation is converted to a free radical.

Another model (Chapman and Gillespie, 1981) considers that radiation can act on the biologically important target molecules, such as DNA, either directly or indirectly—through the action of hydrated electrons, hydroxyl radicals, or other radicals generated by the radiation depositing energy on the aqueous environment. The DNA radicals thus generated can either be repaired by reduction or "fixed" by oxidation (the oxygen effect) (see Fig. 3).

All radiosensitizers mimic some component(s) of the oxygen effect, although their mechanisms may differ. The mechanism by which damage is produced in DNA by ionizing radiation can be explained in terms of damage to bases, main chain, protein, single strand DNA, and double strand DNA as discussed by Myers and Kay (1979). The importance of the membrane as a possible target site for radiosensitization has been emphasized (Alper, 1979).

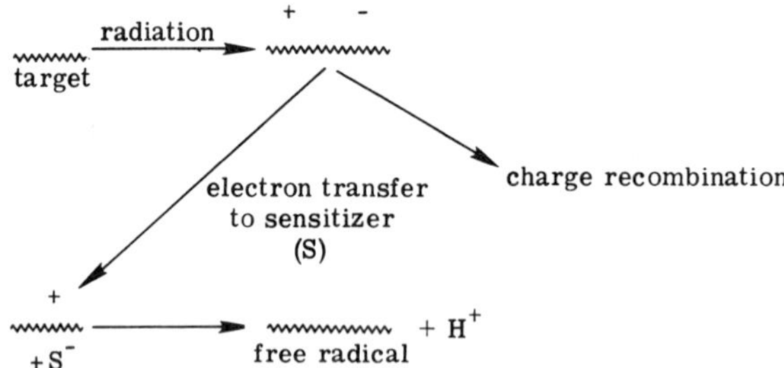

Fig. 2. Direct action model of radiosensitization. This mechanism proposed by Adams and Cooke (1969) involves the interaction of sensitizers directly with the radiant energy deposited in or around the target molecule, or complex, involving DNA. Reprinted with permission of the publisher.

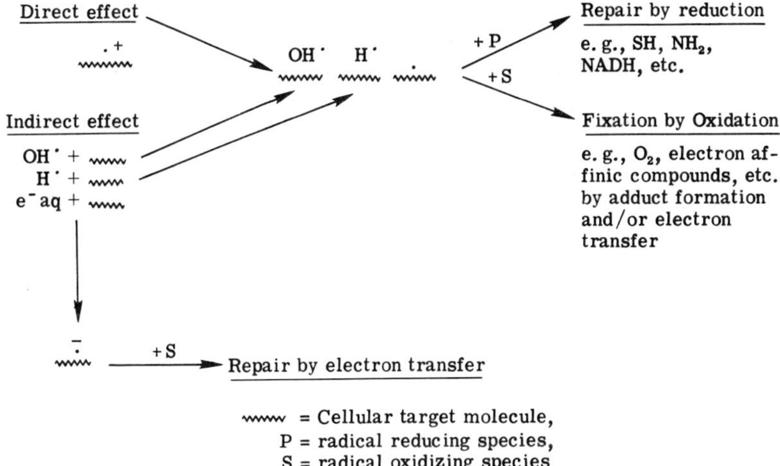

FIG. 3. Diagram of radiation-induced events. This diagram identifies some important intracellular free-radical redox processes. These processes and associated time scales can account for much of the radiobiological oxygen effect, the action of electron-affinic radiosensitizers, and cellular radioprotection by sulfhydryls. From Chapman and Gillespie (1981). Reprinted with permission of the publisher.

E. CRITERIA FOR RADIOSENSITIZERS

In addition to having the proper electron affinity for effective radiosensitization, the hypoxic cell radiosensitizers must possess other properties in order to be clinically useful (see DCT Linear Array, 1978). Ideally they must be (1) selective in sensitizing only hypoxic cells and not oxic cells to any significant degree; (2) transported to the hypoxic tumor cells; (3) metabolized at such a rate that effective radiosensitizing concentrations can be achieved; (4) effective against cells at all stages of the cell cycle; (5) nontoxic at therapeutically useful dose levels; (6) and effective with fractionated radiation.

III. Structure Activity/Toxicity Determinants

A. ELECTRON AFFINITY (REDOX POTENTIAL)

1. *Relation to Radiosensitization*

In 1963, Adams and Dewey suggested that the electron affinity is related qualitatively to radiosensitization effectiveness. Many additional studies supported this relationship. Adams *et al.* (1976, 1979b) have demonstrated that *in vitro* radiosensitizing effectiveness can be correlated quantitatively with electron affinity. For a variety of organic compounds they obtained a straight line plot of radiosensitizing effectiveness versus the electron affinity according to the equation:

$$-\log C = a + b\, E_7^1$$

where C is the concentration required to achieve a standard level of radiosensitizing effectiveness, E_7^1 is the one-electron reduction potential measured at pH 7, a measure of the electron affinity, and a and b are constants. They showed that this correlation is valid for 44 compounds including 2-, 4-, and 5-nitroimidazoles, nitrofurans, and nitrobenzenes as well as oxygen. Among the imidazoles, the electron affinity decreased in this order: 2-nitro > 5-nitro > 4-nitroimidazole.

Meisel and Neta (1975) have reported E_7^1 values for nitro derivatives of imidazoles, furans, benzene, pyridine, and thiophene as well as nitrouracil and 9,10-anthraquinone-2-sulfonate. These E_7^1 values correlated well with radiosensitization effectiveness and with the spin densities of the nitro radical anions.

Sancier (1980), in an attempt to develop a rapid and reliable method for determining radiosensitizing effectiveness, has studied the correlation between photolysis and radiolysis of compounds using electron spin resonance (ESR) of nitroaromatic radical anions.

Measuring E_7^1, one electron reduction potentials, by pulse radiolysis (Wardman, 1977; Meisel and Czapski, 1975) under equilibrium conditions requires costly equipment, such as a linear accelerator or a Van der Graaf generator, not readily available to most laboratories. A convenient alternative measure of redox properties of compounds is the polarographic half-wave reduction potential ($E_{1/2}$), which has been shown to correlate well with electron affinity for many hydrocarbons (Dewar *et al.*, 1970). Ruddock and his colleagues (Ruddock and Greenstock, 1977; Greenstock *et al.*, 1976) correlated half-wave potentials with radiosensitization effectiveness. They suggested that nitroheterocyclic sensitizers with half-wave potentials more positive than -0.5 V (measured against the standard calomel electrode) may have promise as clinically useful radiotherapeutic agents. The more positive the $E_{1/2}$ or E_7^1 values, the greater is the electron affinity of the compound. Breccia *et al.* (1979) have correlated cyclic voltametric results with pulse radiolysis data for radiosensitizers. Chapman *et al.* (1974) have also suggested that the electron affinity of nitrobenzene ($E_7^1 = -486$ mV, Meisel and Neta, 1975, and $E_{1/2} = -460$ mV, Greenstock *et al.*, 1974) is near the threshold for radiosensitizing effectiveness and that compounds with greater electron affinity would be effective sensitizers. Tables I and II list the E_7^1 and $E_{1/2}$ values for various types of electron affinic compounds and Fig. 4 gives their structures.

TABLE I

ONE ELECTRON REDUCTION POTENTIALS (E_7^1) OF SELECTED NITRO COMPOUNDS AND QUINONES[a]

Number	Compound	E_7^1 (mV)
1	5-Nifuroxime, *9a*	−253
2	5-Nitrofuran-2-CO_2H, *9b*	−317
3	2-Nitrothiophene, *10a*	−395
4	4-Nitropyridine, *11*	−191
5	*p*-Nitroacetophenone, *12b*	−356
6	Nitrobenzene, *12a*	−486
7	2-Nitrobenzimidazole, *13a*	−300
8	Duroquinone, *14*	−244
9	Menadione, *15*	−203
10	9,10-Anthraquinone-2-sulfonic acid, *16a*	−375
11	Misonidazole, *5a*	−389
12	Metronidazole, *4*	−486

[a] See Meisel and Neta (1975) for compounds 1–6; Wardman *et al.* (1980) for compound 7; Wardman (1977) for compounds 8–10; Adams *et al.* (1976) for compounds 11 and 12.

TABLE II

HALF-WAVE REDUCTION POTENTIAL ($E_{1/2}$) OF SELECTED CLASSES OF COMPOUNDS[a]

Number	Compound	$E_{1/2}$ (V)
1	5-Nitrofuran-2-CHO, *9c*	−0.25
2	2-Nitrothiophene, *10a*	−0.45
3	3-Nitrothiophene, *10b*	−0.52
4	2-Nitropyrrole, *17*	−0.67
5	2-Nitro-5-pyridinylthiazole, *18a*	−0.31
6	2-Br-5-Nitrothiazole, *18b*	−0.40
		−0.30
7	4-NO_2-Isothiazole, *19*	−0.45
8	5-CN-1,3-Me_2-4-NO_2-pyrazole, *20*	−0.45
9	2-NH_2-5-NO_2-thiazole, *18c*	−0.50
10	3-NO_2-triazole, *21*	−0.55
11	2-NO_2-5-Pyridinylthiadiazole, *22a*	−0.20
12	2-NO_2-5-NH_2-thiadiazole, *22b*	−1.16
13	Misonidazole, *5a*	−0.36
		−0.30
14	Metronidazole, *4*	−0.60

[a] See Biaglow *et al.* (1978) for compounds 1–6, 13, and 14; Ruddock and Greenstock (1977) for compounds 1 and 6–13. Where two values are given, the top one is from Biaglow *et al.* (1978).

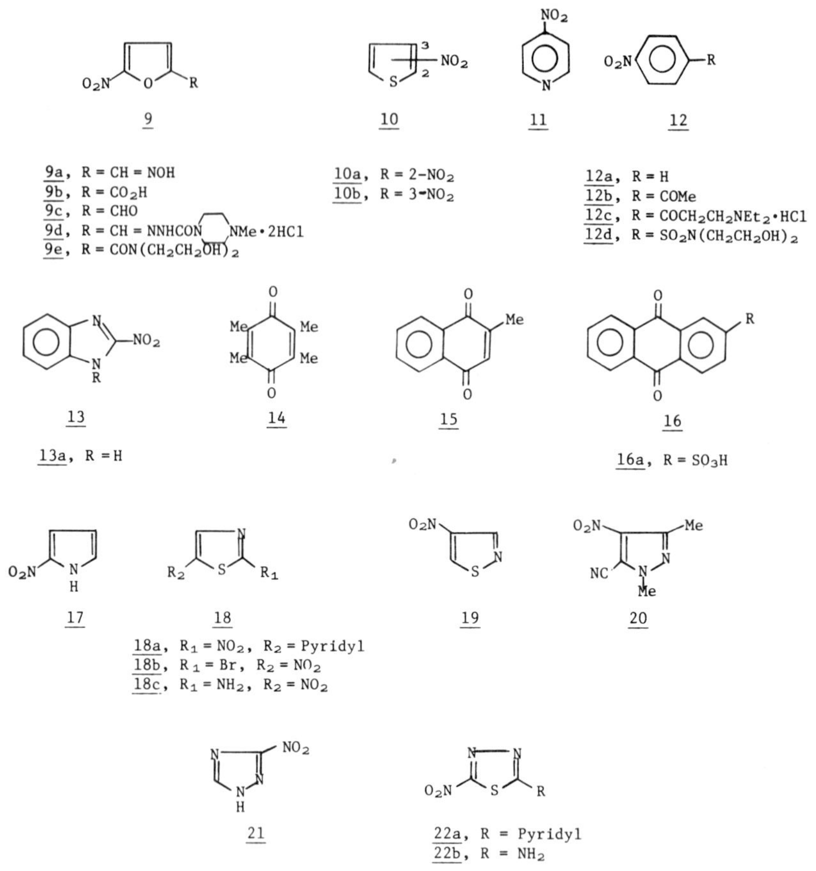

FIG. 4. Chemical structures.

Note that half-wave reduction potentials vary with experimental conditions such as solvent composition (Jaworski *et al.*, 1979), pH, ionic strength, buffer, and, of course, reference electrode. As an example see the variations in the $E_{1/2}$ values reported in the literature for metronidazole in Table III. Therefore, any comparison and ranking of various compounds should be based on measurements performed under identical conditions. To compare two sets of compounds, some cross-check measurements are necessary.

2. *Substituent Effects*

The electron affinity of nitrobenzenes is affected by the electron-withholding or electron-releasing nature of other substituents on the ben-

TABLE III

HALF-WAVE REDUCTION POTENTIALS REPORTED FOR METRONIDAZOLE

$E_{1/2}$ (V)	Reference
−0.415	Chien *et al.* (1978)
−0.500	Cavalleri *et al.* (1978)
−0.500	Goldstein *et al.* (1977)
−0.600	Biaglow *et al.* (1978)
−0.408 at pH 6 −0.556 at pH 7.4	de Carneri *et al.* (1976)

zene ring. Raleigh *et al.* (1973) have demonstrated a quantitative relationship between the radiosensitizing efficiency [as measured by the enhancement ratio (ER) of the drug] and the Hammett sigma values (σ) of a series of nitrobenzenes. Wardman (1979) has similarly demonstrated the usefulness of Hammett's sigma values (σ^-) in correlating the radiosensitizing efficiency of a series of 5-substituted-1-methyl-2-nitroimidazoles (*23*).

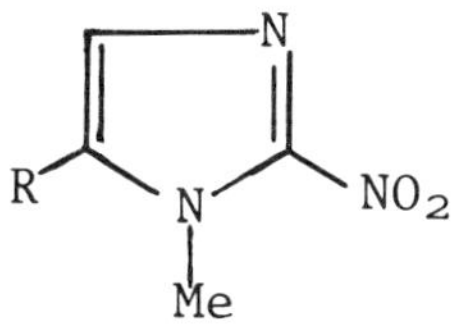

R N NO2 Me

23

23a, R = CHO

3. *Relation to Toxicity*

For nitroheterocycles in general, electron affinity parallels not only radiosensitizing effectiveness but also cytotoxicity to oxic cells (Adams *et al.*, 1979a) and mutagenicity (Chessin *et al.*, 1978; Chin *et al.*, 1978). Therefore the development of nitroimidazoles with improved therapeutic indices will not be easy and straightforward. However, there is no reason to believe that a similar correlation should extend to other classes of compounds as well. Thus, Adams *et al.* (1980b) have demonstrated that for quinones the toxicity toward hypoxic mammalian cells *in vitro* did not correlate well with the one-electron reduction potential, in contrast to nitro compounds.

B. Lipophilicity and Aqueous Solubility

To exert its radiosensitizing effect, the drug must be transported to the site of hypoxic cells; preferentially it should be selectively concentrated in the hypoxic cells. The tissue distribution of the radiosensitizer is primarily a function of both its lipophilicity and aqueous solubility.

Adams and his colleagues (Adams *et al.*, 1976, 1979b) found that lipophilicity, as measured by log P (Fujita *et al.*, 1964), did not influence the *in vitro* radiosensitization effectiveness in their monolayer cell culture systems. They noted that log P, although not a factor *in vitro*, should be of considerable importance *in vivo*. However, Anderson and Patel (1979) found that even *in vitro* radiosensitization did depend on P as well as E^1_7 if P were higher than 3.5. More recently, Anderson *et al.* (1981) plotted the relationship of log P to sensitization effectiveness in two bacterial systems. For *E. coli* they obtained a parabola with a sensitization maximum when log P was about 1.0, whereas for *S. lactis* no such relationship was noted. This finding was attributed to differences between the membrane properties of *E. coli* which resembled a multicompartment model, and *S. lactis* which resembled a two-compartment model.

The work of Brown and Lee (1980) discussed later, clearly demonstrated the importance of achieving an optimum balance of hydrophilicity to lipophilicity in determining *in vivo* radiosensitizing effectiveness. For nitroimidazoles Brown and Lee (1980) and Brown and Workman (1980) have shown that the partition coefficient plays a significant role in determining the relative drug concentration in tumor versus other tissues (see Fig. 5). Uniform distribution of the compound throughout all tissues is not always achieved. For example, using Lewis Lung carcinoma in mice, Donnelli *et al.* (1977) found that the drugs were concentrated mostly in the viable regions and were practically absent in the necrotic region.

Radiosensitizers must possess high water solubility because of the high doses that have to be delivered to rapidly achieve peak drug concentration in the hypoxic cell site. Misonidazole is soluble only to the extent of 26 mg/ml, whereas metronidazole is even less soluble. Should an analog as effective as misonidazole but one-third as toxic be developed, it would need to be administered at three times the dose of misonidazole, and therefore would need to be more water soluble. Increasing water solubility generally follows increasing hydrophilicity (decreasing log P), but there are exceptions.

In designing clinically improved analogs, particular emphasis must be placed on the synthesis of compounds of high water solubility since the hydrophilic compounds can be expected to be less neurotoxic than misonidazole (Brown and Lee, 1980). Soloway and colleagues (1958, 1960)

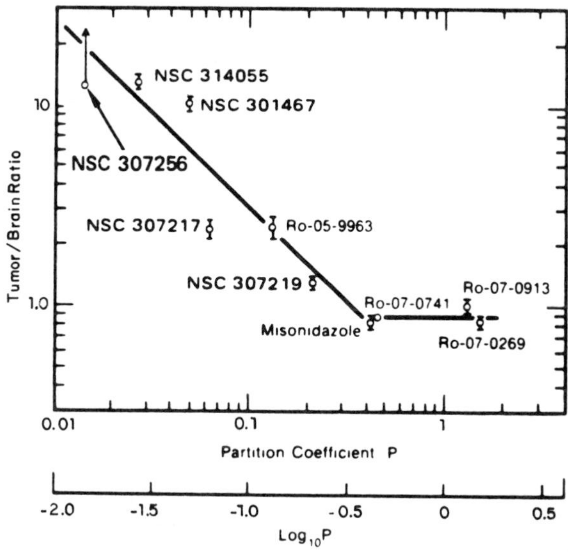

FIG. 5. The tumor/brain ratio as a function of partition coefficient. From Brown and Workman (1980). Reprinted with permission of the publisher.

have shown that the degree of lipophilicity of drugs is the major determinant of their ability to penetrate the blood–brain barrier. It should be noted that metronidazole ($\log p = -0.02$) is known to penetrate well into all body fluids including cerebrospinal fluid (CSF) (Jokipii *et al.,* 1977).

C. TOXICITY

The clinical utility of these agents is determined by factors such as toxicity, metabolism, and aqueous solubility. For example, the recommended radiosensitization dose for metronidazole is around 94 g (Karim, 1978), whereas the maximum dose of the same drug administered for the treatment of trichomoniasis (Goldman, 1980) is around 7.5 g. To be effective with fractionated radiation, the dose of drug for each fraction must be sufficiently high to produce effective radiosensitization without causing accumulative toxicity. Because of neurotoxicity, the total dose recommended for misonidazole does not give maximum radiosensitization when distributed over the fractionated doses of X rays. In order to minimize toxicity at therapeutically useful dose levels, the clinical dose of misonidazole is limited to 0.05–0.5 mmol/kg even though in animal experiments, up to 5 mmol/kg has been used to achieve the maximum radiosensitizing effect. If the neurotoxicity of misonidazole were lower, higher clinical doses, closer to effective radiosensitization doses, could have been used (the recommended total clinical dose is 12 g/m^2 over 3 weeks, or 24 g for a 75-kg person, Wasserman *et al.,* 1979).

In early clinical trials with the nitroimidazole hypoxic cell sensitizers neurotoxicity was found to be dose limiting. With single high doses, convulsions may occur; with multiple doses, peripheral neuropathy (fingers tingling, numbness) appears first followed by symptoms of central nervous system toxicity. Therefore a workshop was sponsored by the DCT in January 1978 to stimulate the development of test systems to measure neurotoxicity. Subsequently, a number of investigators reported their results at a conference (DCT, 1980).

Neurotoxicity models were developed utilizing, for example, the dog (Brown, above conference; White *et al.,* 1980), the rat (M. S. Edwards *et al.* and Griffin, above conference; Griffin *et al.,* 1979), and the mouse (R. J. R. Johnson and P. Conroy, above conference; Subjeck *et al.,* 1980). In the mouse model, Conroy *et al.* (1980) found that after the chronic administration of misonidazole (0.3 mg/g/day, 5 times weekly) for a period of 3–4 weeks a sequence of toxic effects appeared, and the resultant neurotoxicity could be correlated with the performance of the mice on a rotating rod (rotarod performance). Most recently Conroy and Shaw (1981) and Passalacqua *et al.* (1981) using a mouse model have shown that the hearing loss at high frequencies is an indicator of neurotoxicity. These hearing losses were correlated with histological changes in the CNS.

A quantitative cytochemical method has been developed (C. Clarke, above conference; Clarke *et al.,* 1980) that measures the increases in lysosomal enzyme activity that accompany the development of peripheral neuropathy. These quantitative estimates of the changes in the level of enzyme activity are useful indices of the degree of neuropathy and are of value in ranking compounds in structure–activity relationship studies. Figure 6 from Clarke *et al.* (1980) shows the gradual increase in β-glucuronidase activity as neuropathy develops and the subsequent decrease as recovery takes place.

Mutagenicity, a property shared by many nitro compounds, is cause for concern in the long-term use of radiosensitizers. The general relationship of mutagenicity to electron affinity was mentioned earlier. Miller and Hall (1980) have summarized their studies of oncogenic transformations produced by both chemotherapeutic agents and by the new generation of radiosensitizers. The carcinogenic potential of the sensitizers, while not negligible, is considerably less than that associated with many chemotherapeutic agents in common use. Furthermore, 2-nitroimidazoles that are equivalent in radiosensitization efficiency may differ significantly in their rates of producing oncogenic transformations.

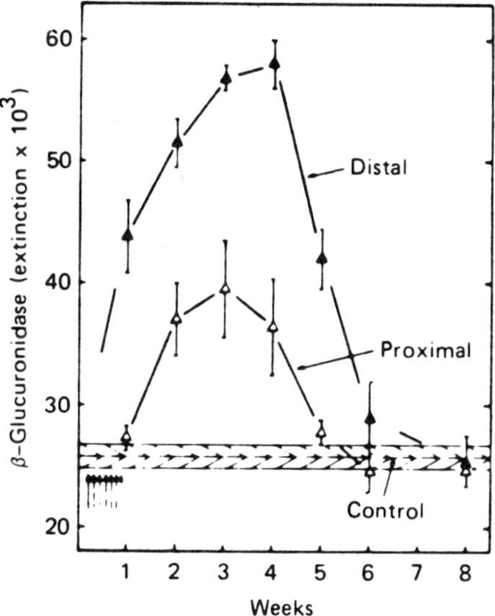

FIG. 6. Cytochemical assay for neurotoxicity. β-Glucuronidase activity in the sciatic nerves of mice following 0.5 mg/g misonidazole, daily for 7 days. Control data are pooled from 14 mice, both distal and proximal portions of nerve. All other points represent the mean of six mice. Standard errors of the mean are shown. From Clarke *et al.* (1980). Reprinted with permission of the publisher.

D. METABOLISM

The rate of metabolism of a radiosensitizer determines both its radiosensitizing effectiveness and its toxicity. For effective radiosensitization the drug must be present at the maximum concentration only at the moment of irradiation. However, the toxicity of the compound depends on the total exposure (concentration × time). Therefore, to enhance the therapeutic index, the radiosensitizer should be eliminated rapidly or metabolized immediately after reaching peak concentration at the time of irradiation. This will minimize the total exposure and consequent toxicity. Martin and Lee (1980) have discussed this criterion using two hypothetic drugs, A and B (see Fig. 7). The drugs A and B both give the same maximum drug concentration in the tumor and other tissues at the time of irradiation. However, A after reaching its maximum concentration is cleared much more rapidly than B thus accounting for the lower toxicity of A. Another case of reduced toxicity results when a drug preferentially concentrates in the tumor tissue (curve B) in contrast to normal tissues (curve BB).

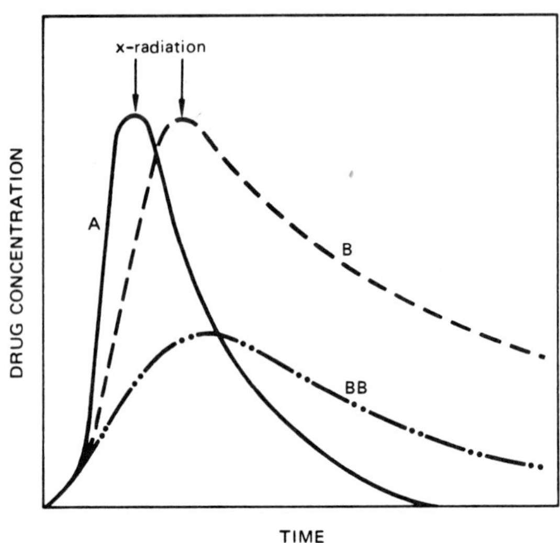

FIG. 7. Maximum concentration and clearance time.

E. STRATEGY FOR DESIGNING NOVEL RADIOSENSITIZERS

We have discussed above some of the critical structure activity/toxicity parameters that determine radiosensitization effectiveness. Methods for predicting and measuring these factors have now become available and are invaluable tools for the rational design and development of novel radiosensitizers.

For example, through the synthesis and evaluation of a limited number of compounds of a specific structural class, taking into consideration the Hammett sigma values of substituents and measurement of their redox potentials, we can design and synthesize new members of the class having the desired redox potential for achieving maximum radiosensitizing effectiveness.

Such a design logic can be extended to include other relevant parameters (e.g., lipophilicity, toxicity) that we have discussed earlier leading ultimately to novel radiosensitizers possessing the optimum balance of the desirable properties.

These approaches have been successfully employed by both the NCI contractors and by other investigators for the design and development of novel radiosensitizers potentially superior to misonidazole.

One such approach is to design and synthesize compounds with greater electron affinity and therefore greater radiosensitization than misonidazole. This would require either (1) a search for other classes of nitroheterocycles or compounds with higher electron affinity or (2) placing electron-withdrawing substituents on the nitroimidazole ring to increase the electron affinity as for example *23*, with R being some electron-withdrawing substituent.

The second approach involves the design and synthesis of analogs with the same electron affinity as misonidazole but with better pharmacological properties, and lower toxicity, such as *24*. The unique feature of com-

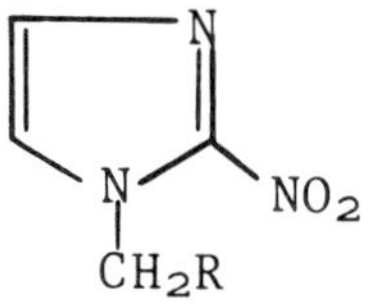

CH_2R NO_2

<u>24</u>

pounds of type *24* is the fact that broad changes in the nature of the R group does not alter the electron affinity appreciably since the substituents are insulated from the ring nitrogen by the methylene bridge. Therefore each of these analogs should radiosensitize as effectively as misonidazole *in vitro* as well as *in vivo* if it can be delivered at the equivalent concentration to the site of the hypoxic tumor cells. However, the tissue distribution of these compounds will depend upon their solubility and lipophilicity which are determined in turn by the nature of the R group in *24*.

IV. Medicinal Chemistry of Electron-Affinic Radiosensitizers

A. Early Studies

Until 1970, reports on the radiosensitization of hypoxic mammalian cells by chemicals were limited to two classes of compounds. The first class included conjugated carbonyl compounds such as menadione (*15*), and glyoxal *25a*, or other 1,2-dicarbonyl derivatives *25* (Ashwood-Smith *et al.*, 1967; Adams and Cooke, 1969). The second class of compounds was exemplified by the stable free radical (TAN) *1* (Parker *et al.*, 1969), mentioned earlier.

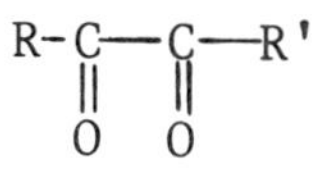

R–C(=O)–C(=O)–R'

<u>25</u>

<u>25a</u>, R = R' = H

B. Nitrobenzenes

p-Nitroacetophenone (PNAP, *12b*) was one of the first nitrobenzene compounds studied (Chapman *et al.*, 1971; Adams *et al.*, 1971). The compound was effective as a radiosensitizer against mammalian cells *in vitro*, but it was too insoluble for further development. A water-soluble compound, 4′-nitro-3-(dimethylamino)propiophenone hydrochloride (NDPP, *12c*) (Adams *et al.*, 1972) was found to be more effective than PNAP *in vitro*. Unfortunately, the compound showed only modest radiosensitization in mice and at the same time caused marked kidney abnormalities (Sheldon and Hill, 1975). The lack of high radiosensitization can be rationalized on the basis that in the cell, NDPP can be metabolically activated and then undergo reaction with SH compounds like glutathione (GSH) to form $GSCH_2CH_2COC_6H_4NO_2(p)$ (Wong and Whitmore, 1977).

Rauth and Kaufman (1975) have compared the relative radiosensitization effectiveness of several nitrobenzenes (including NDPP) with two nitroimidazoles *in vivo* and have shown that the nitrobenzenes are inferior to the nitroimidazoles.

Recently, Stratford *et al.* (1981b) have reported that *26*, CB 1954, a monoalkylating agent, has $E^1_7 = -385$ mV, very close to that of misonidazole, $E^1_7 = -389$ mV. However, *26* radiosensitized hypoxic cells *in vitro* more effectively than misonidazole. (The enhancement ratio for *26*

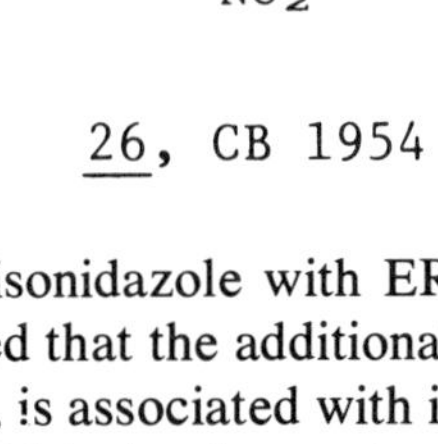

CONH2 NO2 N NO2

26, CB 1954

was 2.2, as contrast to misonidazole with ER = 1.45.) Through further experiments they concluded that the additional sensitizing action of *26*, as compared to misonidazole, is associated with its alkylating activity. However, the effectiveness of *26* in *in vivo* systems could not be determined because of its poor water solubility.

In summary, nitrobenzenes are found to be poor radiosensitizers *in vivo* even though many have shown good activity *in vitro* [see above references and Chapman *et al.* (1972a)]. Since nitrobenzene derivatives with suitable electron affinity can be easily synthesized, the critical limitation is the incorporation of the other necessary properties—e.g., aqueous solubility, stability, low toxicity—in the nitrobenzene derivative to obtain a clinically useful radiosensitizer. With this objective in mind we prepared the more soluble and more hydrophilic *12d,* NSC 711432 (SR 2586). Unfortunately, it was found to be less effective than misonidazole and the compound was also unstable (undergoes a Smiles type of rearrangement). Thus nitrobenzenes as a class do not show much promise.

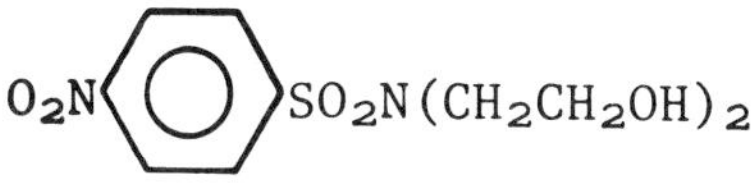

12d

C. Nitrofurans

The readily available nitrofurans *9* are more electron affinic (see Table I, *9a* and *9b*; Table II, *9c*) than their corresponding nitrobenzene derivatives (Sasaka, 1954). Extensive studies have shown that nitrofurans are effective radiosensitizers *in vitro* (Chapman *et al.,* 1972b, 1973), exceeding that of the nitroimidazoles (Hall *et al.,* 1978). The nitrofuran *9d* was found to act by two different mechanisms—one related to misonidazole and other electron-affinic radiosensitizers, and the other involving a shoulder effect (Watts, 1977). Unfortunately nitrofurans proved to be less effective radiosensitizers *in vivo* than the nitroimidazoles. For example, in an epidermal cell survival *in vivo* assay the nitrofuran *9c* and misonidazole (*5a*) were found to be equally effective as radiosensitizers at doses of 0.2 mg/g. However, misonidazole was less toxic and could bc uscd at a higher dose for greater radiosensitization effectiveness than the nitrofurans (Denekamp *et al.,* 1974).

In general, nitrofurans are found to be quite toxic and are metabolized rapidly. These findings can be rationalized on chemical grounds since many of the compounds in the series are aldehyde derivatives and as such can be expected to be hydrolyzed back to the parent aldehyde. In addition they can also undergo metabolic reduction of the nitro function (to hydroxylamine and then to the amine) with concomitant ring cleavage (Swaminathan and Lower, 1978). Based on these facts and our experience with nitroimidazoles, we synthesized the 5-nitrofuran, *9e,* (NSC 328806; SR 2581) as a potential radiosensitizer. We rationalized that the *N,N*-dihydroxyethylamide group should increase water solubility and reduce toxicity. At the same time, since R is no longer an aldehyde derivative it should increase the stability of the compound as well. In fact, *9e* was found to be more soluble, more stable and less toxic than many nitrofuran aldehyde derivatives. It was almost as effective a radiosensitizer as misonidazole *in vitro* ($ER_{1.6}$ = 3.5 and 2.6 for *9e* and misonidazole, respectively). However it was not active *in vivo*.

From these results and those of earlier investigators, we conclude that nitrofurans in general do not appear to show potential for further development.

D. Nitroimidazoles, General

Nitroimidazoles as a class have been extensively investigated previously as antibacterial and antiprotozoan agents and recently the potential of nitroimidazoles as radiosensitizers has been discovered. Metronidazole (Flagyl; *4*) and misonidazole (*5a*) were found to be effective radiosensitizers not only *in vitro* but also *in vivo*. Metronidazole was soon tried in humans and misonidazole followed [see Fowler and Denekamp (1979) and Adams (1977) for more detailed discussions]. Much radiosensitization study has centered on developing the necessary knowledge to exploit these two compounds clinically. Clinical trials (Dische, 1978) with metronidazole and misonidazole were encouraging but neuropathy was dose limiting (Dische *et al.*, 1978; Walker *et al.*, 1980; Bradley *et al.*, 1977; Phillips, 1981). A metabolite of misonidazole formed by the cleavage of the methyl ether, desmethylmisonidazole (NSC 261036; *5b*) is more soluble and more hydrophilic ($\log P = -1.53$) than misonidazole ($\log P = -0.37$), and promises to be less neurotoxic than misonidazole as evidenced in early clinical trials.

The redox potentials and radiosensitization effectiveness of some of the nitroimidazoles that have been synthesized earlier are shown in Table IV (Adams *et al.*, 1976, 1979b; Hall *et al.*, 1978). It is seen that both redox potential and radiosensitization efficiency decrease in the order: 2-nitro > 5-nitro > 4-nitroimidazoles. In the case of N-substituted 2-nitroimidazoles, if the changes in the N-substituent are insulated from the nitrogen by at least one carbon atom, the substitutions can be varied considerably without changing the E^1_7 values significantly.

In the expectation of generating compounds with greater radiosensitization effectiveness, the study of 2-nitroimidazoles that are more electron affinic than misonidazole has been explored. For example *23a* (compound 1, Table IV) is more electron affinic than misonidazole and radiosensitizes *in vitro* as effectively as misonidazole at less than one-tenth the molar

TABLE IV

REDOX AND RADIOSENSITIZING PROPERTIES OF SOME NITROIMIDAZOLES

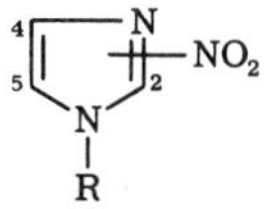

NO_2 at	Substituents at 1	Substituents at 2 or 5	E^1_7 (mV)	$[S]_{1.6}$[a] (mV)
2	Me	CHO	−243	0.02
2	Me	$CH{=}CH_2$	−392	0.18
2	CH_2CH_2OH		−398	0.3
2	$CH_2CHOHCH_2OMe$		−389	0.3
2	$CH_2CH_2SO_2Et$		−368	0.3
2	$CH_2CH_2OC_6H_5$		−391	0.25
2	CH_2CO_2Me		−355	0.17
2	CH_2COMe		−358	0.4
2	$CH_2CH_2N(C_2H_4)_2O$		−390	1.5
5	$CH_2CH_2SO_2Et$	Me	−464	2.7
5	CH_2CH_2OH	Me	−496	4.0
5	$CH_2CH_2N(C_2H_4)_2O$		−457	2.4
4	$CH_2CH_2N(C_2H_4)_2O$		−554	14

[a] $[S]_{1.6}$ is the concentration necessary to achieve the standard radiosensitization level; in this case, an enhancement ratio of 1.6 *in vitro* with Chinese hamster cells.

concentration. However, it has been found to be far more cytotoxic to mammalian cells and afforded no therapeutic advantage over misonidazole.

E. N-SUBSTITUTED 2-NITROIMIDAZOLES

Recently Adams *et al.* (1980a) have systematically studied several series of nitroimidazoles. Compounds of structure *27a* were synthesized with varying chain length (n = 2–11). As expected the electron affinities remained essentially constant. On the other hand, sensitization of mammalian cells increased with increasing n until it reached a maximum at n = 5 and then decreased; however the chronic aerobic toxicity to the mammalian cells increased with increasing chain length. Consequently, the "sensitization effectiveness," which corresponds to the therapeutic ratio *in vivo,* reaches a maximum in *27a* at n = 5 (NSC 313396, RSU 1032). In the related series where the morpholino group was replaced by the

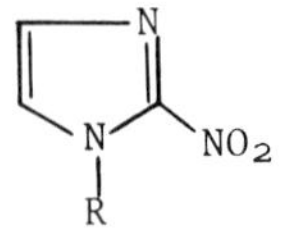

27

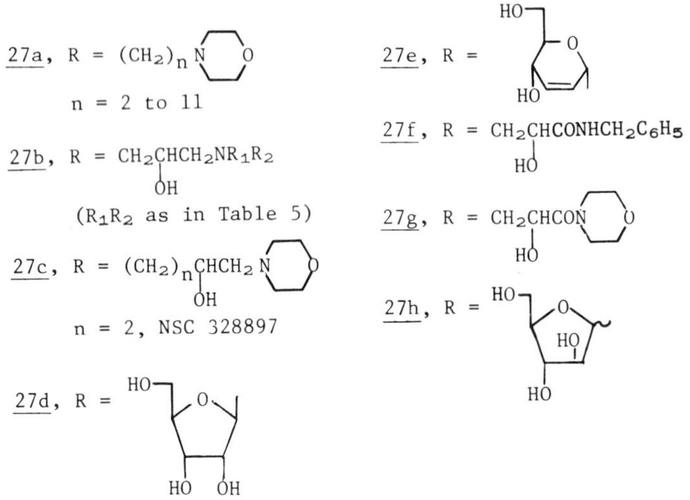

27a, R = $(CH_2)_n$N O (morpholino)
n = 2 to 11

27b, R = $CH_2CH(OH)CH_2NR_1R_2$
(R_1R_2 as in Table 5)

27c, R = $(CH_2)_nCH(OH)CH_2$N O (morpholino)
n = 2, NSC 328897

27d, R = (HO–CH₂ furanose ring with O, HO, OH)

27e, R = (HO–CH₂ dihydropyran ring with O, HO)

27f, R = $CH_2CH(OH)CONHCH_2C_6H_5$

27g, R = $CH_2CH(OH)CO$N O (morpholino)

27h, R = (HO–CH₂ furanose ring with O, HO, HO)

piperidino or the pyrrolidino group, the same dependence on chain length was observed (see Fig. 8).

When these compounds are administered to mice iv or ip the acute toxicity or "gross" toxicity (LD_{50} for deaths in 2 days) increased with increasing *n* (Adams *et al.*, unpublished). All had LD_{50}/2 days $\leq$ 2 μmol/g; they were more toxic than misonidazole with LD_{50}/2 days ~ 8.9 μmol/g. After oral administration, toxicity decreased as the chain length increased from $n = 2$ to $n = 5$ and thereafter increased with increasing *n*. The least toxic compound of the series, with $n = 5$, had LD_{50}/2 days ~ 7 μmol/g. The neurotoxicity as measured by lysosomal activity, paralleled the gross toxicity, and the "radiosensitizing effectiveness" peaked at $n = 4$ (Adams *et al.*, unpublished). These results prompted the synthesis and testing of more water-soluble hydroxy analogs *27c*. One of these, NSC 328897 (RSU 1047), *27c* with $n = 2$, has shown sufficient promise in *in vivo* tests to be selected for more extensive evaluation by NCI.

Smithen *et al.* (1980) have prepared and evaluated in Chinese Hamster V79-379A cells 34 2-nitroimidazoles of structure *27b*. They used the ratio, $C_c/C_{1.6}$, as an indication of the *in vitro* "therapeutic index" where C_c and $C_{1.6}$ are the concentrations of drug for a given level of chronic aerobic cytotoxicity and of sensitization effectiveness, respectively. Five of their

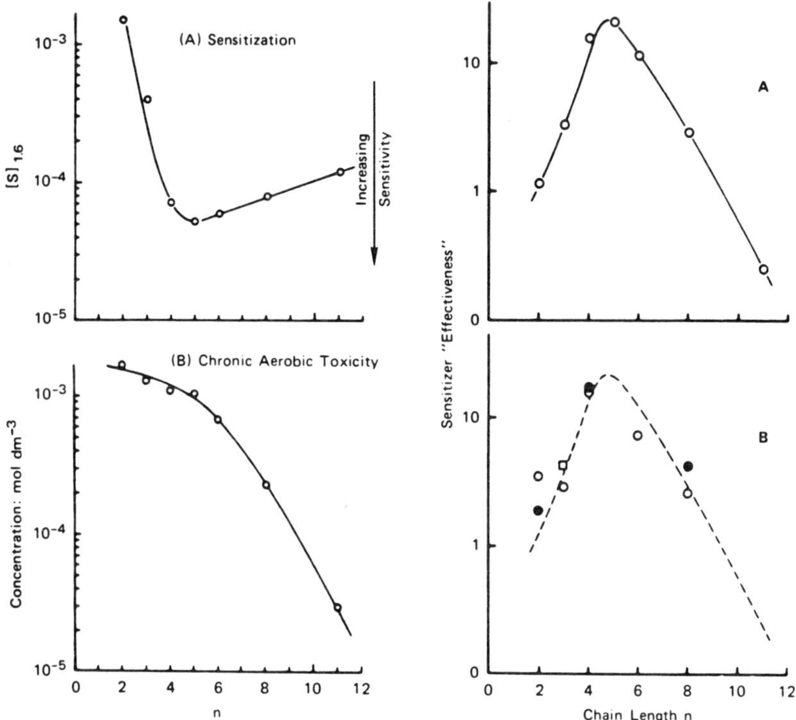

FIG. 8. Effect of chain length on sensitizing efficiency, aerobic toxicity, and sensitizer "effectiveness." (a) (A) Dependence of sensitizing efficiency, $S_{1.6}$; and (B) chronic aerobic toxicity on the length of the N1 side chain when the terminal group is a morpholine group. (b) Sensitizer "effectiveness" as a function of chain length for (A) the morpholine series of compounds; (B) ○, piperidine series; ●, pyrrolidine series; □, misonidazole. From Adams *et al.* (1980). Reprinted with permission of the publisher.

compounds (see Table V) are currently being evaluated *in vivo*. Of these, the most promising is considered to be the piperidinyl compound (Ro3-8799) (Williams *et al.*, 1981).

With the objective of finding analogs with better water solubility, improved transport properties, and less CNS toxicity, Sakaguchi *et al.* (1980) prepared nucleosides of 2-nitroimidazole from 1-β-D-glucopyranose, 1-β-D-5-thioglucopyranose, sialic acid, and 1-β-D-ribofuranose (*27d*). Of these, only *27d* was found to be cytotoxic to Chinese hamster cells (V-79). More recently Sakaguchi *et al.* (1981) have prepared additional nucleosides of 2-nitroimidazole including both the α- and β-anomers (*27h*) from arabinofuranose and *27e* and its β-anomer. Of these compounds *27e* (RA-263) was found to be the best (Agrawal *et al.*, 1981b).

TABLE V

RADIOSENSITIZING EFFECTIVENESS OF SOME 2-NITROIMIDAZOLES OF STRUCTURE *27b*

NR_1R_2 in *27b*	$C_c/C_{1.6}$[a]
3-Hydroxypiperidinyl	8.9
p-Methoxybenzylamino	5.8
Piperidinyl	5.0
Benzylamino	4.2
Morpholino	3.5
Misonidazole	3.0

[a] $C_{1.6}$ is the concentration of drug that gives an enhancement ratio of 1.6 (ER = 1.6).

Preliminary *in vivo* studies show *27e* to be an effective sensitizer (Agrawal *et al.*, 1981c).

Based on the report (Lee *et al.*, 1980) of exceptionally low toxicity of the amides of 2-nitroimidazoles, Agrawal *et al.* (1981a) have also prepared a series of 3-(2-nitro-1-imidazole)lactic acid amides such as *27f* and *27g*; they confirmed that the amides, as a class, had low toxicity. The best was amide *27g* (S-193) which was found to have about the same log *P* value (−0.49) as misonidazole (−0.37) but was 2.5 times less toxic to mice (Agrawal *et al.*, 1981a).

Posteseu *et al.* (1979) have converted metronidazole to a phosphate ester *28*. This modification increases the solubility considerably, but reduces the electron affinity only slightly (to $E_7^1 = -509$ from $E_7^1 = -489$). However, the compound may not be an effective radiosensitizer because it cannot penetrate the cell membrane and reach the hypoxic target site because of the presence of the charged phosphate group.

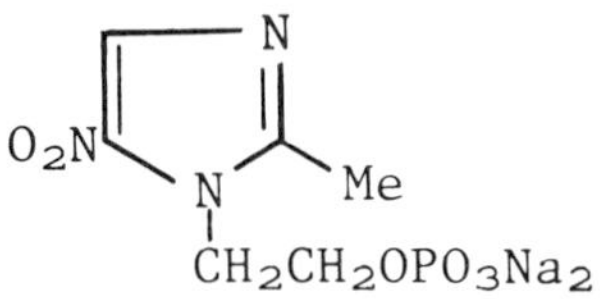

O_2N N Me N $CH_2CH_2OPO_3Na_2$

28

F. N- AND C-SUBSTITUTED NITROIMIDAZOLES

Electron-withdrawing substituents on the ring can increase the electron affinity and therefore the potential radiosensitization effectiveness. However, the effects of such substitution cannot always be predicted accurately, as discussed below. For example, Agrawal *et al.* (1977) have prepared seven nitroimidazoles with substituents ranging from electron-withdrawing to electron-releasing groups. As expected the 2,5-dinitro derivative, *29a,* was most interesting; but it was, in turn, less so than the 2,4-dinitro analog *30.* Both *29a* and *30* were formed by treatment of 1,4(5)-dinitroimidazole with ethylene oxide. In addition, major amounts of *33a* and *34a* were formed from internal displacement of the 2-nitro group by the hydroxyl group. Similarly, treatment with substituted ethylene oxides gave analogs corresponding to *29a, 30, 33,* and *34.* (Sehgal and

O_2N N N R CH_2CH_2OH

29

29a, R = NO_2
29b, R = CO_2Me
29c, R = NH_2

R' N N NO_2 R

	R	R'
30,	CH_2CH_2OH	NO_2
31,	$CH_2CH(OH)CH_2OMe$	NO_2
32,	"	COMe

O_2N N N O R

33, 4-NO_2
33a, 4-NO_2, R = H
34, 5-NO_2
34a, 5-NO_2, R = H

Agrawal, 1979; Sehgal *et al.,* 1981). Their design and synthesis of congeners was based on the feedback of *in vitro* radiosensitization results from earlier compounds. Thus 2,4(5)-dinitroimidazole initially seemed the most promising. It sensitized more effectively than misonidazole (Rupp *et al.,* 1978; Rockwell, 1978) and was less mutagenic (Rupp *et al.,* 1978). Compound *30* represented further improvement (Agrawal *et al.,* 1979a,b). The optimum compound in their series was *31* (less toxic than *30*) (Sehgal *et al.,* 1981).

Adams *et al.* (1980a) studied 4-nitroimidazoles of structure *35* with thioether or sulfonyl substituents at C-5. Surprisingly, some of these were found to be many times more effective as radiosensitizers in mammalian cell culture systems than would be predicted on the basis of their electron affinity. For example, *35a* NSC 38887 (E^1_7 = −490 mV) and metronidazole (E^1_7 = −486 mV) are equally electron affinic, but NSC 38887 radiosensitizes much more effectively *in vitro.* The more potent radiosensitizers had good leaving groups. One of these *35b* NSC 38087 (E^1_7 = −345 mV) gave the same level of radiosensitization *in vitro* as misonidazole at much lower concentrations (≈10^{-2}). Additional details of the *in vitro* radiosensitization by 5-substituted 4-nitroimidazoles have been reported (Adams *et al.,* 1981). Stratford *et al.* (1981a) found that *35b* was more toxic to aerobic cells than to hypoxic cells *in vitro.* Consequently it offers little therapeutic advantage over misonidazole. Moreover, little or no *in vivo* radiosensitization was observed for *35b* (Adams, unpublished; Brown, unpublished).

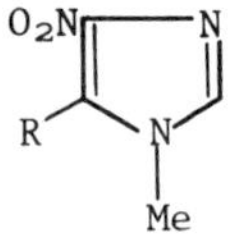

35

R = –S (2-amino-purin-6-yl)

36

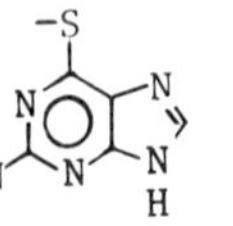

35a, NSC 38887

35b, NSC 38087

R = $SO_3C_6H_5$

35c, R = SO_2NH_2

35d, R = Cl

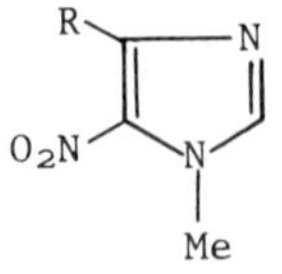

36a, R = SO_2NH_2

The 4-nitroimidazoles were compared with the corresponding 5-nitroimidazoles of structure *36* in which the R groups were R = Br, I, SO_2NH_2, $SO_2N(CH_2CH_2)_2O$, $SO_2C_6H_5$, and $SO_3C_6H_5$ (Adams *et al.*, unpublished). Even though the 5-nitroimidazoles had higher electron affinities, they were less effective radiosensitizers *in vitro* than the similarly substituted 4-nitroimidazoles. Astor *et al.* (1980) have also compared *35c* ($E_7^1 = -395$ mV) with *30a* ($E_7^1 = -336$ mV), and their results agreed with those of Adams' group. Astor *et al.* (1981) have suggested two mechanisms of action for *35c* through electron affinity and through alkylation of sulfhydryl groups.

The *in vitro* results from the nitroimidazoles containing strongly electron-withdrawing groups in the *ortho* position suggest that electron affinity may not be the only factor affecting radiosensitization efficiency. Clarke and Wardman (1980) suggested that these compounds, like Teicher and Sartorelli's (1980) nitrobenzyl halides, may represent new types of radiation-induced alkylating agents. They postulated that within the hypoxic cells, the nitro groups of the benzyl halide compounds can be reduced, thereby enhancing the release of the leaving groups and providing an alkylating agent at the hypoxic tumor site. Clarke and Wardman (1980) have shown that *35d* (CMNI) gave radiosensitization equal to other 4-nitroimidazoles but at 100 times lower concentration. They found that *35d* formed the expected normal radical anion ($ArNO_2^- \cdot$) on one-electron reduction. They plan further experiments to establish whether *35d* and related *ortho*-substituted nitroaromatic compounds can synergize radiosensitization through bioreductive alkylation.

Thus far, these nitroimidazoles with good leaving groups in the *ortho* position have not been extensively evaluated *in vivo* and the few that were tested have not met expectations based on *in vitro* results. Possibly these compounds may be effective sensitizers only *in vitro*. They, like NDPP, and some nitrofurans, may be too toxic and too reactive *in vivo* to traverse all the different host compartments and hence may not reach the hypoxic cell site at the required drug concentration. Therefore in designing effective radiosensitizers with two or more strong electron-withdrawing or good leaving groups, one should bear in mind the fact that one of these groups may be easily displaced by nucleophilic reagents [see March (1968) for dinitrobenzene; see Kleb (1968) for $O_2NC_6H_4SO_2NHCH_2CH_2OH$; Truce (1970) for the Smiles rearrangement; and Sehgal *et al.* (1981) for the formation of *33* and *34* by internal displacement of the NO_2 group]. Goldman and Wuest (1981) have shown that the nitro group of metronidazole, *4*, also can be displaced in nucleophilic substitutions. Displacement by nucleophilic reagents like SH, NH, and OH groups of biomolecules can prevent the potential radiosensitizer from reaching the target.

Both NCI contractors have also investigated a series of 5-R-1-Me-2-nitroimidazoles *23* with electron-withdrawing R groups designed to increase the electron affinity. Adams and co-workers (unpublished) have obtained *in vitro* sensitization data for over 20 aldehyde derivatives of structure *23*. Some examples are the oximes *37*, and the hydrazones *38*. Only the oximes *37* show higher electron affinity and greater radiosensitizing effectiveness than misonidazole. Generally *37* and *38* do not show the degree of increased radiosensitization effectiveness beyond that predicted by their electron affinity. In this respect they differ from the 4- and 5-nitro series of structures *35* and *36* described earlier.

Nine compounds of structure *23* were prepared by the team headed by Lee and Brown and found to be equal to or more effective than misonidazole as sensitizers *in vitro* (Brown *et al.*, 1981a). Although more electron affinic than misonidazole, none of the three, *39*, NSC 307220, *40*, NSC 207260, and *41*, NSC 314054, that were examined *in vivo* was as efficient a radiosensitizer as misonidazole.

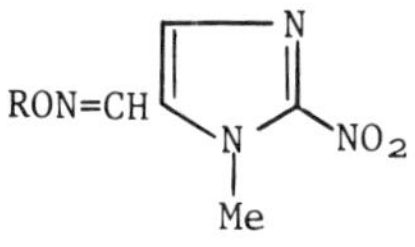

RON=CH (1-Me-2-nitroimidazol-5-yl) — 37

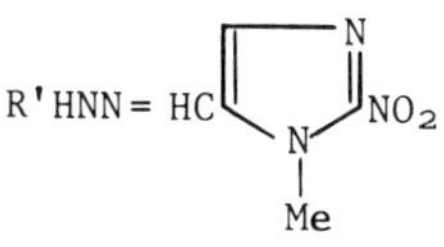

R'HNN=HC (1-Me-2-nitroimidazol-5-yl) — 38

RC(=O) (2-nitroimidazole)

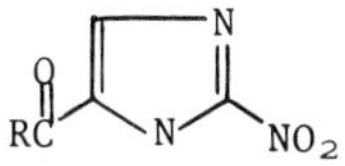

39, R = OMe

40, R = $NHCH_2CH_2OH$

41, R = $NHCH_2CH(OH)CH_2OH$

The basic question as to whether these more electron-affinic compounds will be more effective radiosensitizers *in vivo* than misonidazole remains to be answered. Perhaps, the greater electron affinity confer such high chemical reactivity to these compounds that they metabolize too rapidly or cause excessive toxicity before they can reach the site of the hypoxic tumor cells. If so, this raises other questions such as: Is there a ceiling or maximum level of electron affinity for radiosensitizers above which they are too reactive and too toxic to be effective sensitizers *in vivo*? Would this ceiling be the same for all classes of electron affinic compounds? These questions need to be investigated further.

G. Nitroimidazoles, *in Vivo* Studies

The radiosensitization of nitroimidazoles has been extensively investigated using *in vitro* methods. However, *in vivo* studies are much more limited except for misonidazole and metronidazole and a few related analogs. Rauth and Kaufman (1975) had compared two nitroimidazoles—metronidazole and tinazole *42* with some nitrofurans, and nitrobenzenes using the KHT transplantable tumor of C3H mice. In this test system the nitroimidazoles were found to be equal to each other in potency and superior to the other classes. Rauth *et al.* (1978) compared 12 2-, 4-, and 5-nitroimidazoles and found that the 2-nitroimidazoles gave the best radiosensitization. This represented the first systematic evaluation of the effects of partition coefficient and plasma concentrations on *in vivo* radiosensitization.

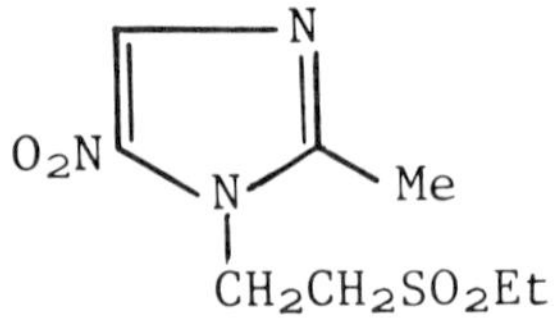

N
O_2N N Me
$CH_2CH_2SO_2Et$

42

Flockhart *et al.* (1978) have demonstrated that NSC 261036, desmethylmisonidazole *5b*, is an effective radiosensitizer *in vivo*. The *in vivo* results for *35a* and *35b* by Adams' group have already been mentioned. Pederson *et al.* (1981) recently have reported that azomycin (*27d*) is not as active *in vivo* as *in vitro*.

The inadequacy of the *in vitro* assay systems in identifying compounds of clinical promise was recognized early by the group at Stanford University and SRI. Their strategy for the design and development of novel radiosensitizers relied heavily on *in vivo* evaluation. This approach, initiated several years ago (Brown *et al.*, 1978), has been sponsored by the NCI since 1978.

The bulk of their effort was directed toward the synthesis of analogs of misonidazole with the same electron affinity but with better pharmacological properties, and decreased toxicity. Their strategy involved the design, synthesis, and evaluation of compounds of structure *24*.

The unique feature of compounds of this series is the fact that broad changes in the nature of the R group does not alter the electron affinity appreciably since the substituents are insulated from the ring nitrogen by the methylene bridge. Therefore each of these analogs should radiosensitize as effectively as misonidazole *in vitro* and also *in vivo* provided they can be delivered at the same concentration to the site of the hypoxic tumor cells. The tissue distribution of these compounds will of course depend upon their solubility and lipophilicity which in turn are determined by the nature of the R group in *24*.

A specific objective was to design and synthesize compounds more hydrophilic than misonidazole, first, to minimize possible neurotoxicity, and second, to extend the range of hydrophilicity for 2-nitroimidazoles. It should be noted that most of the 2-nitroimidazoles that had been synthesized earlier were designed to be more lipophilic than misonidazole.

Compounds of structure *24* were prepared by N-alkylation of azomycin, followed by further sidechain modifications. Over 40 such compounds were synthesized at SRI with mono- and difunctional groups to achieve a wide range of solubility, lipophilicity, and reduced toxicity (Lee *et al.*, 1980). Some representative compounds are shown in Table VI. As predicted, the half-wave reduction potentials and *in vivo* radiosensitization effectiveness of these compounds did not vary significantly. However, these compounds showed great variations in short-term toxicity, lipophilicity, and solubility. For example, analysis of these structures revealed that amine groups afforded high solubilities (when prepared as salts), but they generally were more toxic than other functional groups such as hydroxyl, acids and their derivatives, sulfoxides, sulfones, etc.

The amides *43* had high solubility and showed low acute toxicity. From an extensive structure–activity analysis of many amides prepared at SRI,

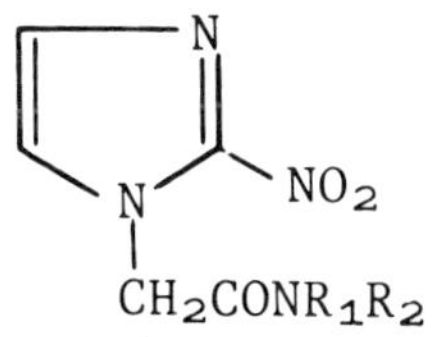

N

NO_2

N

$CH_2CONR_1R_2$

43

43a, $R_1 = H$, $R_2 = CH_2CH_2OH$

43b, $R_1 = R_2 = CH_2CH_2OH$

TABLE VI

REPRESENTATIVE 1-SUBSTITUTED 2-NITROIMIDAZOLES

(Structure 24: 1-(CH_2R)-2-nitroimidazole, N, NO_2, N, CH_2R)

24

NSC number	R	MW	Sol. (mg/ml)	Log P	$E_{1/2}$ (mV)	LD_{50} (mmole/kg)	Radiosensitization[a] In vitro $[ER_{1.6}]$ (mM)	Radiosensitization[a] In vivo (R/S)
	Alcohol and derivatives							
261037	$CH(OH)CH_2OMe$ (misonidazole)	201.2	25.7	−0.37	−350 (−389)[b]	8.7	1–3	3
292930	$CH(OH)Me$	175.7	35	−0.16		7.5		3
SR 1370	CH_2OH	157.1	>30	−0.47	(−398)[b]	1.5–2.0		
261036	$CH(OH)CH_2OH$	187.2	208	−0.89		17.4	4	2
307258	$CH_2CH(OH)CH_2OH$	201.2	>41	−0.90	−370	10–20		3
307222	$CH(OMe)CH_2OMe$	(233.3)[c]	>74.5	0.06		5.0		

307997	$CH(OAc)CH_2OMe$	243.2	>50	−0.04		5–10		
302983	$CH(OAc)CH_2OAc$	271.2	16.4	−0.07	−327	>10		3–4
331618	$CH(OH)CH_2OAc$	222.9	>46.3	−0.37			~2	
	Amines and derivatives							
307215	$CH_2NMe_2 \cdot HCl$	(256.7)[c]	>47.5	−0.97		0.3–0.6		
307219	CH_2N (ring) $O \cdot HCl$	262.7	>54.1	−0.68		2.2–4.3		
	Other							
292930	$CH(OH)CH_2F$	189.2	20	−0.36		4.5		3
307217	CH_2SOMe	203.2	>40.7	−1.27	−360	10.0		3
307218	CH_2SO_2Me	219.2	3.8	−1.11		>0.85		
SR 1371	$COCH_2OMe$	199.2	>40	−0.26		5.0		3
	Acids and esters							
302984	CO_2R, R = Et	199.2	26.4	0.33		>10.0		1–2
302986	CO_2R, R = Me	185.1	13.6	−0.14		>7.0		

[a] Radiosensitization *in vitro* is given as $[ER_{1.6}]$, the concentration (mM) required to achieve an enhancement ratio of 1.6. Radiosensitization (R/S) *in vivo* is given on an arbitrary scale of 0–4 where misonidazole is ranked at 3, and those superior to misonidazole at 4.

[b] E^1_7 from Wardman and Clarke (1976).

[c] Solvated molecule. Unsolvated MW = 215.2 for NSC 307222 and 220.7 for NSC 307215.

two compounds, *43a* NSC 301467 (SR 2508) and *43b* NSC 314055 (SR 2555), emerged as prime candidates for further studies. They were as effective as misonidazole *in vivo* and found to be less toxic. At the same time, these compounds were much more soluble. The better therapeutic index in mice of *43a* and *43b* lends hope that these compounds will be more useful clinically than misonidazole.

A comparison of the properties of *43a* and *43b* with several other amides and with misonidazole, *5a*, is given in Table VII (Brown *et al.*, 1981b).

Among 2-nitroimidazoles *43a* and *43b* seem to have the optimum range of properties for effective radiosensitization. Their log P values (-1.34 and -1.58) are sufficiently negative that they concentrate 10 times more in tumor tissue than in brain tissue. Figure 5 shows that misonidazole and other 2-nitroimidazoles, with log P equal to -0.37 (or greater), are distributed equally between tumor and brain tissues. When log P becomes even more negative than that of *43b* the compound becomes too polar to be transported from the blood to the hypoxic cells of the tumor. For example, *43f* (log $P = -1.86$) was found to be ineffective as a radiosensitizer both *in vitro* and *in vivo*. However, more extensive recent results (Brown *et al.*, 1981b) suggest that even *43b* may be too hydrophilic and less efficient as an *in vivo* sensitizer than *43a*. These results suggest that the synthesis of other analogs with log P values falling between that of *43a* and *5a* should be investigated to see at what log P the sensitizing effectiveness reaches a maximum. A possible approach is to provide more lipophilic prodrug forms of *43a* and *43b* (Coleman *et al.*, 1981).

Recent rotarod studies at Stanford University show both that *43a* and *43b* are less toxic, and can be administered at doses 5 to 7 times that of misonidazole (Brown *et al.*, 1981a,b).

Most recently Conroy and Shaw (1981) and Passalacqua *et al.* (1981) have measured hearing loss at high frequencies in mice as an indicator of neurotoxicity. They found that neurotoxicity decreases in the following order: misonidazole > desmethylmisonidazole > metronidazole > *43a* > *43b*. Because neurotoxicity, rather than short-term toxicity, is dose limiting, *43a* and *43b* may offer considerable advantages over misonidazole. The National Cancer Institute is now proceeding with preclinical toxicology studies of *43a* prior to initiating clinical trials.

In summary, improved analogs of 2-nitroimidazole radiosensitizers have been designed through a systematic evaluation of the parameters critical to achieving effective radiosensitization *in vivo*. We believe that a new generation of novel radiosensitizers that are more effective and useful clinically can be designed and developed through a similar systematic investigation of other classes of electron-affinic compounds.

TABLE VII

Comparison of Some 2-Nitroimidazole-1-acetamides

$$\text{1-}(CH_2CONR_1R_2)\text{-2-}NO_2\text{-imidazole}$$

43

Cpd	NSC number	R_1	R_2	Log *P*	R/S *in vivo*[a]	LD_{50} (mmole/kg)	Equitoxic dose LD_{50}	Equitoxic dose Rota-rod
5a	Misonidazole			−0.37	3	8.7	1	1
43c	307998	H	CH_2CH_2OMe	−0.77	3	>20		
43d	314056	H	$CH(Me)CH_2OH$	−1.02	3	>10		
43a	301467	H	CH_2CH_2OH	−1.34	3	23 ± 3	2.6	>9.3
43b	314055	$R_1 = R_2 =$	CH_2CH_2OH	−1.58	3 (iv) 2 (ip)	>34 ± 4	>3.9	>11.6
43e	328805	H	$C(CH_2OH)_3$	−1.78	1 (iv)	>10		
43f	307256	H	$CH_2CH(OH)CH_2OH$	−1.86	1–2	>20		

[a] Arbitrary scale from 0 to 4 for increasing radiosensitization (R/S). If R/S = 3, equal to *5a*; if R/S = 4, better than *5a*.

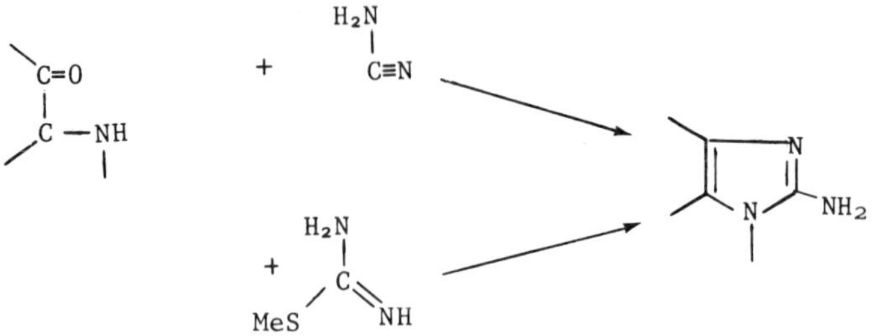

SCHEME I.

H. NITROIMIDAZOLES, SYNTHESIS

The general synthesis of imidazoles is described in a number of articles (Grimmitt, 1970, 1980; Schipper and Day, 1957; Hofman, 1953; Townsend, 1967). Mooney *et al.* (1981) recently reviewed the synthesis of nitroimidazole radiosensitizers, and only a few observations pertinent to the synthesis of specific nitroimidazoles will be presented here.

Nitration, like other electrophilic reactions, proceeds quite readily with N-substituted imidazole to provide a mixture of 4- or 5-nitro derivatives. However, 2-nitroimidazoles cannot be prepared by direct nitration but have to be synthesized from 2-aminoimidazoles by a Gatterman type reaction. The 2-aminoimidazoles are formed by cyclization of the appropriate intermediates such as those shown in Scheme I. If the 2-amino carbonyl intermediate has substituents on the carbon or the nitrogen atoms, cyclization affords substituted aminoimidazoles.

The synthetic route and the conversion of the NH_2 to the NO_2 is illustrated by the preparations of azomycin (II-5) in Scheme II, and of *23a* in

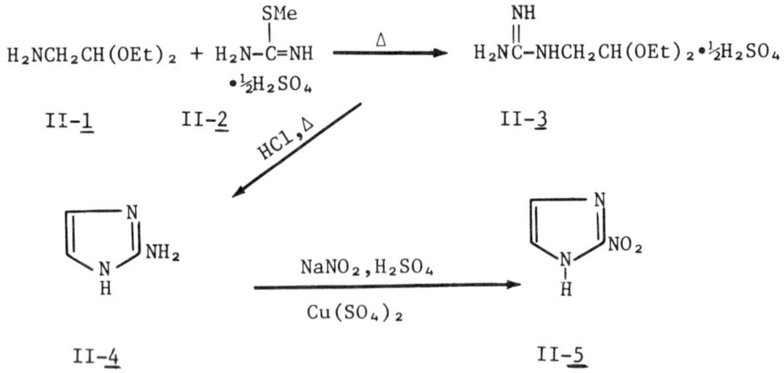

SCHEME II. From Story *et al.* (1964), Beaman *et al.* (1965), and Agrawal *et al.* (1979a) (used HBF_4).

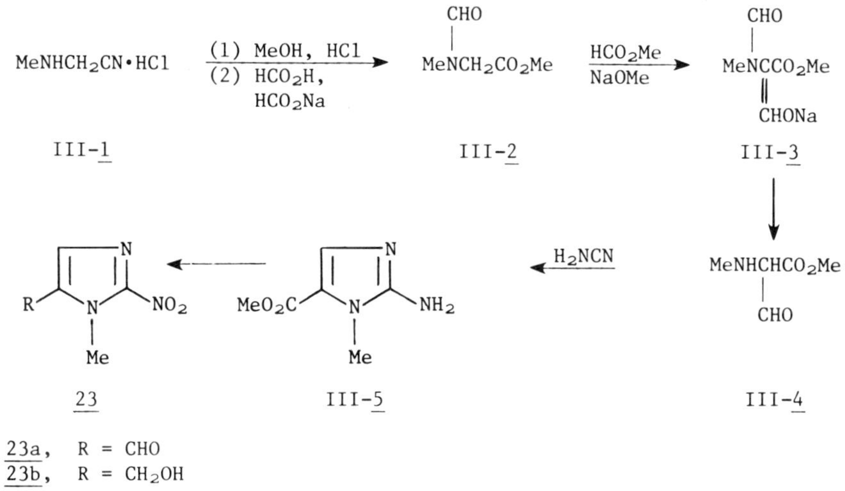

$MeNHCH_2CN \cdot HCl$ (III-1) $\xrightarrow{(1)\ MeOH,\ HCl;\ (2)\ HCO_2H,\ HCO_2Na}$ $MeN(CHO)CH_2CO_2Me$ (III-2) $\xrightarrow{HCO_2Me,\ NaOMe}$ $MeN(CHO)C(=CHONa)CO_2Me$ (III-3) $\rightarrow$ $MeNHCH(CHO)CO_2Me$ (III-4) $\xrightarrow{H_2NCN}$ III-5 (MeO_2C, NH_2, N-Me imidazole) $\rightarrow$ 23 (R, NO_2, N-Me imidazole)

23a, R = CHO
23b, R = CH_2OH

SCHEME III.

Scheme III. Azomycin and the carboxaldehyde are key intermediates to many of the 2-nitroimidazoles discussed earlier.

Because the above Gatterman type reaction gives variable yields and requires a laborious workup, several investigators (Story *et al.*, 1964; Beaman *et al.*, 1965; Agrawal *et al.*, 1979a; Lee *et al.*, 1980) have attempted various modifications of the process (Scheme II) but with limited success. The preferred route for the synthesis of *23a* which represents a combination of the routes reported by Cavalleri *et al.* (1979) and by Asato and Berkelhammer (1972) is outlined in Scheme III. This sequence gave the intermediate ester III-*5*, from which is derived all the other compounds of structure *23* discussed earlier: the alcohol *23b* by reduction, the aldehyde *23a* by oxidation of the alcohol, the hydrazones and oximes from aldehydes, and the amides by aminolysis of the ester, III-*5*.

The 4-nitro and 5-nitro-1-substituted-imidazoles IV-*2* and IV-*3* can be prepared in several ways, as shown in Scheme IV. Alkylation of a 4(5)-nitroimidazole (IV-*1*) gives the 4-nitro-1-substituted-imidazole (IV-*2*) when the sodium salt of the imidazole is utilized. If the alkylation is performed in acid, the 5-NO_2 isomer (IV-*3*) is the major product (Butler *et al.*, 1967; Kajfez *et al.*, 1968).

Nitration of a 1-substituted imidazole (IV-*4*) gives a mixture of the 4- and 5-nitro isomers, IV-*2* and IV-*3*. If the imidazole already has a 4- or 5-substituent as in IV-*6* and IV-*7*, then the nitro group will enter the adjacent position to afford compounds IV-*5* and IV-*8*, respectively. No nitration occurs at the 2-position.

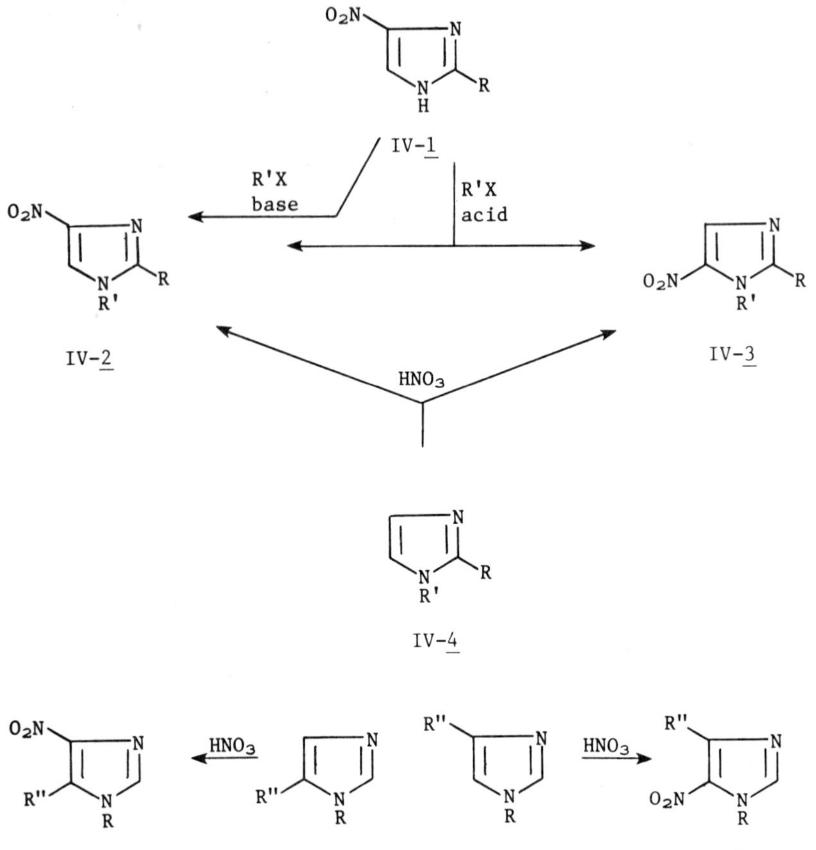

SCHEME IV.

A variety of N-1-substituted nitroimidazoles can be synthesized by reaction with suitable electrophilic reagents as shown in Scheme V.

Beaman and his colleagues (1967) have reacted azomycin with various epoxides. Sehgal and Agrawal (1979) have cyanoethylated 4(5)chloro-5(4)nitroimidazole to obtain a 1-cyanoethyl-5-chloro-4-nitroimidazole. The Michael reaction of 2-nitroimidazole with ethyl acrylate and methyl propiolate has been achieved (Lee *et al.*, unpublished). The imidazole nucleosides have been synthesized using the general methods reported in the literature (Rosseau *et al.*, 1967; Townsend, 1967). In general the reaction conditions for the synthesis of the 2-nitroimidazole nucleosides have to be mild and carefully controlled.

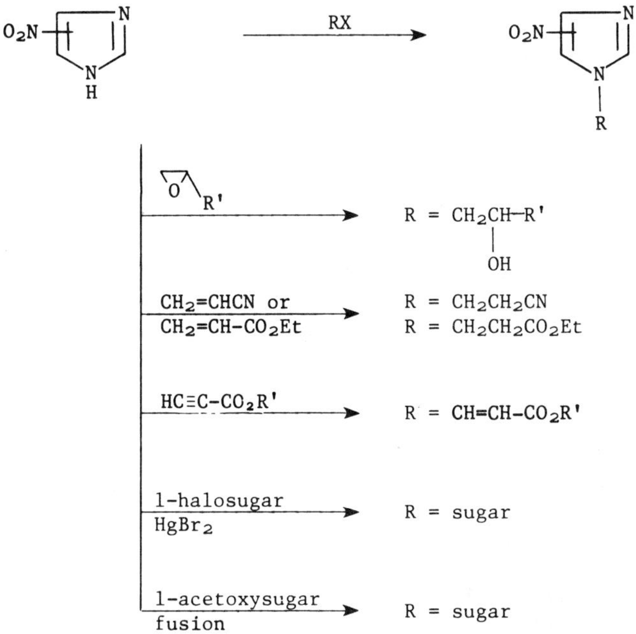

O_2N-imidazole (N-H) $\xrightarrow{RX}$ O_2N-imidazole (N-R)

Reagent	Product
epoxide (R')	R = $CH_2CH(OH)-R'$
$CH_2{=}CHCN$ or $CH_2{=}CH{-}CO_2Et$	R = CH_2CH_2CN; R = $CH_2CH_2CO_2Et$
$HC{\equiv}C{-}CO_2R'$	R = $CH{=}CH{-}CO_2R'$
1-halosugar, $HgBr_2$	R = sugar
1-acetoxysugar, fusion	R = sugar

SCHEME V.

The reactivity of imidazoles in electrophilic reactions falls between that of pyrrole and pyridine, being closer to that of pyrrole. For instance an imidazole that has one electron-withdrawing substituent can still undergo further electrophilic reactions. The following examples involving nitroimidazoles are illustrative [see Scheme VI which is mostly the work of Lancine *et al.* (1963), and Scheme VII, of Sharnin and his colleagues (1977a,b,c)].

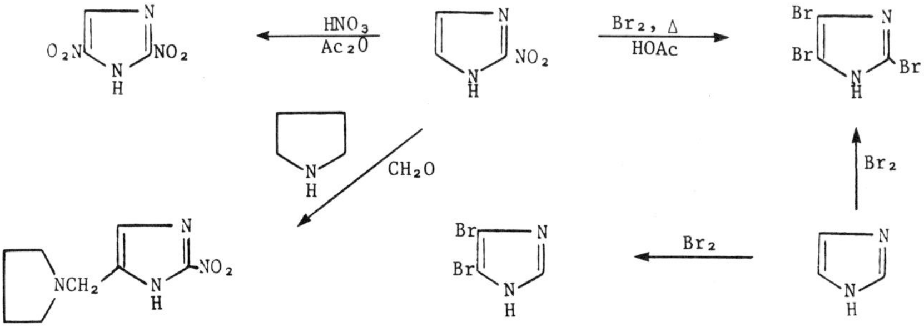

SCHEME VI.

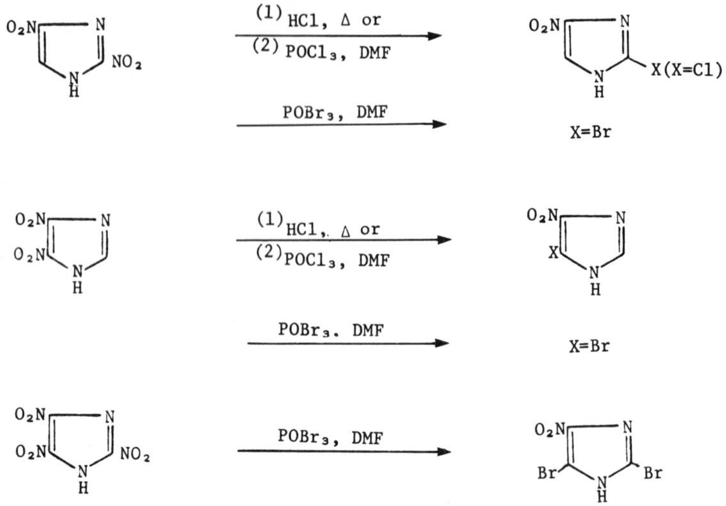

(1) HCl, Δ or (2) $POCl_3$, DMF → X (X=Cl)

$POBr_3$, DMF → X=Br

(1) HCl, Δ or (2) $POCl_3$, DMF → X

$POBr_3$, DMF → X=Br

$POBr_3$, DMF →

SCHEME VII.

Scheme VIII, from Iradyan *et al.* (1978), demonstrates the relative reactivity of a nitroimidazole versus that of a halogen-substituted benzene.

I. OTHER NITROHETEROCYCLIC COMPOUNDS

Only limited studies have been undertaken on other classes of nitroheterocyclic compounds as potential radiosensitizers. For several types of compounds redox potentials have been reported (see Table I). Utilizing these redox values one can design and synthesize derivatives with the proper electron affinities.

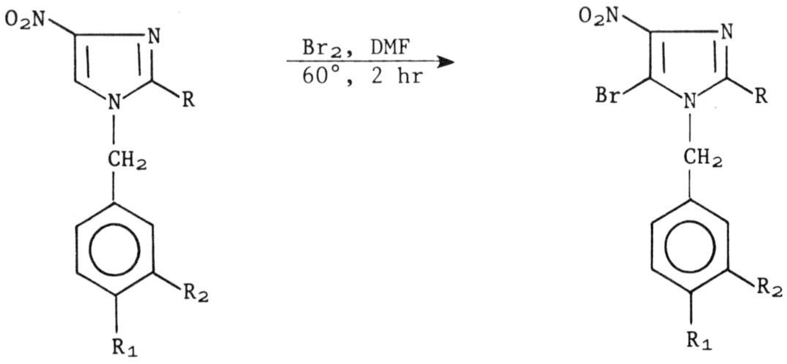

Br_2, DMF, 60°, 2 hr →

R = H, Me; R_1 = H, F, Cl, MeO; R_2 = H, Br, Cl

SCHEME VIII.

For example, it is possible to raise the $E_{1/2}$ value of nitropyrrole ($E_{1/2}$ = −0.67 V; Table II) to that of misonidazole by N-substitution and introduction of the proper electron-withdrawing substituents on the ring. Such nitropyrroles have been synthesized and studied by Raleigh *et al.* (1978). Using Chinese hamster V-79 cells for the *in vitro* assay, they showed that radiosensitizing efficiency of *44* increased with electron affinity, and that the sensitizing efficiency of *44a* approached that of oxygen. However, in *in vivo* systems, even the two best compounds of the series, *44a* and *44b* ($E_{1/2}$ = −0.35 and −0.35 V, respectively, and $E_{1/2}$ = −0.30 V for misonidazole) gave enhancement ratios (ER) of only 1.4–1.5 and 1.2–1.4 as compared to misonidazole with ER = 2.0. Based on these results, the nitropyrroles do not seem to warrant additional study.

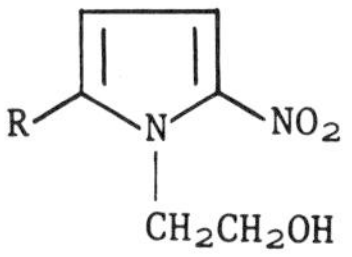

R N NO_2 CH_2CH_2OH

44

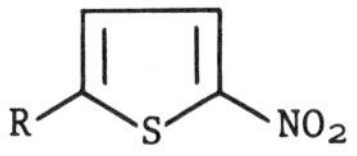

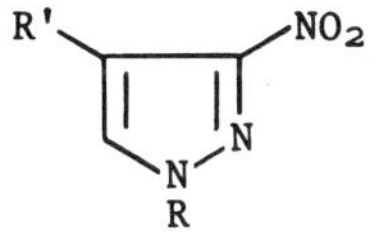

44a, R = CN
44b, R = $CONH_2$

R S NO_2

45

45a, R = H
45b, R = Br

R' NO_2 N N R

46

46a, R = R' = H
46b, R = Me, R' = CO_2H
46c, R = CH_2CH_2OH, R' = CO_2H

The 2-nitrothiophenes *45* represent another class of compounds with suitable electron affinities. For example Ruddock and Greenstock (1977) have reported that *45a, 45b,* and misonidazole have $E_{1/2}$ = −0.46, −0.30, and −0.30 V, respectively. On this basis, other derivatives with $E_{1/2}$ approximating that of misonidazole can be designed. At SRI we have prepared several 2-nitrothiophenes with electron-withdrawing groups. However, none provided a suitable combination of solubility, lipophilicity, and low acute toxicity to match the properties of the nitroimidazoles. Thus nitrothiophenes do not appear to have good prospects as radiosensitizers.

Nitropyrazoles, *46,* are another prospective class of radiosensitizers. 3-Nitropyrazole, *46a,* has $E_{1/2}$ = −0.53 V as compared to $E_{1/2}$ = −0.52 for metronidazole. Proper N- and ring-substitution should increase the electron affinity. Kimler *et al.* (1979) have examined some nitropyrazoles and a series of other heterocyclic compounds. In their *in vitro* assay using Chinese hamster lung fibroblasts (V-79), the 3-nitropyrazoles *46b* and *46c* were found to be the most active compounds [dose modification factors (DMF) of 1.8 and 1.6, respectively, as compared to misonidazole with DMF = 2.8]. Earlier Asquith *et al.* (1974) in a comparative study of misonidazole with other nitroimidazoles and three 4-nitropyrazoles, concluded that in both hypoxic bacterial and mammalian cell culture systems the nitropyrazoles were inferior to the nitroimidazoles. Thus, the nitropyrazoles do not appear to warrant further study.

Besides the above, several other nitroheterocyclic classes of compounds are available and should be considered for their radiosensitizing potential. A preliminary investigation of other classes has begun at SRI including the nitrobenzimidazoles and nitropyridines (see Table I for $E_{\frac{1}{2}}$), and nitrothiazoles and nitrotriazoles.

We found that the 2-nitrobenzimidazole, *47*, was very electron affinic ($E_{1/2} = -90$ mV vs $E_{1/2} = -350$ mV for misonidazole), but had low solubility (2.77 mg/ml). Gupta and Agrawal (1981) have investigated some 2-nitrobenzimidazoles (*48*) and other benzimidazoles with the nitro group in the aromatic ring (*49*). In addition, they also studied 5(6)-nitrobenzimidazoles, *49*, with another electron-withdrawing group at the 2-position in order to examine their effect on electron affinity and radiosensitization efficiency. In the synthesis of *48*, they isolated the cyclic by-product *50* that was formed by the internal displacement of the leaving group when X = NO_2 and SO_2Me. They also compared some nonnitrobenzimidazoles of structure *48b* to *48g* with *48a*. Their prelimi-

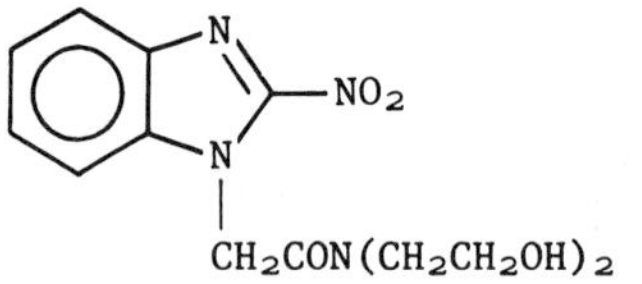

$CH_2CON(CH_2CH_2OH)_2$

47

$CH_2CH(OH)CH_2OMe$

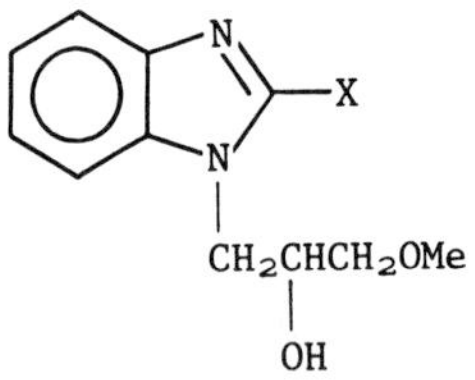

48

48a, X = NO_2 48e, X = CN
48b, X = COMe 48f, X = CF_3
48c, X = CO_2Me 48g, X = SO_2Me
48d, X = $CONH_2$

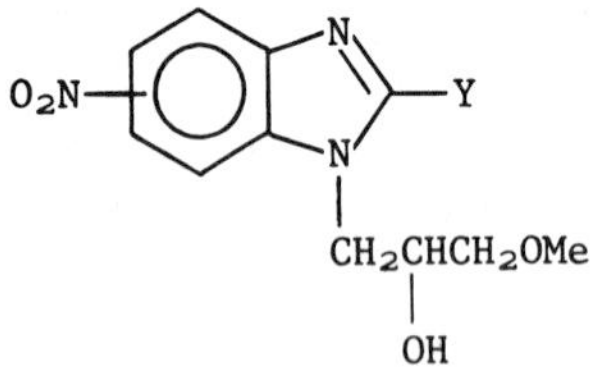

O_2N ... Y

$CH_2CH(OH)CH_2OMe$

49

OMe

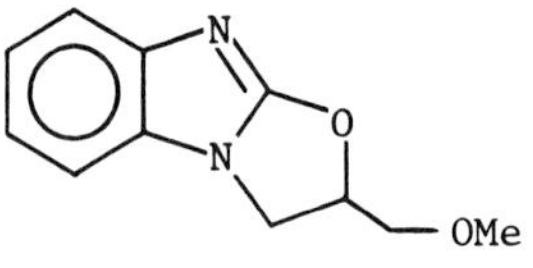

50

nary results show that only nitrobenzimidazoles produced radiosensitization. The necessity of the nitro group has been previously demonstrated in the benzene series (Chapman *et al.,* 1972a), and most recently in imidazoles and other compounds (Wardman *et al.,* 1981).

In summary, the 5- and 6-nitrobenzimidazoles have low electron affinity, comparable to that of the nitrobenzenes, as well as low water solubility and hydrophilicity. They are poor prospects as radiosensitizers. The 2-nitrobenzimidazoles, on the other hand, possess higher electron affinity than the corresponding 2-nitroimidazoles, but have much lower water solubility and hydrophilicity. Unless the 2-nitrobenzimidazoles can radiosensitize *in vivo* as efficiently as expected from their high electron affinity, their low water solubility and low hydrophilicity will limit the possibility of designing analogs that will be effective *in vivo.*

J. Other Classes of Compounds

Among the earliest compounds examined as potential radiosensitizers were glyoxal derivatives and quinones. Later studies provide additional hints of radiosensitization for these compounds. However, compounds with the optimal combination of properties have not yet been designed. Thus, Astudillo *et al.* (1974) and Cabildo *et al.* (1976) have evaluated some benzoquinones, naphthoquinones, and anthraquinone *in vitro,* and diphenylquinone, both *in vivo* and *in vitro.* Astudillo *et al.* (1974) also investigated some arylglyoxals and reported that these showed radiosensitization in *S. cerevisiae* cell culture system. See the above authors for reference to earlier work in glyoxal and related compounds. Some of these classes are worthy of further investigation with the objective of discovering compounds with the optimum combination of electron affinity, water solubility, lipophilicity, and low toxicity.

The simple benzoquinones as a class are too reactive, too toxic, and too electron-affinic (E^1_7 = 99 mV; Neta, 1981). However, modified benzoquinones have potential as radiosensitizers provided they are designed to have substituents that appropriately reduce the electron affinity, minimize 1,4-additions, and increase water solubility.

Naphthoquinones on the other hand are less electron affinic than benzoquinones. One of the early compounds studied, menadione *15* was effective in bacteria but too toxic and insoluble for mammalian radiosensitization studies (Adams and Cooke, 1969). Again, naphthoquinones with electron-releasing groups and solubilizing groups and naphthoquinone imides may be worth considering.

Anthraquinones such as *16a* (E^1_7 = −375 mV) have electron affinity similar to that of misonidazole (E^1_7 = −389 mV). Hence anthraquinones with solubilizing groups are worthy of investigation. For example, dihydroxyanthracenedione dihydrochloride, *51* NSC 301739, now in clinical trials as a chemotherapeutic agent, and related compounds are worthy of investigation as potential radiosensitizers since they can bind to DNA and be localized close to the site of the DNA radiation damage.

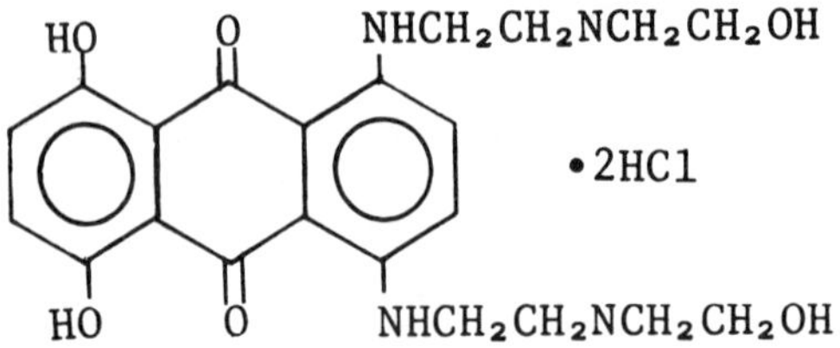

HO O $NHCH_2CH_2NCH_2CH_2OH$

•2HCl

HO O $NHCH_2CH_2NCH_2CH_2OH$

51, NSC 301739

Another class of potential radiosensitizers, the isoindole quinones, have been reported by Correa *et al.* (1980) and Infante *et al.* (1981a,b) to radiosensitize effectively *in vivo* and further development of more water-soluble analogs is anticipated. The methods of preparing these isoindole quinones by the Diels Alder route have recently reported by Myers *et al.* (1980, 1981):

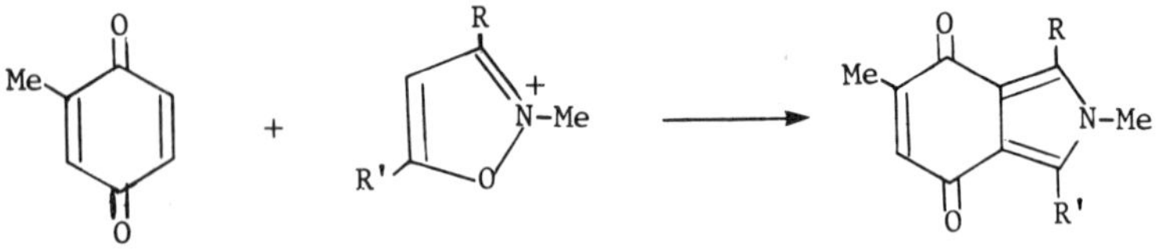

mixture of isomers
(R and R' inverted)

V. Summary and Perspectus for the Future

In summary, in this article we have integrated the concepts and research results available on the subject of electron-affinic radiosensitizers from the physicochemical, radiobiological, structure–activity, synthesis, and pharmacological points of view as they relate to the discovery of clinically useful effective agents. We now have a better understanding of the relationship between molecular structure and radiosensitization effectiveness, thus providing the basis for the rational design and synthesis of novel radiosensitizers.

For example in the nitroimidazole class, systematic study of the critical structure–activity/toxicity parameters that underlie radiosensitizing effectiveness has enabled us to design and develop compounds like NSC 301467 with clinical potential.

The strategy, as extensively discussed in this article, involves the optimization through synthesis of a limited number of specific 2-nitroimidazoles, taking into consideration the Hammett sigma values of the substituents and measurement of their redox potentials.

In this design logic, other relevant parameters like lipophilicity, aqueous solubility, and toxicity were also considered to be critical. Thus, compounds with optimum balance of these properties to achieve maximum therapeutic effectiveness were arrived at.

We believe that this strategy can be applied to other classes of compounds. The nitroimidazoles have been fully exploited, and future efforts should be directed to other areas, using the principles and approaches we have learned from the systematic study of the nitroimidazoles.

Some other classes of nitro compounds appear to have low potential as a source for the development of clinically useful radiosensitizers. These include nitrobenzenes, nitrofurans, nitrothiophenes, nitropyrroles, and nitrobenzimidazoles.

Other nitroheterocyclic classes that may have potential but have not been sufficiently explored include nitropyridines, nitro-*s*-triazoles, nitrothiazoles, nitrothiadiazoles, and probably many others. We believe that the electron affinity, aqueous solubility, and lipophilicity can be modified to achieve a suitable balance in these classes of compounds.

The greater challenge is the design and development of compounds without the nitro group as electron-affinic radiosensitizers. For example, members of the following classes hold promise and are worthy of systematic structure–activity relationship (SAR) study: (1) compounds containing other electron-withdrawing groups (e.g., SO_2NH_2, $-SO_2R$, $-CN$, $N \rightarrow O$, $-O_2CCF_3$) that by virtue of the presence of these additional groups become sufficiently reducible; (2) quinones: both aromatic (such as benzoquinones and naphthoquinones) and heteroaromatic (such as isoindoloquinones, quinoxaline-5,8-diones, etc.) with proper substituents; and (3) 1,2-dicarbonyl compounds (such as glyoxals and pyruvates) with proper substituents.

In exploring these new areas we believe it is essential to establish effective teamwork between chemists and radiobiologists with rapid feedback of developing data. Such a participatory approach will enable the research team to address the questions that are fundamental for the design and development of novel electron-affinic radiosensitizers with clinical potential.

1. Is there a ceiling or maximum level of electron affinity for radiosensitizers above which they are too reactive and too toxic to be effective sensitizers *in vivo?*
2. Would this ceiling be the same for all classes of electron-affinic compounds?

We close with one final question. Are there classes of compounds, acting by mechanisms different from those of the electron-affinic radiosensitizers, that can be developed and exploited as clinically effective radiosensitizers?

References

Adams, G. E. (1977). *In* "Cancer" 6 (F. F. Becker, ed.), Vol. 6, p. 181. Plenum, New York.

Adams, G. E. (1979). *In* "Radiosensitizers of Hypoxic Cells" (A. Breccia, C. Rimondi, and G. E. Adams, eds.), p. 13. Elsevier/North Holland, Amsterdam.

Adams, G. E. (1981). *Cancer* **48,** 696.

Adams, G. E., and Cooke, M. S. (1969). *Int. J. Radiat. Biol.* **15,** 457.

Adams, G. E., and Dewey, D. L. (1963). *Biochem. Biophys. Res. Commun.* **12,** 473.

Adams, G. E., and Jameson, D. G. (1980). *Radiat. Environ. Biophys.* **17,** 95.

Adams, G. E., Asquith, J. C., Dewey, D. I., Foster, J. I., Michael, B. D., and Willson, R. E. (1971). *Int. J. Radiat. Biol.* **19,** 575.

Adams, G. E., Asquith, J. C., Watts, M. E., and Smithen, C. E. (1972). *Nature (London) New Biol.* **239,** 23.

Adams, G. E., Flockhart, I. R., Smithen, C. E., Stratford, I. J., Wardman, P., and Watts, M. E. (1976). *Radiat. Res.* **67,** 9.

Adams, G. E., Clarke, E. D., Gray, P., Jacobs, R. S., Stratford, I. J., Wardman, P., Watts, M. E., Parrick, J., Wallace, R. G., and Smithen, C. E. (1979a). *Int. J. Radiat. Biol.* **35,** 151.

Adams, G. E., Clarke, E. D., Flockhart, I. R., Jacobs, R. S., Sehmi, D. S., Stratford, I. J., Wardman, P., Watts, M. E., Parrick, J., Wallace, R. G., and Smithen, C. E. (1979b). *Int. J. Radiat. Biol.* **35,** 133.

Adams, G. E., Ahmed, I., Fielden, E. M., O'Neill, P., and Stratford, I. J. (1980a). *Cancer Clin. Trials* **3,** 37.

Adams, G. E., Stratford, I. J., Wallace, R. G., Wardman, P., and Watts, M. E. (1980b). *J. Natl. Cancer Inst.* **64,** 555.

Adams, G. E., Fielden, E. M., Hardy, C., Millar, B. C., Straford, I. J., and Williamson, C. (1981). *Int. J. Radiat. Biol.* **40,** 153.

Agrawal, K. C., Bears, K. B., and Sehgal, R. K. (1977). *Natl. Meet. Am. Chem. Soc. 173rd 1977, Washington, D.C.* (Abstr. Medi-70).

Agrawal, K. C., Bears, K. B., Sehgal, R. K., Brown, J. N., Rist, P. E., and Rupp, W. D. (1979a). *J. Med. Chem.* **22,** 583.

Agrawal, K. C., Millar, B. C., and Neta, P. (1979b). *Radiat. Res.* **78,** 532.

Agrawal, K. C., Webb, M. W., and Sehgal, R. K. (1980). *AACR Abstr.* 304.

Agrawal, K. C., Gupta, R. P., Sakaguchi, M., Larroquette, C. A., Casey, M. A., and Yates, R. D. (1981a). *Annu. Meet. Radiat. Res. Soc., 29th 1981, Minneapolis* (Abstr. Be-8).

Agrawal, K. C., Larroquette, C. A., and Sakaguchi, M. (1981b). *Int. Cong. Pharmacol. IUPHAR 8th 1981, Tokyo* (Abstr.)

Agrawal, K. C., Sakaguchi, M., and Rockwell, S. (1981c). *Conf. Chem. Mod.: Radiat. Cytotoxic Drugs 1981 Key Biscayne* (Abstr. 54).

Alper, T. (1979). "Cellular Radiobiology." Cambridge Univ. Press, Cambridge.
Anderson, R. F., and Patel, K. B. (1979). *Br. J. Cancer* **39,** 705.
Anderson, R. F., Patel, K. B., and Sehmi, D. S. (1981). *Radiat. Res.* **85,** 496.
Asato, G., and Berkelhammer, G. (1972). *J. Med. Chem.* **15,** 1086.
Ashwood-Smith, M. J., Robinson, D. M., Barnes, J. H., and Bridges, B. A. (1967). *Nature (London)* **216,** 137.
Astor, M. B., Hall, E. J., Alonso, B. P., and Abrams, S. A. (1980). *Annu. Meeting Radiat. Res. Soc. 28th, New Orleans, 1980* (Abstr. Gc-2).
Astor, M., Hall, E. J., Martin, J., *et al.* (1981). *Conf. Chem. Modification: Radiat. Cytotoxic Drugs Key Biscayne, 1981* (Abstr. 121).
Astudillo, M. D., Sanz, F., Alvarez, M. V., and Partida, P. G. (1974). *In* "Advances in Chemical Radiosensitization," p. 77. Internat. Atomic Energy Agency, Vienna.
Asquith, C., Watts, M. E., Patel, K., Smithen, C. E., and Adams, G. E. (1974). *Radiat. Res.* **60,** 108.
Bagshaw, M. A., Doggett, R. L., Smith, K. C., *et al.* (1967). *Am. J. Roentgenol.* **99,** 886.
Beaman, G. A., Tautz, W., Gabriel, T., and Duschinsky, R. (1965). *J. Am. Chem. Soc.* **87,** 389.
Beaman, A. G., Tautz, W., and Duschinsky, R. (1967). *Antimicrobial Agents Chemother.* 520.
Biaglow, J. E., Greenstock, C. L., and Durand, R. E. (1978). *Br. J. Cancer* **37,** Suppl. III, 145.
Bradley, W. G., Karlsson, J. J., and Rassol, C. G. (1977). *Br. Med. J.* **2,** 610.
Breccia, A., Berrilli, C., and Roffia, S. (1979). *Int. J. Radiat. Biol.* **36,** 85.
Brown, J. M. (1977). *Radiat. Res.* **72,** 469.
Brown, J. M. (1979). *Br. J. Radiat.* **52,** 650.
Brown, J. M., and Lee, W. W. (1980). *In* "Radiation Sensitizers: Their Use in the Clinical Management of Cancer" (L. W. Brady, ed.), p. 7. Masson, New York.
Brown, J. M., and Workman, P. (1980). *Radiat. Res.* **82,** 171.
Brown, J. M., and Yu, N. Y. (1980). *Br. J. Radiol.* **53,** 915.
Brown, J. M., Yu, N. Y., Cory, M. J., Bicknell, R. B., and Taylor, D. L. (1978). *Br. J. Cancer* **37,** Suppl. III, 206.
Brown, D. M., Yu, N. Y., Brown, J. M., and Lee, W. W. (1981a). *Conf. Chem. Modification: Radiat. Cytotoxic Drugs Key Biscayne, 1981* (Abstr. 115).
Brown, J. M., Yu, N. Y., Brown, D. M., and Lee, W. W. (1981b). *Int. Rad. Oncol. Biol. Phys.* **7,** 695.
Bush, R. S., Jenkin, R. D. T., Allt, W. E. C., Beale, F. A., Bean, H., Dembo, A. J., and Pringle, J. F. (1978). *Br. J. Cancer* **37,** Suppl III, 302.
Butler, K., Howes, H. L., Lynch, J. E., and Pirie, D. K. (1967). *J. Med. Chem.* **10,** 891.
Cabildo, M. P., Smeyers, Y. G., Astudillo, M. D., and Alvarez, M. V. (1976). *Anal. Quimica* **72,** 517.
Cavalleri, B., Ballotta, R., and Lancini, G. C. (1979). *J. Heterocycl. Chem.* **9,** 979.
Chapman, J. D. (1979). *New Engl. J. Med.* **301,** 1429.
Chapman, J. D., and Gillespie, C. J. (1981). *Adv. Radiat. Biol.* **9,** 143.
Chapman, J. D., Webb, R. G., and Borsa, J. (1971). *Int. J. Radiat. Biol.* **19,** 561.
Chapman, J. D., Raleigh, J. A., Borsa, J., Webb, R. G., and Whitehouse, R. (1972a). *Int. J. Radiat. Biol.* **21,** 475.
Chapman, J. D., Reuvers, A. P., Borsa, J., Petkau, A., and McCalla, D. R. (1972b). *Cancer Res.* **32,** 2616.
Chapman, J. S., Reuvers, A. P., and Borsa, J. (1973). *Br. J. Radiol.* **26,** 623.
Chapman, J. D., Reuvers, A. P., Borsa, J., Henderson, J. S., and Migliore, R. D. (1974). *Cancer Chemother. Rep. Part 1* **58,** 559.

Chessin, H., McLaughlin, T., Mroczkowski, Z., Rupp, W. D., and Low, K. B. (1978). *Radiat. Res.* **75,** 424.

Chin, J. B., Sheinin, D. M. K., and Rauth, A. M. (1978). *Mut. Res.* **58,** 1.

Clarke, C., Dawson, K. B., Sheldon, P. W., *et al.* (1980). *In* "Radiosensitizers. Their Use in the Clinical Management of Cancer" (L. W. Brady, ed.), p. 245. Masson, New York.

Clarke, E. D., and Wardman, P. (1980). *Int. J. Radiat. Biol.* **37,** 463.

Clement, J. J., Gorman, M. S., Wodinsky, I., Catane, R., and Johnson, P. K. (1980). *Cancer Res.* **40,** 4165.

Coleman, C. N., Brown, J. M., and Lee, W. W. (1981). *Conf. Chem. Modification: Radiat. Cytotoxic Drugs Key Biscayne, 1981* (Abstr. 117).

Conroy, P. J., and Shaw, A. B. (1981). *Annu. Meeting Am. Assoc. Cancer Res. 72nd Washington, D.C.* (Abstr. 951).

Conroy, P. J., Von Burg, R., Passalacqua, W., Penney, D. P., and Sutherland, R. M. (1979). *Int. J. Radiat. Oncol. Biol. Phys.* **5,** 983.

Correa, J., Infante, G. A., Santos, A., Gonzalez, P., Alvarez, R., Myers, J., and Moore, L. D. (1980). *Annu. Meeting Radiat. Res. Soc. 28th, New Orleans, 1980* (Abstr. B-8).

Denekamp, J., Michael, B. D., and Harris, S. R. (1974). *Radiat. Res.* **60,** 119.

Denekamp, J., Fowler, J. F., and Dische, S. (1977). *Int. J. Radiat. Oncol. Biol. Phys.* **2,** 1227.

Dewar, M. J. S., Hashmall, J. A., and Trinajstic, N. (1970). *J. Am. Chem. Soc.* **92,** 5555.

Dische, S. (1978). *Int. J. Radiat. Oncol. Biol. Phys.* **4,** 157.

Dische, S., Saunders, M. I., Anderson, P., Urtasun, R. C., Karcher, J. H., Kogelnik, H. D., Bleehen, N., Phillips, T. L., and Wasserman, T. H. (1978). *Br. J. Radiol.* **51,** 1023.

Division of Cancer Treatment, National Cancer Institute, (1978). Treatment Linear Array, Radiosensitizers, February 1978.

Division of Cancer Treatment (1980). Proceedings of a Conference on Neurotoxicity of Hypoxic Cell Radiosensitizers at Bethesda, Maryland, March 26, 1980.

Donelli, M. G., Broggini, M., Colombo, T., and Garattini, S. (1977). *Eur. J. Drug Metabol. Pharmacokin.* 63.

Durand, R. E., and Olive, P. L. (1981). *Adv. Radiat. Biol.* **9,** 75.

Flockhart, I. R., Sheldon, P. W., Stratford, I. J., and Watts, M. E. (1978). *Int. J. Radiat.* **34,** 91.

Fowler, J. F. (1980). *In* "Cancer Research" (R. E. Myen and H. R. Withers, ed.), p. 533. Raven, New York.

Fowler, J. F., and Denekamp, J. (1979). *Pharmac. Ther.* **I,** 413.

Fowler, J. F., Adams, G. E., and Denekamp, J. (1976). *Cancer Treat. Rev.* **3,** 227.

Fu, K. K., Phillips, T. L., Rayner, P. A., and Ross, G. Y. (1981). *Annu. Meeting Radiat. Res. Soc. 29th, Minneapolis, 1981* (Abstr. Ff-9).

Fujita, T., Iwasa, J., and Hansch, C. (1964). *J. Am. Chem. Soc.* **86,** 5175.

Goldin, A., Wodinsky, I., Merker, P. C., and Venditti, J. M. (1978). *Int. J. Radiat. Oncol. Biol. Phys.* **4,** 25.

Goldman, P. (1980). *Johns Hopkins Med. J.* **147,** 1.

Goldman, P., and Wuest, J. D. (1981). *J. Am. Chem. Soc.* **103,** 6224.

Greenstock, C. L., Chapman, J. D., Raleigh, J. A., Sherman, E., and Reuvers, A. P. (1974). *Radiat. Res.* **59,** 556.

Greenstock, C. L., Ruddock, G. W., and Neta, P. (1976). *Radiat. Res.* **66,** 472.

Griffin, J. W., Price, D. L., Kuethe, D. O., and Goldberg, A. M. (1979). *Neurotoxicology* **1,** 653.

Grimmitt, M. R. (1970). *Adv. Heterocyclic Chem.* **12,** 104.

Grimmitt, M. R. (1980). *Adv. Heterocyclic Chem.* **27,** 242.

Hall, E. J., Miller, R., Astor, M., and Rini, F. (1978). *Br. J. Cancer* **37,** Suppl. III, 120.
Hansch, C., and Leo, A. (1979). "Substituent Constants for Correlation Analysis in Chemistry and Biology." Wiley, New York.
Hofmann, K. (1953). *In* "The Chemistry of Heterocyclic Compounds" (A. Weissberg, ed.). Interscience, New York.
Infante, G. A., Correa, J. N., Gusman, P., *et al.* (1981a). *Annu. Meeting Radiat. Res. Soc. 24th Minneapolis, 1981* (Abstr. Gc-5).
Infante, G. A., Correa, J. N., Guzman, P., *et al.* (1981b). *Conf. Chem. Modification: Radiat. Cytotoxic Drugs Key Biscayne, 1981* (Abstr. 136).
Iradyan, M. A., Iradyan, N. S., and Avetyan, Sh. A. (1979). *Chem. Abstr.* **89,** 197409.
Jaworski, J. C., Lisniewska, E., and Kalinowski, M. K. (1979). *J. Electroanal. Chem.* **105,** 329.
Jokipii, A. M. M., Myllala, E. H., and Jokipii, L. (1977). *J. Antimicrob. Chemother.* **3,** 239.
Kajfez, F., Sunjic, V., Kolbah, D., Fajdiga, T., and Oklobdzija, M. (1968). *J. Med. Chem.* **11,** 167.
Kallman, R. F., and Rockwell, S. (1977). *In* "Cancer" (F. F. Becker, ed.), Vol. 6, p. 225. Plenum, New York.
Karim, A. B. M. F. (1978). *Br. J. Cancer* **37,** Suppl. III, 299.
Kimler, B. F., Sinclair, W. K., and Elkind, M. M. (1977). *Radiat. Res.* **71,** 204.
Kimler, B. F., McDonald, T., Cheng, C. C., Podrebarac, E. G., and Mansfield, C. M. (1979). *Radiology* **133,** 515.
Kleb, K. G. (1968). *Angew. Chem. Int. Ed.* **7,** 29.
Klein, L., Presant, C. A., Vogel, C. L., Gams, R., and Johnson, R. (1981). *Conf. Chem. Modification: Radiat. Cytotoxic Drugs Key Biscayne, 1981* (Abstr. 68).
Lancini, G. C., Maggi, N., and Sensi, P. (1963). *Farmaco (Pavia)* **18,** 390. *Chem. Abstr.* **59,** 10032.
Law, M. P., Hirst, D. G., and Brown, J. M. (1981). *Br. J. Cancer* **44,** 208.
Lee, W. W., Martinez, A. P., Bicknell, R. B., Taylor, D. L., Cory, M. J., and Brown, J. M. (1980). *Chem. Congress N. Am. Continent, 2nd, Las Vegas, 1980* (Abstr. Medi-30).
McNally, N. J., and DeRonde, J. (1978). *Br. J. Cancer* **37,** Suppl. III, 90.
McNally, N. J., Denekamp, J., Sheldon, P. W., and Flockhart, I. R. (1978). *Br. J. Radiol.* **51,** 317.
Mahood, J. S., and Willson, R. L. (1981). *Br. J. Cancer* **43,** 35a.
March, J. (1968). *In* "Advanced Organic Chemistry: Reactions, Mechanisms, and Structure," p. 498 ff. McGraw-Hill, New York.
Martin, W. M. C., McNally, N. J., and DeRonde, J. (1981). *Br. J. Cancer* **43,** 756.
Meisel, D., and Czapski, G. (1975). *J. Phys. Chim.* **79,** 1503.
Meisel, D., and Neta, P. (1975). *J. Am. Chem. Soc.* **97,** 5198.
Michael, B. D., Harrup, H. A., Maughan, R. L., and Patel, K. B. (1978). *Br. J. Cancer.* **37,** Suppl. III, 29.
Millar, B. C., Fielden, E. M., and Smithen, C. E. (1978). *Br. J. Cancer* **37,** Suppl. III, 73.
Millar, B. C., Fielden, E. M., and Steele, J. J. (1980). *Radiat. Res.* **83,** 57.
Miller, R. C., and Hall, E. J. (1980). *In* "Radiation Sensitizers. Their Use in the Clinical Management of Cancer" (L. W. Brady, ed.), p. 146. Masson, New York.
Mitchell, J. S. (1965). *In* "Progress in Biochemistry and Pharmacology," Vol. 1, p. 335. Karger, Basel.
Mooney, H., Parrick, J., and Wallace, R. G. (1981). *Pharm. Ther.* **14,** 197.
Mulcahy, R. T., Siemann, D. W., and Sutherland, R. M. (1981). *Br. J. Cancer* **43,** 93.
Mullenger, L., Singh, B. B., Ormerod, M. G., and Dean, C. J. (1967). *Nature (London)* **216,** 372.

Myers, J. A., Moore, L. D., Whitter, W. L., *et al.* (1980). *J. Org. Chem.* **45,** 1202.
Myers, J. A., Whitter, W. L., Ahmad, M. F., Infante, G. A., Santos, A., and Correa, J. (1981). *Natl. Meeting Amer. Chem. Soc. 181st Atlanta, 1981* (Abstr. Orgn-26).
Myers, L. S., Jr., and Kay, E. (1979). *Int. J. Radiat. Oncol. Biol. Phys.* **5,** 1055.
Neta, P. (1981). *J. Chem. Educ.* **58,** 110.
Parker, L. Skarsgard, L. D., and Emmerson, P. T. (1969). *Radiat. Res.* **38,** 493.
Passalacqua, W., Reich, K., Meritt, J., and Conroy, P. G. (1981). *Annu. Meeting Radiat. Res. Soc. 29th Minneapolis, 1981* (Abstr. Be-9).
Pederson, J. E., Barron, G., and Chapman, J. D. (1981). *Conf. Chem. Modification: Radiat. Cytotoxic Drugs Key Biscayne, 1981* (Abstr. 127).
Phillips, T. L. (1977a). *Cancer* **39,** 987.
Phillips, T. L. (1977b). *In* "Cancer Research" (R. E. Meyn and H. R. Withers, eds.), p. 588. Raven, New York.
Phillips, T. L. (1981). *Seminars Oncol.* **8,** 165.
Postescue, I. D., Mustia, I., Sucin, D., Comes, R., Erikson, I., Sjoberg, L., Revesz, L., and Littbrand, B. (1979). *Strahlentherapie* **155,** 358.
Radiosensitizer/ Radioprotector Working Group, DCT, NCI. (1979). Conference at Banff, Alberta, Canada, April 2, 1979.
Raleigh, J. A., Chapman, J. D., Borsa, J., Kremer, S. W., and Reuvers, A. P. (1973). *Int. J. Radiat. Biol.* **23,** 377.
Raleigh, J. A., Chapman, J. D., Reuvers, A. P., Biaglow, J. E., Durand, R. E., and Rauth, A. M. (1978). *Br. J. Cancer* **37,** Suppl. III, 6.
Rasey, J. S., and Nelson, N. J. (1980). *Br. J. Cancer* **41,** Suppl. IV, 217.
Rauth, A. M., and Kaufman, K. (1975). *Br. J. Radiol.* **48,** 209.
Rauth, A. M., Chin, J., Marchow, L., and Paciga, J. (1978). *Br. J. Cancer* **37,** Suppl. III, 202.
Rockwell, S. (1978). *Br. J. Cancer* **37,** Suppl. III, 212.
Roizin-Towle, L. A., and Hall, E. J. (1981). *Annu. Meeting Radiat. Res. Soc. 29th Minneapolis, 1981* (Abstr. Ff-6).
Ruddock, G. W., and Greenstock, G. W. (1977). *Biochim. Biophys. Acta* **496,** 197.
Sakaguchi, M., Webb, M. W., and Agrawal, K. C. (1980). *Natl. Meeting Am. Chem. Soc. 179th Houston, 1980* (Abstr. Medi-54).
Sakaguchi, M., Larroquette, C. A., and Agrawal, K. C. (1981). *Natl. Meeting Am. Chem. Soc., 181st Atlanta, 1981* (Abstr. Medi-39).
Sancier, K. M. (1980). *Radiat. Res.* **81,** 487.
Sapora, O., Fielden, E. M., and Loverock, P. S. (1977). *Radiat. Res.* **69,** 293.
Sasaki, T. (1954). *Pharm. Bull. Tokyo* **2,** 104.
Schipper, E. S., and Day, A. R. (1957). *In* "Heterocyclic Compounds" (R. C. Elderfield, ed.), Vol. 5, Chap. 4. Wiley, New York.
Sehgal, R. G., and Agrawal, K. C. (1979). *J. Heterocyclic Chem.* **16,** 871.
Sehgal, R. K., Webb, M. W., and Agrawal, K. C. (1981). *J. Med. Chem.* **24,** 601.
Sharnin, G. P., Fassakhov, R. Kh., Eneikina, T. A. (1977a). *U.S.S.R.* Pat. 565,913; *Chem. Abstr.* **87,** 184504.
Sharnin, G. P., Fassakhov, R. Kh., Eneikina, T. A., and Orlov, P. P. (1977b). *Khim. Geterotsikl. Soedin.* (5), 653; *Chem. Abstr.* **87,** 84886.
Sharnin, G. P., Fassakhov, R. Kh., and Eneikina, T. A. (1977c). *Khim. Geterotsikl. Soedin* (12), 1666; *Chem. Abstr.* **88,** 121050.
Sheldon, P. W., and Hill, S. A. (1977). *Br. J. Cancer* **35,** 797.
Sheldon, P. W., and Smith, A. M. (1975). *Br. J. Cancer* **31,** 81.
Smithen, C. E., Clarke, E. D., Dale, J. A., Jacobs, R. S., Wardman, P., Watts, M. E., and

Woodcock, M. (1980). *In* "Radiation Sensitizers. Their Use in the Clinical Management of Cancer" (L. Brady, ed.), p. 22. Masson, New York.
Soloway, A. H. (1958). *Science* **128,** 1572.
Soloway, A. H., Whitman, B., and Messer, J. R. (1960). *J. Pharmacol. Exp. Ther.* **129,** 130.
Story, B. T., Sullivan, W. W., and Moyer, C. L. (1964). *J. Org. Chem.* **29,** 3118.
Stratford, I. J., Williamson, C., and Hardy, C. (1981a). *Br. J. Cancer* **44,** 109.
Stratford, I. J., Williamson, C., Hoe, S., and Adams, G. E. (1981b). *Br. J. Radiol.* **54,** 368.
Sutherland, R. M. (1980). *Pharmacol. Ther.* **8,** 105.
Sutherland, R. M., and Franko, A. J. (1980). *Int. J. Radiat. Oncol. Biol. Phys.* **6,** 117.
Subjeck, V. R., Chao, C. F., Johnson, R. J. R., Dreschel, R. and E. Repasky (1980). *In* "Radiation Sensitizers. Their Use in the Clinical Management of Cancer" (L. W. Brady, ed.), p. 478. Masson, New York.
Swaminathan, S., and Lower, G. M., Jr. (1978). *In* "Carcinogenesis, Vol. 4: Nitrofurans" (G. T. Bryan, ed.), p. 59. Raven, New York.
Teicher, B. A., and Sartorelli, A. C. (1980). *J. Med. Chem.* **23,** 955.
Tomasik, P., and Johnson, C. D. (1976). *Adv. Heterocyclic Chem.* **20,** 1.
Townsend, L. B. (1967). *Chem. Rev.* **67,** 533.
Truce, W. E., *et al.* (1970). *Org. React.* **18,** 99.
Twentyman, P. R. (1981). *Br. J. Cancer* **43,** 745.
Walker, M. D., Strike, T. A., and BTSG. (1980). *Cancer Clin. Trials* **3,** 105.
Wardman, P. (1977). *Current Topics Radiat. Res. Quart.* **11,** 347.
Wardman, P. (1979). *In* "Radiosensitizer of Hypoxic Cells" (A. Breccia, C. Rimondi, and G. E. Adams, eds.), p. 91. Elsevier/North Holland, Amsterdam.
Wardman, P., and Clarke, E. D. (1976). *J. Chem. Soc. Trans. Faraday Soc. I* **72,** 1377.
Wardman, P., Clarke, E. D., Jacobs, R. S., Minchinton, A., Stratford, M. R. L., Watts, M. E., Woodcock, M., Moazzan, M., Parrick, J., Wallace, R. G., and Smithen, C. E. (1980). *In* "Radiation Sensitizers. Their Use in the Clinical Management of Cancer" (L. W. Brady, ed.), p. 83. Masson, New York.
Wardman, P., Anderson, R. F., Parrick, J., *et al.* (1981). *Conf. Chem. Modification: Radiat. Cytotoxic Drugs Key Biscayne, 1981* (Abstr. 48).
Wasserman, T. H., Phillips, T. L., Johnson, R. J., *et al.* (1979). *Int. J. Radiat. Oncol. Biol. Phys.* **5,** 775.
Wasserman, T. M., Stetz, J., and Phillips, T. L. (1981). *Cancer* **47,** 2382.
Watts, M. E. (1977). *Int. J. Radiat. Biol.* **31,** 237.
White, R. A. S., Workman, R., and Brown, J. M. (1980). *Radiat. Res.* **84,** 542.
Williams, M. V., Denekamp, J., Minchinton, A. L., and Stratford, M. R. L. (1981). *Conf. Chem. Modification: Radiat. Cytotoxic Drugs Key Biscayne, 1981* (Abstr. 43).
Wong, T. W., and Whitmore, G. F. (1977). *Radiat. Res.* **71,** 132.

ADVANCES IN PHARMACOLOGY AND CHEMOTHERAPY, VOL. 19

The Effects of Antineoplastic Therapy on Growth and Development in Children

UDO BODE* AND ALLEN OLIFF†

* *Universitaetskinderklinik*
Bonn, Federal Republic of Germany
and
† *Laboratory of Tumor Virus Genetics*
National Cancer Institute
Bethesda, Maryland

I. Introduction . . . 207
II. Antineoplastic Therapy . . . 209
 A. Surgery . . . 209
 B. Radiotherapy . . . 209
 C. Chemotherapy . . . 212
III. Central Nervous System Toxicity . . . 215
 A. Radiotherapy . . . 215
 B. Chemotherapy . . . 218
 C. Combined Modality Treatment . . . 225
IV. Endocrine Organ Toxicity . . . 229
 A. Hypothalamic–Pituitary . . . 229
 B. Thyroid–Parathyroid . . . 232
 C. Gonadal . . . 233
V. Skeletal Growth . . . 236
VI. Psychosocial Development . . . 237
VII. Concluding Remarks . . . 239
 References . . . 239

I. Introduction

In the last 20 years a dramatic change in the prospects for long-term survival of patients with a number of malignancies has occurred. Improved surgical techniques, supportive care strategies, and the introduction of megavoltage radiotherapy have each contributed greatly to the modern successes of antineoplastic therapy (Holland, 1981; Sutow, 1980; Altman and Schwartz, 1978). In addition the advent of combination chemotherapy has been pivotal in combating several malignancies. In the case of pediatric hematologic tumors combination chemotherapy frequently results in cure rates as high as 50% (Van Eys and Sullivan, 1980). Multimodality therapy (radiation and/or surgery plus chemotherapy) has

ISBN 0-12-032919-0

also become increasingly popular as evidence of the effectiveness of these strategies has accumulated.

The potent nature of these therapeutic modalities is evident from their success, however, only recently have we begun to appreciate that many of these forms of therapy can also have adverse long-term effects upon normal tissues. Ironically, it has been the very success of modern antineoplastic therapy in combating the growth and spread of tumor tissues which has allowed us to document the chronic side effects of these therapies upon normal tissues. These long-term adverse effects can take from months to years to manifest themselves and frequently occur only in a minority of the patients receiving a particular form of treatment. Therefore, these delayed side effects become evident only as greater numbers of cancer patients achieve long-term survival.

Late effects of antineoplastic therapy range in severity from minor abnormalities of laboratory test values to catastrophic disorders such as severe encephalopathy and death. As more patients are cured of their malignancies, it is likely that the scope of this problem will continue to enlarge. Certainly, many more patients will continue to develop the complications already described. In addition, as the present population of "cured" patients becomes older, other, as yet unidentified, late effects of therapy will undoubtedly become evident. Recent trends in antineoplastic therapy have emphasized the use of more intensive treatment protocols in order to improve the remission rates and hopefully the cure rates associated with these therapies. It is likely that these newer treatment strategies will produce even more damage to normal tissues as well as greater antineoplastic effects. It is clear that we have only begun to analyze the "tip of the iceberg" in dealing with these late effects of therapy. Therefore, it is of primary importance that we begin to identify the principal offending agent(s) producing these complications. Hopefully, effective alternative agents will then be found to replace the specific drug or treatment modality associated with these adverse effects.

This review deals with the complications of antineoplastic therapy in children, and emphasizes the effects of therapy upon normal growth and development. Pediatric populations are particularly at risk for adverse effects from therapy due to the presence of immature and developing normal tissues. Children frequently also have a better prognosis than adults with a given malignancy, and therefore are more likely to survive long enough to develop late complications. Thus the influence of these late effects upon the quality of life of the pediatric oncology patient requires careful consideration. Normal growth can be affected by direct physical damage to skeletal structures such as the surgical removal of long bones or by the radiotherapeutic destruction of growth plates. Indirect inhibition of growth and development can be produced by antineoplastic therapies aimed at the central nervous system and/or the neuroendocrine glands. Radiotherapy for tumors involving the head can cause damage to the pituitary and/or the hypothalamus with resulting endocrine insufficiency. The effect of cytotoxic therapy upon normal neuropsychological development is also of concern. Finally, normal growth and development is frequently subject to interruption by the mere diagnosis of childhood malignancy. The threat of death to a child and his family may force major changes upon the family structure and relationships. These social adjustments can totally derange the patient's social maturation.

We will attempt to detail the late effects of therapy upon the central nervous system, the hypothalamic–pituitary axis, and the endocrine organs. Where possible we will indicate which agents have been implicated as the primary cause of these adverse effects, and what steps can be taken to minimize the risk of developing these complications.

II. Antineoplastic Therapy

A. Surgery

Although surgical treatment is not the dominant form of therapy in pediatric oncology, local resections are performed in some cases of solid tumors, e.g., osteosarcoma, Ewing's sarcoma, rhabdomyosarcoma, Wilms tumor, and tumors of the central nervous system. In the case of soft tissue sarcomas the effects of surgery upon growth and development are generally limited to the anatomic distribution of the bones involved. However, limb amputations and/or disfiguring resections can have a devastating impact upon the child's psychological development. Adolescents are particularly susceptible to the emotional trauma associated with these procedures (Hersh, 1978). Surgical intervention is also a primary treatment modality for brain tumors of childhood. The major late effects associated with these procedures are dependent upon the amount of local damage incurred by the surrounding normal nervous tissues. Residual motor paralysis and/or damage to associative capacities will obviously impair the patient's normal development.

B. Radiotherapy

In order to understand the complications associated with radiotherapy, the different forms of radiation treatment and the various modes of ionizing radiation in use today must be understood. X-Ray and γ radiation are the forms of electromagnetic energy commonly used to kill tumor tissue.

These forms of energy exert their lethal biologic effect by transferring sufficient energy to some of the atoms they encounter in order to produce ions. The ion pairs (a free electron and a positively charged nucleus) generated in this fashion can interact with other atoms and ions resulting in the formation of charged free radicals within the irradiated tissues. The free radicals then interact with and alter the structure of the cell's nucleic acids by modifying bases and producing single and/or double strand breaks in the cellular DNA (Altman *et al.,* 1970, and references cited therein). Free radicals can also impair cytoplasmic functions such as oxidative phosphorylation (Alexander *et al.,* 1965; Phillips *et al.,* 1972). The effects of ionizing radiation are summarized in Fig. 1.

The overall effect of radiation upon biologic material is to impair the proliferative capacity of treated tissues. However these effects may not be immediately apparent and radiation-induced cell lysis frequently will occur several generations after irradiation. Presumably this delay is due to the persistence of nonviable cells whose static metabolic functions have remained temporarily intact despite therapy (Court-Brown *et al.,* 1965; Tolmach, 1961). Chromosomal abnormalities may also become evident during later mitosis (Little, 1968). The factors governing the effectiveness of radiotherapy and its potential for damage to normal tissues are complex, and the effects of a particular dose of radiation may vary in different tissues. The rate and effectiveness of the normal radiation damage repair mechanisms can be variable in different tissues. Similarly, the effects of radiotherapy may vary depending upon the stages (G_0,G_1,G_2,S, or M) of the cell cycle (Terasima and Tolmach, 1963; Sinclair, 1968). The degree of oxygenation of a particular tissue is also important since oxygen can have a potentiating effect upon ionizing radiation (Gray, 1961).

Each of these factors can be manipulated in order to enhance the effectiveness of a particular course of treatment. Fractionation of the total dose of radiation is done in part because many tumor tissues are poorly vascularized and therefore are poorly oxygenated (Powers and Tolmach, 1963). Fractionation allows for revascularization and thus better oxygenation of tumor tissue between treatments. Fractionation also allows the normal tissues which have suffered sublethal damage to repair themselves. While tumor cells also undergo some repair, normal tissues may have more efficient repair mechanisms and thus possess a selective advantage over malignant cells (Hanawalt *et al.,* 1978). Recently, radiosensitizers have been used to potentiate the effects of radiotherapy. These agents (e.g., BUdR, metronidazole, and actinomycin D) have shown enhanced antitumor effects in animals at a given dose of radiation (Brady, 1980). However, until now the clinical trials of these agents in conjunction with radiation have been disappointing due to increased toxicity from these

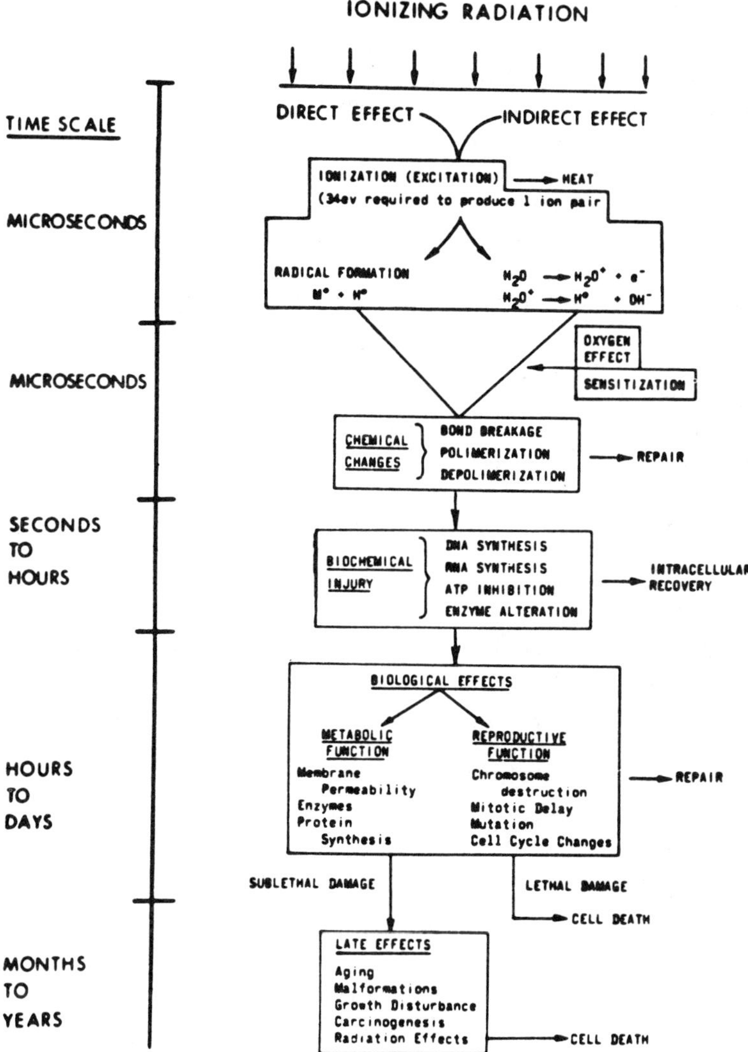

FIG. 1. Schematic representation of the instantaneous, acute, and chronic effects of ionizing radiation upon biological tissues. Adapted from Perez (1977).

regiments which parallels the enhanced antitumor effects (Adams, 1978). Similarly, hyperthermia has been shown to increase the effectiveness of radiotherapy in animal studies (Robinson and Wizenberg, 1974; Hahn, 1974) but trials in humans have not been encouraging (Brenner and Har-Kedar, 1977).

More effective radiation treatments have been made possible in recent years by the development of megavoltage radiotherapy equipment. Older orthovoltage equipment produced radiation which had its maximum effect at the skin surface and thus often produced severe damage to superficial tissues without adequately treating deep lying tumor tissue. ^{60}Co source irradiators may be suitable for deeper lesions, but the maximum ionization produced by these apparatuses occurs approximately 0.5 cm below the skin. Modern megavoltage linear accelerators produce radiation with a maximum ionization effect several centimeters below the skin and thus allow for effective treatment of deep-seated malignancies. The use of this newer equipment has resulted in much more effective therapy for a number of malignancies. In particular megavoltage radiotherapy has been useful for treating such pediatric malignancies as Ewing's sarcoma or rhabdomyosarcoma where orthovoltage radiation previously resulted in a preferential absorption of energy in bone tissue which frequently produced bone necrosis.

C. Chemotherapy

Virtually all chemotherapeutic agents interfere with the capacity of cells to proliferate. Many of these agents have been in clinical use since the 1950s (Smyth, 1976), but we are still far from understanding their basic mechanisms of action. Although a myriad of differences have been described between the metabolic functions of normal and malignant cells, few of these differences have been successfully exploited to selectively promote the death of tumor cells. Nonetheless, it is clear that some forms of chemotherapy do preferentially destroy malignant cells. The successful use of these agents is directly related to the balance struck between tumor cell kill and toxicity to normal tissues. Many chemotherapeutic agents exert their lethal effects at the level of nucleic acid metabolism (e.g., methotrexate, 6-mercaptopurine, and cytosine arabinoside) by interfering with the events required for synthesis of DNA and normal cell division. These agents are predictably toxic to the most rapidly dividing normal tissues in the body, i.e., hematopoietic and gastrointestinal tissues. Other agents have nuclear and/or cytoplasmic effects which can affect cells in different stages of the cell cycle (Fig. 2). These agents often have toxic effects upon selective normal tissues, e.g., cyclophosphamide—hemorrhagic cystitis (Anderson *et al.*, 1967), anthracyclines—cardiomyopathy (von Hoff *et al.*, 1977), and bleomycin—pulmonary fibrosis (Chabner *et al.*, 1975). The mechanisms responsible for these specific organ toxicities are not well understood. Recently, a number of agents have been described which can ameliorate the toxic effects of some of

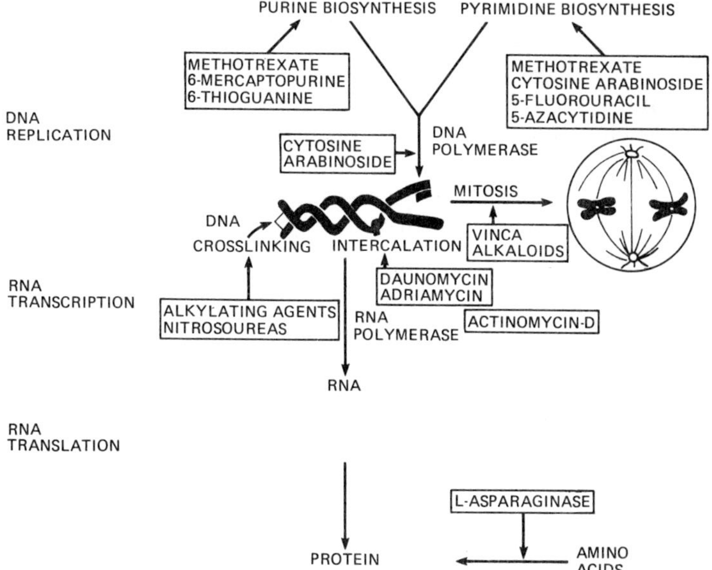

FIG. 2. Commonly used chemotherapeutic agents. Mechanism of action and corresponding phase of the cell cycle where maximum tumor cell kill occurs. Adapted from Altman and Schwartz (1978).

these agents. Cyclophosphamide-induced cystitis can be reduced in animals by the use of chemicals containing sulfhydryl groups (e.g., cysteamine) which interfere with the oxidative effects of the metabolites of cyclophosphamide (Primack, 1971). The use of tocopherol can prevent the cardiotoxicity associated with anthracycline administration in dogs (Myers *et al.*, 1976). A major issue in the use of these agents is the question of whether the reduced toxicity associated with their use will be accompanied by an equally diminished antitumor effect. In each case the effectiveness of the chemotherapy must be reevaluated in the presence of the antitoxicity agent(s). It is notable that one such agent, citrovorum factor, has been shown to effectively prevent the toxic effects of methotrexate without reducing the antitumor effects of therapy (Tattersall *et al.*, 1975). Citrovorum factor bypasses the metabolic blockade caused by methotrexate, and can be effective in rescuing normal cells up to 40 hours after the start of methotrexate therapy (Goldie *et al.*, 1972). Fortunately, many tumor cell types are not capable of being rescued from methotrexate's effects by this agent (Frei *et al.*, 1975).

The use of combination chemotherapy has become the mainstay of modern antineoplastic therapy. This reliance on multiagent chemotherapy has developed in large measure due to the success of this form of therapy in the treatment of several malignancies (e.g., acute lymphocytic leukemia and Hodgkin's disease). The use of multiple cytotoxic drugs can also present new problems for the clinician concerned with the long-term effects of cancer therapy. Carter (1975) divided the potential effects of combination chemotherapy into four categories. Multiple agents might act independently, additively, synergistically, or antagonistically. Vincristine has been reported to inhibit the egress of intracellular methotrexate, and thus may serve to potentiate methotrexate's antitumor effects (Bender *et al.*, 1975). The use of radiosensitizers represents the analogous phenomenon of multimodality treatments which may work synergistically. Actinomycin D plus radiotherapy enhance one another's effects in the treatment of Wilms tumor (D'Angio, 1969). Vinblastine and radiation have also been reported to act synergistically in the therapy of rhabdomyosarcomas in rats (Barendson and Janse, 1977). Synergistic effects such as these are thought to occur via synchronization of the tumor cell populations within a particular phase of the cell cycle. Actinomycin D can arrest cell growth in G_1 or G_2 where tumor cells are sensitive to radiation. (Elkind and Sakamdo, 1969). Radiotherapy has relatively less effect upon cells in S phase. However cells in S phase are sensitive to the effects of actinomycin D (Griem and Malkinson, 1969). Thus the use of these agents in combination results in both additive and synergistic tumor cell death. Other radiosensitizers (e.g., cyclophosphamide, nitrosoureas, and antimetabolites) are believed to exert their potentiating effect by stopping tumor cell populations in the G_2 phase of growth where they are particularly sensitive to radiation damage (Elkind and Sakamdo, 1969). Antagonistic combinations have been reported as well; the use of L-asparaginase following methotrexate apparently reduces the effectiveness of the methotrexate therapy by rescuing the tumor cells from the methotrexate (Capizzi, 1975).

Similarly, the toxicities of multiagent chemotherapy and/or multimodality therapy may be considered to fall into these four classifications. However, the mechanisms responsible for the toxic effects of these agents are not fully understood, and the recognition of this problem as it relates to the effects of therapy has only recently become widespread. Therefore little has been done with the multiagent therapies to dissect out the contribution of individual agents to the chronic complications of therapy. The residual effects of the tumor itself must also be considered in attempting to identify the cause of a particular dysfunction which arises many months or years after the completion of therapy. We and others (Peylan-Ramu *et al.*, 1978; Ochs *et al.*, 1980; Oliff *et al.*, 1979) have attempted to correlate the effects of specific forms of central nervous system prophylaxis for acute lymphocytic leukemia with the subsequent development of particular anatomic abnormalities or laboratory conditions (see below). More studies of this nature are necessary if we are to acquire the data necessary to identify the precise causes of the chronic complications associated with multiagent antineoplastic therapy.

III. Central Nervous System Toxicity

Malignancies involving the central nervous system may arise as either primary tumors of nerve cells or their supporting tissues, or they may develop as metastatic lesions from sites outside the nervous system. Primary tumors are generally treated by surgical resection when possible while metastatic disease is dealt with by chemotherapy and/or radiotherapy. In addition certain hematologic malignancies (e.g., acute lymphocytic leukemia) can also involve the central nervous system. These patients require cranial irradiation and/or intrathecal chemotherapy directed at the central nervous system (Hustu *et al.*, 1973; Willoughby, 1976). The adverse effects of surgical resection are mainly due to the local tissue damage which occurs at the time of surgery and they are generally apparent within a few weeks following resection. Radiation and/or chemotherapy on the other hand frequently produce both acute and late adverse effects upon the nervous system. The use of systemic chemotherapy directed at malignancies located outside the central nervous system can also have adverse effects upon the nervous system.

A. Radiotherapy

Nervous tissue per se is generally considered to be resistant to damage by ionizing radiation (Allen, 1978). However, the surrounding glial and vascular tissues limit the tolerance of nerve cell containing tissues to between 1400 and 1800 rets[1] depending upon the location of the irradiated structures. The incidence of persistent central nervous system toxicity after radiation in this range is approximately 5% (Allen, 1978). Acute toxicity during radiotherapy of the brain occurs to some extent in most patients, and consists of nausea, vomiting, headache, and anorexia. EEG changes and elevations of brain tissue enzymes (e.g., CPK and LDH) in the CSF can be demonstrated at this time. These signs and symptoms

[1] Rets or nominal standard dose (NSD) is a unit of biological radiation effects which can be calculated from the radiation dose in rads by dividing the dose of radiation by the product of the specific tissue fraction and the time of therapy. $NSD = RAD/(N^{0.24} \times T^{0.11})$ where N = fraction number, and T = time of radiation.

probably represent a mild form of self-limited damage (Simila *et al.*, 1977; Maas, 1977). A more serious form of acute toxicity has recently been reported shortly after the initiation of radiation therapy for meningeal leukemia. Oliff *et al.* (1978) reported a series of patients who developed a lethal encephalopathy within 3–30 hours following the initiation of radiotherapy. While the precise etiology of this syndrome was unclear, transient cerebral edema may have been responsible. Subacute toxicity frequently occurs in the form of the "somnolence syndrome" which develops from 4 to 8 weeks following cranial radiation. Additional signs consist of lethargy and irritability. Occasionally, fever and SCF pleocytosis may accompany this syndrome and create a diagnostic dilemma in distinguishing between this syndrome and meningitis or early meningeal leukemia. Up to 50% of all patients receiving cranial radiation (2400 rads) as prophylaxis for acute lymphocytic leukemia will experience some form of this syndrome (Freeman *et al.*, 1973; Hustu *et al.*, 1973). Fortunately, this disorder is self-limited and treatment is not usually required. In severe cases the administration of corticosteroids is effective in reversing these signs and symptoms. Children receiving higher doses of radiation for brain tumors develop this syndrome more frequently and routinely receive steroids in order to allow the continuation of their radiotherapy (Van Eys, 1977). The etiology of this syndrome is believed to be increased intracranial pressure secondary to the reactive edema which accompanies radionecrosis of tumor cells and the neighboring normal tissues. Studies on the nature of acute radionecrosis in animals have revealed that the major effect of radiotherapy is to damage the blood–brain barrier by causing separation of the vascular endothelial cells from one another which allows the subsequent extravasation of proteins. In addition direct cellular damage to the nervous tissue can be demonstrated by alterations in the protein and carbohydrate metabolism of these cells resulting in increased deposition of glycogen in the supporting glial cells.

Davis (1979) has described another toxic effect of radiotherapy which he terms an "early delayed" reaction. This is a rare disorder which begins abruptly about 10 weeks following radiation therapy of extracranial disease. Signs of brain stem involvement progress rapidly to death in the majority of patients. At autopsy the pathologic findings reveal extensive areas of demyelinization with reactive proliferation of glial and astrocytic elements. A perivascular lymphocytic infiltration is also present, but little evidence of neuronal damage can be found (Lampert and Davis, 1964).

Chronic radiation toxicity can occur several months to years following the course of radiotherapy. These delayed effects generally develop over many months and may present difficulties in distinguishing between the late effects of radiotherapy and the recurrence of the primary tumor (Mikhael, 1978). The signs and symptoms of this toxicity vary greatly, ranging from minimal brain dysfunction to frank dementia or encephalopathy. Bloom (1978) reported dementia in 10% of a series of patients treated with cranial radiation for medulloblastoma. An additional 10% of these patients exhibited other neurologic deficiencies. Similar results were reported by Sheline (1975). Jenkin (1969) found that 6% of their patients treated with radiotherapy (3000 to 3500 rads) for medulloblastoma developed ataxia and/or nystagmus within 5–20 years following therapy. Even higher rates of complications have been found by Bamford (1976) who reported that the majority of his long-term survivors of brain tumors had evidence of physical and/or mental handicaps with 17/30 (56%) demonstrating subnormal intelligence.

The precise contribution of the radiation therapy to the development of these abnormalities is difficult to dissect out from the damage caused by the malignancies themselves. However a number of pathologic studies have found that progressive abnormal changes can occur following cranial radiation. Parenchymal coagulation and white matter necrosis combined with ectatic growth of blood vessels and amyloid formation have been reported (Llena *et al.,* 1976; Martins *et al.,* 1977). In each of these studies the neuronal elements were relatively spared while the majority of damage was confined to the glial supporting structures. Recently, other studies have claimed that residual damage may eventually express itself in the nerve cell populations as well (Wheeler and Lett, 1974; Lett *et al.,* 1978). Parenchymal damage to the nervous tissues may occur as a secondary phenomenon due to the effects of radiotherapy upon the vascular components of the central nervous system. Radiation therapy can lead to stenosis of major vessels and premature arteriosclerosis (Hayward, 1972). These vascular changes can lead to vascular occlusions and cerebral vascular accidents years following radiotherapy (Conomy and Kellermeyer, 1975; Wright and Bresnam, 1976; Bladin and Royle, 1977; Silverberg *et al.,* 1978).

Radiation myelopathy can be a progressive complication of local radiotherapy. The onset of symptoms generally occurs within 5–30 months following therapy (Reagon, 1968; Littman, 1978; Verity, 1968). The early symptoms include numbness and paresthesias followed by weakness and paralysis. Damage to the autonomic nervous functions can occur causing bladder and bowel dysfunction. Asymmetrical changes may produce a Brown Sequard like syndrome (Locksmith, 1968; Dynes and Smedel, 1960). Pathologic examinations have revealed vascular alterations including intimal thickening and fibroid necrosis (Godwin *et al.,* 1975; Palmer, 1972; Itabashi *et al.,* 1957). Lesions of this nature can be expected in 1–5% of patients within 5 years after spinal radiation doses of 5000 rads (Phillips and Buschke, 1969; Kramer *et al.*, 1972; Rubin and Casarott, 1972). However, myelitis may occur with lower doses. The prognosis for this disorder is poor with progressive impairment, paralysis, and/or death being the general outcome, but stabilization of the deterioration has occurred in some cases (Solheim, 1971).

Radiation can produce both sensory and/or motor neuropathies. Local radiotherapy is an uncommon cause of peripheral neuropathy, but it can cause permanent damage when it does effect local nerves. Radiation damage of peripheral nerves frequently requires months to years to manifest itself, with the latency period for developing neurologic dysfunction being inversely related to the radiation dosage. Clinically significant nerve damage has been noted following radiation doses of 5,500–12,000 rads. These neuropathies are most commonly seen among the cranial nerves. Both direct damage to the nerve trunk and radiation-induced perineural fibrosis are thought to contribute to the development of this disorder (Cheng and Schultz, 1975; Berger and Bataini, 1977; Davis, 1979).

B. Chemotherapy

1. *Alkylating Agents*

Nitrogen mustard in large doses can damage the VIII cranial nerve producing signs of tinnitus and hearing loss (Lawrence *et al.*, 1961). This predilection for the VIII nerve has been documented in animal experiments where radiolabeled nitrogen mustard has been found to localize specifically to the VIII nerve (Mahaley, 1961). Animal experiments have produced seizures, cerebral dysfunction, coma, and death following intracarotid infusion (Ariel, 1961). However, since lower doses of nitrogen mustard have become widely used, only one case of severe neurotoxicity has been reported (Bethlenfalvay and Bergin, 1972). In this instance the patient developed fever, hemiplegia, and coma within 1 week of receiving intravenous mustard therapy. At autopsy this patient had no signs of tumor infiltration of his central nervous system but did exhibit areas of focal gliosis.

Chlorambucil is generally not neurotoxic. However, cases of accidental overdoses have been reported where the patient developed ataxia followed by seizures and coma (Wolfson and Olney, 1957; Green and Naiman, 1968).

Cyclophosphamide is considered not to be neurotoxic (Bland *et al.*, 1961), although early reports that it did not enter the CNS in its active form have been disproved (Skipper *et al.*, 1964). Both cyclophosphamide and its metabolites can be detected in the CSF of patients receiving the drug (Egorin *et al.,* 1981). De Fronzo *et al.* (1973) suggested that the water retention seen with cyclophosphamide administration was caused by inappropriate ADH secretion. However, newer data (Bode *et al.,* 1980a) indicate that vasopressin levels remain unchanged during cyclophosphamide therapy. The antidiuretic effect of cyclophosphamide is therefore most likely a nephrotoxic not a neurotoxic effect.

2. *Other Agents*

Procarbazine can produce four classes of CNS side effects: altered state of consciousness, ataxia, peripheral neuropathy, and effects secondary to procarbazine's monoamine oxidase inhibitory activity. Somnolence, confusion, lethargy, and stupor have occurred in patients receiving standard therapy (Brunner and Young, 1965; Stolinsky *et al.,* 1970; Samuels *et al.,* 1967; De Conti, 1971). Agitation, hallucinations, and manic psychosis have also been described (Mann and Hutchison, 1967). Ataxia, paresthesias, depressed reflexes, and muscle pains occur in 10–20% of patients. Many of these side effects including somnolence, weakness, dizziness, and paresthesias are dose dependent (Chabner *et al.,* 1973). Procarbazine readily crosses the blood–brain barrier, but it must be metabolically altered before it can act as an MAO inhibitor (Oliverio *et al.,* 1964). Its ability to inhibit enzymatic reactions accounts for its synergistic effects in conjunction with phenothiazines, barbituates, and narcotics (Sicher and Backhouse, 1965; Billmeyer and Holton, 1969; Falkson *et al.,* 1965). Similarly, orthostatic hypotension, and a "flushing syndrome" after ingestion of alcohol have been related to procarbazine's antienzymatic activities (Mathe *et al.,* 1963).

Interestingly, nitrosoureas which are effective in the treatment of brain tumors because of their lipophilic nature and their ability to penetrate into the CNS, are not neurotoxic (Vietti and Valeriole, 1976).

L-Asparaginase hydrolyzes the amino acids asparagine and glutamine to their amino acid analogs aspartic acid and glutamic acid. Since some malignant tumors lack the synthesizing enzymes necessary for the manufacture of asparagine, the depletion of this amino acid by L-asparaginase can be lethal to these tumors. However, 20 to 60% of the patients receiving this drug experience symptoms ranging from drowsiness and lethargy to disorientation and coma (Oettgen *et al.,* 1970; Moure *et al.,* 1970; Ohnuma *et al.,* 1970; Land *et al.,* 1972). Organic brain dysfunction and seizures have also been reported (Zubrod, 1970; Haskell *et al.,* 1969). Those effects are generally self-limited and subside quickly after therapy is discontinued, but at least one case of prolonged encephalopathy has been noted where this disorder persisted for several weeks after therapy (Ohnuma *et al.*, 1970).

3. *Vinca Alkaloids*

Vincristine and vinblastine are the commonly used agents from this class of drugs, and in both cases neurologic toxicity is the dose-limiting factor governing their use (Weiss *et al.*, 1974). These drugs arrest cell growth in metaphase by inhibiting microtubule formation which is required for construction of the mitotic spindle. Clinically their major toxicity is peripheral neuropathy. The first signs of this disorder are depression of the deep tendon reflexes. In particular the Achilles tendon reflex is depressed in from 60 to 100% of all patients receiving multiple doses of vincristine (Holland *et al.*, 1973; Casey *et al.*, 1973). Maximum depression of these reflexes occurs about 17 days following the administration of a single dose of vincristine, and complete recovery may take from 2 to 10 weeks. Muscle weakness of the extensors in the distal extremities is frequently seen, and may progress to frank "foot drop" resulting in a slapping gait if the vinca alkaloid therapy is not curtailed (Casey *et al.*, 1973; Bradley *et al.*, 1970). Other symptoms of neurologic toxicity include jaw pain, numbness, and paresthesias of the fingers and toes which occur in approximately 50% of patients (Weiden and Wright, 1972; Mushabir and Bart, 1972; Holland, 1981). Vibration, pin prick, and position senses generally remain intact, and the neuropathies that do exist tend to be symmetrical. Cranial nerve palsies including vocal cord paralysis and optic neuropathy have been reported (Bohanon *et al.*, 1963; Brook and Schreiber, 1971; Sanderson *et al.*, 1976; Albert *et al.*, 1967). The autonomic nervous system may be affected as well. Illeus and bladder atonia are frequent complications, and impotence is a potential problem (Hancock and Naysmith, 1975; Holland *et al.*, 1973; Gottlieb and Cuttner, 1971). Interestingly, orthostatic hypotension is rarely encountered (Carmichael *et al.*, 1970; Aisner *et al.*, 1974). The CNS is also subject to the neurotoxic effects of these drugs. Seizures and even coma have been reported several days after vincristine therapy in the absence of any obvious metabolic derangements (Johnson *et al.*, 1973; Hardisty *et al.*, 1969; Whittaker *et al.*, 1973). Inappropriate ADH secretion can occur from 5 to 20 days following therapy, and generally correlates with the presence of other signs of neurotoxicity (Robertson *et al.*, 1973; Haggard *et al.*, 1968; Fine *et al.*, 1966; Cutting, 1971; Wakem and Bennet, 1975).

The pathophysiologic basis for these abnormalities remains unclear. Electromyograms can be abnormal in patients exhibiting vincritine neurotoxicity, but nerve conduction velocity studies and neuromuscular transmission studies are generally unchanged (Casey *et al.*, 1973; Bradley *et al.*, 1970; Tobin and Sandler, 1968; McLeod and Penny, 1969; Sieber and Adamson, 1975; Uy *et al.*, 1967). Pathologically the primary lesion associated with these neuropathies is distal axonal degeneration which appears to be secondary to neurofilament proliferation (Moress *et al.*, 1967; Gottschalk *et al.*, 1968; Shelanski and Wisniewski, 1969; Schochet *et al.*, 1968; Journey *et al.*, 1969).

While most studies concerning vinca alkaloid-induced neurotoxicities have been performed with vincristine, vinblastine produces basically the same effects (Hertz *et al.*, 1960; Frei *et al.*, 1961; Brook and Schreiber, 1971). Finally, it should be noted that although many of these complications are reversible, recovery can require many months and may not be total.

4. *Antimetabolites*

Cytosine arabinoside (Ara-C) is used in both the treatment and the prophylaxis of acute lymphocytic leukemia within the intrathecal space. A syndrome of arachnoiditis can accompany this treatment. Symptoms include headache, nausea, vomiting, and nuchal rigidity, and may be more common when doses of Ara-C exceed 30 mg/m^2. The occurrence of paraplegia following intrathecal Ara-C has been described (Wolff *et al.*, 1979; Saiki *et al.*, 1972; Band *et al.*, 1973) and will be discussed in connection with intrathecal methotrexate (see below).

5-Fluorouracil has been associated with the development of cerebellar dysfunction in approximately 1% of patients. Fortunately, this syndrome is generally mild and rarely requires the interruption of therapy (Riehl and Brown, 1964; Gottlieb and Luce, 1971; Koenig and Patel, 1970).

6-Mercaptopurine is a major component in the maintenance therapy of childhood leukemia in many treatment protocols. Neurotoxic symptoms have not been clearly associated with this drug (Pizzo *et al.*, 1979).

5. *Folic Acid Antagonists*

Aminopterin and methotrexate exert their cytotoxic effect by inhibiting the enzyme dihydrofolate reductase which normally converts folic acid into tetrahydrofolic acid. This blockade results in the depletion of the reduced folates needed for the *de novo* synthesis of purines and pyrimidines in most cells. Since these compounds are needed for DNA synthesis, the major cytotoxic effect of the folic acid antagonists occurs upon cells that are in the S phase of the cell cycle and will have little effect upon dormant cell populations in the G_0 phase (Ernst and Killmann, 1971). Reduced folates are also needed for the conversion of glycine to methionine and homocysteine to methionine. In this manner methotrexate may interfere with protein synthesis as well (Bleyer, 1977a,b, 1981). In recent years the use of methotrexate has gained renewed interest due to the development of rescue agents such as citrovorum factor which can by-pass the enzymatic blockade established by the folic acid antagonists. Preliminary evidence indicates that citrovorum factor may work selectively on normal and not on tumor cells (Frei *et al.*, 1975). The introduction of these rescue agents has opened the possibility of using much higher doses of methotrexate for longer times without the development of acute toxicities. Goldie *et al.* (1972) have shown that bone marrow can tolerate very high doses of antifolates for periods of up to 40 hours. After this time therapy must be stopped and citrovorum factor must be administered in order to prevent severe hematopoietic toxicity.

Using this strategy drug concentrations up to $10^{-3} M$ may be achieved in the blood. However, since methotrexate is water soluble, it does not penetrate the blood–brain barrier very well, and CSF drug concentrations are only 3–5% of the concomitant blood levels (Shapiro *et al.*, 1973a). Therefore when methotrexate has been used in the treatment of intracranial neoplasms (e.g., meningeal leukemia), the standard route of administration has been by intrathecal injection. CNS prophylaxis in childhood leukemia or lymphoma frequently includes several treatments of intrathecal methotrexate at doses of 10 mg/m^2. CSF methotrexate concentrations of greater than $10^{-6} M$ can be obtained in this way for prolonged periods of time (Bleyer, 1977a,b, 1981).

Acute neurotoxicity has been associated with the use of intrathecal methotrexate. Headache, vomiting, and nuchal rigidity can occur in from 4 to 40% of patients within the first 12 hours after receiving intrathecal methotrexate as prophylaxis against meningeal leukemia (Geiser *et al.*, 1974; Concord Trail, 1971). Lumbar puncture at this time may reveal an elevated opening pressure, pleocytosis, and increased CSF protein. These symptoms generally subside within a few days, but they may persist for a week or longer. The incidence of this syndrome tends to increase with increasing numbers of intrathecal injections and with the presence of meningeal leukemia (Duttera *et al.*, 1973; Sullivan *et al.*, 1969; Naiman *et al.*, 1970). Several factors including the pH, osmolality, ionic strength, and the preservative content of the methotrexate solution used for intrathecal injections have been proposed as the determinants responsible for this syndrome (Geiser *et al.*, 1974; Walker *et al.*, 1969; Duttera *et al.*, 1973). However, this toxicity has been shown to be dose dependent upon methotrexate in both humans and in animal models (Bleyer *et al.*, 1973; Pizzo *et al.*, 1979). The use of commercially available and preservative-free preparations of methotrexate for intrathecal use has also failed to lower the incidence of these complications (Duttera *et al.*, 1973). A more severe acute reaction of intrathecal methotrexate can occur which is characterized by paraplegia, leg pain, and in at least one instance death (Back, 1969).

The majority of patients exhibiting this syndrome had evidence of meningeal leukemia and had received cumulative doses of intrathecal methotrexate of from 100 to 300 mg (Pasquinucci *et al.*, 1970; Baum *et al.*, 1971; Thompson *et al.*, 1971; Luddy and Gilman, 1973). The increased risk of this syndrome in patients with CNS leukemic infiltrates has been confirmed by Bleyer *et al.* (1973) and was shown to correlate with increased concentrations of methotrexate in the CSF. These variations in CSF methotrexate concentration may reflect alterations in the normal cerebral flow of CSF due to leukemic infiltrates. Young *et al.* (1974) has shown that ventricular methotrexate levels are highly variable after intrathecal lumbar injections in the presence of malignant CNS disease. Neurotoxicity has also been reported following intraventricular injections of methotrexate in the presence of intraventricular obstruction to CSF flow (Wilson and Norrell, 1969; Shapiro *et al.*, 1973; Norrell *et al.*, 1974). Thus the local concentration of methotrexate may dictate the occurrence of neurotoxicity. Epidural drug leaks during intrathecal injections could raise the local concentration to toxic levels. In this regard it is notable that Saiki *et al.* (1972) have found demyelination of the spinal cord and the spinal nerve roots in a patient following methotrexate-induced neurotoxicity. These lesions corresponded to the anatomic distribution of the patient's symptoms prior to death.

Subacute methotrexate neurotoxicity consisting of encephalopathy, weakness, leg pain, peripheral anesthesia, and paraparesis, paraplegia, or quadraplegia can occur days to weeks following intrathecal methotrexate. The autonomic nervous system may be affected producing a neurogenic bladder and/or an illeus. This syndrome is usually transient but permanent deficits can result (Sullivan *et al.*, 1969; Saiki *et al.*, 1972; Bagshaw *et al.*, 1969; Luddy and Gilman, 1973; Pasquiucci *et al.*, 1970; Gaglino and Costani, 1976). CSF protein levels are frequently elevated at the time of clinical toxicity in these patients (Luddy and Gilman, 1973). Less frequent complications of intrathecal methotrexate include subdural or subarachnoid hemorrhage, radicular pain and neuritis and seizures (Sullivan *et al.*, 1969; Bagshaw *et al.*, 1969). Recently, cerebellar dysfunction characterized by truncal ataxia, and intention tremors have been described as reversible signs of subacute methotrexate toxicity (Pizzo *et al.*, 1979). Intracarotid artery infusion of methotrexate has resulted in brain damage (Greenhouse *et al.*, 1964). Finally, high dose methotrexate infusion followed by citrovorum rescue has been associated with the sudden onset of hemiparesis, dysphagia, dysarthria, and cranial nerve palsies 10 days following therapy. No evidence of a cerebral vascular accident to account for these symptoms could be detected in this case (Allen and Rosen, 1978).

Chronic encephalopathy is the most common long-term neurotoxicity associated with methotrexate administration. Necrotizing leukoencephalopathy is frequently mentioned in connection with methotrexate therapy, but this disorder is probably the result of combined modality therapy including methotrexate and will be dealt with under that heading. Clinically significant encephalopathy following therapy with methotrexate but without cranial radiation is not commonly described. Meadows and Evans (1976), reporting on a group of 23 children with leukemia who had received methotrexate in addition to other chemotherapeutic agents and had survived for at least 5 years, found that 14 patients had neurologic abnormalities and 4 of these were disabled by their deficits. One of these patients had intractable seizures and spastic quadreplegia. He had received methotrexate both orally and intravenously for 6 years (cumulative dose 1500 mg/kg) without any cranial radiation or evidence of CNS leukemia. A brain biopsy obtained from this patient showed cortical degeneration and white matter gliosis. Another six patients without and two patients with histories of CNS leukemia had abnormal EEGs, psychological tests, and/or minimal brain dysfunction. No abnormal findings were obtained from eight patients who had received mostly oral methotrexate for shorter periods of time. Pizzo *et al.* (1976) have described a case of reversible dementia occurring in a patient with meningeal leukemia. This patient received oral methotrexate for 4 years. At the time of CNS relapse intrathecal methotrexate and cytosine arabinoside as well as intraventricular methotrexate were administered when disorientation and progressive dementia developed. These symptoms abated upon cessation of therapy. Interestingly, these abnormalities occurred despite the fact that this patient's methotrexate and folate levels had always been maintained in the therapeutic range. A similar case was described by Fusner *et al.* (1977) where the patient developed leukoencephalopathy while receiving intraventricular methotrexate and cytosine arabinoside for the treatment of metastatic rhabdomyosarcoma. Following therapy CT scans showed that the leukoencephalopathy had been reversed.

The pathologic changes associated with intrathecal methotrexate include fibrosis of the meninges, fibrillary gliosis, and Alzheimer Type II cells (Hendin *et al.*, 1974). Demyelination was reported in only one patient in this series who had not received radiation in addition to methotrexate. Kay *et al.* (1972) reported on the clinical course of seven patients with encephalopathy following total methotrexate doses of 950–3500 mg. The encephalopathy was believed to have improved after cessation of therapy and the administration of folinic acid. Since the CSF levels of folinic acid were low in these patients, it was assumed that the mechanism responsible for the neurologic deficits was folate deficiency. However, the administration of folic acid to patients with methotrexate-induced encephalopathy is no longer believed capable of reversing this disorder, and little improvement is to be expected in the chronic neurologic deficits exhibited by these patients upon withdrawal of methotrexate therapy.

C. Combined Modality Therapy

The synergistic antitumor effects of radiotherapy and certain chemotherapeutic agents have been mentioned previously. Of concern to us in this section are the possible synergistic toxic effects that these treatment modalities may have on normal tissues. The use of hydroxyurea in combination with radiotherapy has produced extensive tumor necrosis (Irwin *et al.,* 1977; Kagan *et al.,* 1976). However, this combination of agents has also led to a number of precipitous deaths (Irwin *et al.,* 1977). Actinomycin D and radiotherapy combined in the treatment of medulloblastoma have been associated with radiation myelitis (Littman *et al.,* 1978). Additional evidence of adverse effects upon the CNS from the combination of radiotherapy and chemotherapy comes from a number of pathologic studies. Beuer *et al.* (1978) noted multifocal pontine lesions in four patients after treatment with multiagent chemotherapy and cranial radiation. Destruction of axons and myelin was found in the absence of an inflammatory response. Pratt *et al.* (1977) reported a case of cerebral necrosis occurring 4 weeks after radiotherapy (3000 rads) and intravenous actinomycin and methotrexate. Histologic examination revealed coagulation tissue necrosis, vascular thrombosis, and endothelial cell proliferation. Two cases of blindness have been reported occurring in children with acute lymphocytic leukemia in remission. These patients had received 2400 rads of cranial radiation plus intrathecal cytosine arabinoside. A brain biopsy from one patient revealed fibroid necrosis and hyaline degeneration of the vascular structures (Margileth *et al.,* 1977).

The best characterized of these neurotoxic syndromes associated with radiotherapy and chemotherapy is necrotizing leukoencephalopathy. This syndrome is most frequently seen following cranial radiation and systemic or intrathecal methotrexate used in the treatment of CNS leukemia (Fig. 3). More than 50 cases of this disorder have been reported. The clinical pattern begins insidiously as neurologic deterioration which can progress to severe dementia, ataxia, spasticity, dysphagia, seizures, and coma. In greater than 80% of cases the syndrome ends fatally. Autopsy findings include spongy degeneration of the white matter with demyelination and

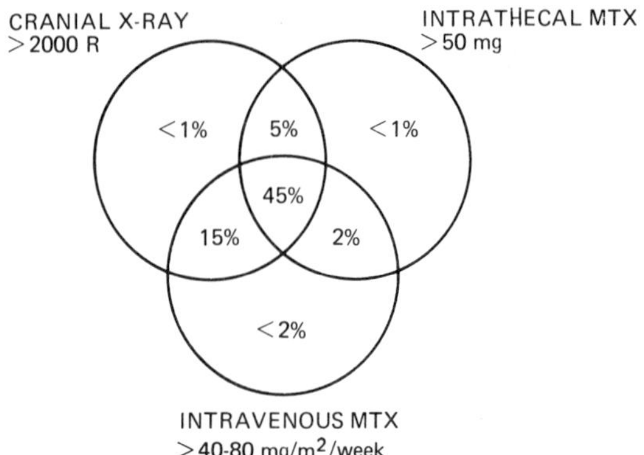

FIG. 3. Approximate risk of clinical leukoencephalopathy as a function of three treatment modalities. Adapted from Bleyer (1977a).

areas of frank necrosis (Flament *et al.,* 1975; Norrell, 1974). The gray matter appears normal (Liu *et al.,* 1978). Early lesions show increases in oligodendroglia (Norrell *et al.,* 1974) which later become pyknotic (Price and Jamieson, 1975). Reactive astrocytosis is also a constant finding while vascular damage appears to be variable. Parenchymal degeneration may lead to perivascular calcification (McIntosh *et al.,* 1976; Flament *et al.,* 1975; Mueller *et al.,* 1976). Axonal swelling is evident in the surrounding necrotic areas, but signs of inflammation are conspicuously absent (Rubinstein *et al.,* 1975). Norrell *et al.* (1974) noted that these lesions resemble those of progressive myelin leukodystrophy except that evidence of oligodendroglial inclusions is missing.

Price and Jamieson (1975) postulated that the development of these lesions was dependent on the dose of cranial radiation (greater than 2000 rads) and the use of high doses of intravenous methotrexate. This study and the work of Norrell *et al.* (1974) seemed to indicate that intrathecal methotrexate was not implicated in this syndrome. However, it has been reported that the intraventricular instillation of methotrexate for the treatment of brain tumors can lead to necrotizing encephalopathy as well (Bresnan *et al.,* 1972; Shapiro *et al.,* 1973b).

McIntosh *et al.* (1977) observed both major and minor neurologic disturbances in her patients with leukemia. Among these patients intracranial calcifications were noted in 2 of 3 of the patients who received more than 4 g/m^2 of methotrexate in contrast to only 2 of 26 patients who received smaller doses. Similarly, Aur *et al.* (1975) reported that 9 of 20 patients receiving methotrexate both intravenously and intrathecally plus cranial radiation developed encephalopathy.

While methotrexate is clearly implicated in the etiology of leukoencephalopathy, a contributory role for intrathecal cytosine arabinoside and/or hydrocortisone cannot be excluded from consideration in some of these cases (Rubinstein *et al.*, 1975). Additionally, it should be noted that many of these patients had meningeal leukemia at some time during their history. The diagnosis of CNS leukemia generally dictates a more aggressive chemotherapeutic approach. Meningeal leukemia may also alter the normal state of the blood–brain barrier making the nervous tissue more accessible to drug penetration and therefore more susceptible to drug toxicity. In summary, the majority of patients who develop necrotizing encephalopathy have received cranial radiation plus intrathecal and/or systemic methotrexate. Many of these patients received intrathecal cytosine arabinoside and/or hydrocortisone, and many patients had evidence of meningeal leukemia at some time during their disease.

As noted Bleyer *et al.* (1973, 1981) have shown that methotrexate neurotoxicity is usually associated with elevated levels of methotrexate in the CSF. Animal experiments with cranial radiation and systemic methotrexate administration have indicated that cerebral drug levels can be increased if preceded by radiotherapy (Griffin *et al.*, 1977). Similar results for other agents have been reported by Clemente and Holst (1954). Elevated levels of CSF methotrexate have been associated with intracranial spread of Burkitt's lymphoma. In this instance elevated intracranial pressure resulted in delayed efflux of methotrexate from the CSF and therefore to elevated CSF methotrexate concentrations (Bode *et al.*, 1980b). Malignant CNS disease has also been associated with destruction of the blood–brain barrier in animal models (Ushio *et al.*, 1977). Electron microscopic studies of the neovascularization which accompanies malignant growth have demonstrated the formation of channels which may enhance the permeability of the meninges (Long, 1970).

From the above data the following statements can be made concerning the etiology of necrotizing leukoencephalopathy. This syndrome appears to be a toxic effect of folate antimetabolites upon the white matter of the brain. In certain patients cranial irradiation, malignant CNS disease, and/or other factors may change the permeability of the blood–brain barrier allowing for increased exposure of neural tissues to these antimetabolites. Whether or not there is a direct contribution of radiation to this toxicity or simply an indirect alteration in the blood–brain barrier has not been determined. However, in most instances no histologic evidence of radiation necrosis (fibrinoid vessel degeneration) has been found (Rubin and Casarett, 1972).

The occurrence of chronic encephalopathy following antineoplastic therapy has stimulated an interest in the toxic effects of CNS therapy. Examinations of the long-term survivors of childhood leukemia have provided ample evidence that this is not the only late effect of therapy upon the CNS. As mentioned previously Meadows and Evans (1976) reported that 14 of 23 survivors of childhood leukemia had evidence of neurologic deficits. These included learning disabilities, minimal brain dysfunction, and EEG abnormalities. McIntosh *et al.* (1976) noted neurologic abnormalities in 12 of 23 children including perceptual problems, motor and language difficulties, and seizures. These children were receiving intravenous methotrexate following radiotherapy as CNS prophylaxis. Other toxic effects of prophylactic therapy directed at the CNS include the detection of elevated levels of normal brain enzymes (e.g., CPK and LDH) in the cerebrospinal fluid following therapy. These elevations are similar to those noted after brain injuries such as contusions (Similae *et al.*, 1977).

Computerized tomographic (CT) scanning of the head has detected specific radiographic abnormalities in patients with overt leukoencephalopathy (Peylan-Ramu *et al.*, 1977). Similar examinations performed upon a series of asymptomatic patients who received cranial radiation (2400 rads) and intrathecal chemotherapy for childhood leukemia demonstrated abnormalities in 53% of cases (Peylan-Ramu *et al.*, 1978). Calcifications and hypodense areas (areas of demyelination) were observed in children who received intrathecal methotrexate, while ventricular dilatation and subarachnoid space occurred in patients treated with either intrathecal methotrexate or intrathecal cytosine arabinoside. A control group which received no cranial radiation but similar systemic chemotherapy had no CT scan abnormalities. One conclusion of this study was that cranial radiation may cause atrophy of the brain parenchyma as evidenced by ventricular dilatation. We therefore examined a series of patients with bone tumors who had received cranial radiation (2000 rads) as CNS prophylaxis. These patients did not exhibit any abnormalities on their CT scans (Bode *et al.*, 1979). These findings were consistent with examinations of the hypothalamic–pituitary functions of these patients which were also normal (see below). These studies appear to indicate that a critical threshold for brain injury may exist between 2000 and 2400 rads of cranial irradiation. Interestingly, a recent report has appeared which states that intrathecal and high dose intravenous methotrexate can be substituted for cranial radiation as the standard regimen for CNS prophylaxis. Patients treated in this manner have not developed CT scan abnormalities, and they have not shown an increased incidence of CNS leukemia (Ochs *et al.*, 1980).

Concern has also been raised concerning the intellectual and psychological effects of combined therapy upon the long-term survivors of malignancy. An examination of 23 5-year survivors of acute lymphocytic leukemia revealed two patients with poor intellectual capacities, two with emotional difficulties, and three with chronic absenteeism from school (Verzosa *et al.*, 1976). Studies from the National Cancer Institute have shown a significant decrease in the intellectual functions of patients who have received CNS prophylaxis compared to their siblings as controls (Pizzo *et al.*, 1979). A similar result was obtained for children between the ages of 2½ through 4½ years who had received antileukemic therapy compared to untreated controls (Eiser and Lansdown, 1977; Eiser, 1978). Interestingly, in the same study children between 5½ through 7 years of age showed no evidence of impaired intellectual function.

The preceding discussion of the long-term effects of antineoplastic therapy upon the CNS has emphasized the most disabling side effects. It should be emphasized that other less dramatic but equally important complications of therapy may yet be uncovered. The availability of newer diagnostic tools (e.g., CT scanning and neuropsychiatric testing) should be used to identify the patients at risk for the development of late complications. In terms of prevention, more prospective studies are needed to identify the individual agents responsible for these side effects. Where possible, changes in the therapeutic regimens of certain malignancies should be made in order to avoid these toxicities (e.g., altering the regimen for CNS prophylaxis in acute leukemia to lessen the use of cranial radiation). If alterations such as these can be made without affecting the therapeutic efficacy of the cancer therapy, pediatric cancer patients in particular could be benefited.

IV. Endocrine Organ Toxicity

A. Hypothalamic–Pituitary

A less dramatic but equally distressing neurotoxic effect of antineoplastic therapy is the development of abnormalities in the neuroendocrine functions of the hypothalamic–pituitary axis. Several groups have reported the delayed onset of hypopituitarism following radiotherapy of nasopharyngeal tumors or brain tumors, when the radiotherapy field has included the hypothalamus and/or the pituitary (Tan *et al.*, 1967; Larkins and Martin, 1973; Samaan *et al.*, 1975; Richard *et al.*, 1976; Perry-Keene *et al.*, 1976). Isolated impairment of growth hormone secretion has also been demonstrated in patients with acute leukemia who have received cranial radiation as part of their CNS prophylaxis (Shalet *et al.*, 1976; Schiliro *et al.*, 1976).

The incidence of neuroendocrine dysfunction following radiotherapy is dependent upon the dose of radiation delivered to the hypothalamic–pituitary axis (Shalet *et al.*, 1976). Muhlendahl *et al.* (1976) found no abnormalities among 22 children with acute lymphoblastic leukemia (ALL) who received CNS prophylaxis with 850–1800 rads of cranial radiation.

Oliff *et al.* (1979) examined 18 patients with ALL who received 2400 rads of prophylactic cranial radiation and found that 50% of these patients had deficient growth hormone responses to hypoglycemia. Samaan *et al.* (1975) reported that 93% (14/15) of patients treated for nasopharyngeal cancer with 500–8300 rads had endocrine deficiencies.

The clinical presentation of endocrine dysfunction among these patients varies according to the hormonal systems affected by their therapy. Abnormalities range from simple growth hormone deficiency to panhypopituitarism with concomitant features of short stature, hypothyroidism, hypogonadism, and Addison's disease (Samaan *et al.*, 1975; Perry-Keene *et al.*, 1976; Oliff *et al.*, 1979). Growth hormone secretion is generally the most susceptible neuroendocrine function. However, short stature does not invariably occur in patients who develop abnormal growth hormone responses even when the radiotherapy is administered in childhood (Shalet *et al.*, 1979). Short stature can be a problem among those patients who receive $\geq$2950 rads cranial radiation during childhood, while children who receive $<$2500 rads rarely develop short stature despite exhibiting abnormal growth hormone responses to pharmacologic stimuli (Shalet *et al.*, 1979; Dickinson *et al.*, 1978). Dickinson *et al.* (1978) have shed some light on this inconsistency by studying growth hormone secretion in response to two types of stimuli in patients who have received varying doses of cranial radiation. Patients who received $\leq$2400 rads had deficient growth hormone responses to hypoglycemia but normal responses to arginine infusions. Patients who received $>$2400 rads had abnormally low growth hormone secretion to both stimuli. Since growth hormone secretion is controlled by several factors which may not be equally susceptible to radiation injury, it may be possible to develop laboratory abnormalities in response to pharmacologic stimuli at lower doses of radiotherapy which do not correlate with clinical growth hormone deficiency.

The precise etiology of these abnormalities is not known. Clearly, radiotherapy of the hypothalamic–pituitary axis is a major factor in the development of neuroendocrine dysfunction, but a contribution from the concomitant use of intrathecal or systemic chemotherapy cannot be ruled out. Several groups have reported that the neuroendocrine abnormalities observed following radiotherapy can be localized to the hypothalamus, the pituitary, or both organs (Larkins and Martin, 1973, Samaan *et al.*, 1975; Perry-Keene *et al.*, 1976).

The diagnosis of neuroendocrine dysfunction rests primarily upon the laboratory demonstration of abnormal baseline and/or abnormal evoked hormone levels in response to specific hormone-releasing stimuli (Martins *et al.*, 1977). However, the clinical signs of hypothyroidism, or hypogonadism in the adult and short stature in the pediatric patient who is off therapy indicate the need for a more thorough work-up (Samaan *et al.*, 1975; Shalet *et al.*, 1979; Swift *et al.*, 1978). The presence of ventricular dilatation on CT brain scanning has also been shown to correlate with abnormal growth hormone responses and may be a useful indicator of hypothalamic–pituitary injury (Fig. 4, Oliff *et al.*, 1979). Treatment of

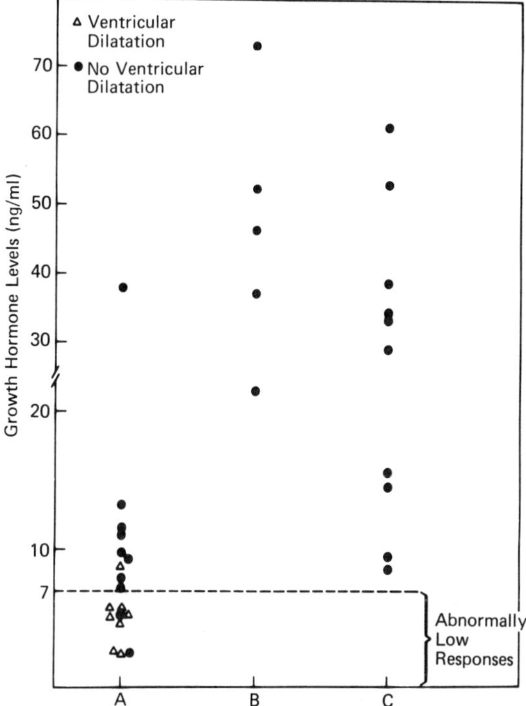

FIG. 4. Graphic representation of the correlation between ventricular dilatation as seen on CT scanning and abnormally low growth hormone responses to insulin-induced hypoglycemia. (A) Childhood leukemia treated with cranial radiation (2400 rads), intrathecal, and systemic combination chemotherapy. (B) Childhood leukemia treated with systemic combination chemotherapy alone. (C) Ewing's sarcoma treated with cranial radiation (2000 rads) and systemic combination chemotherapy.

these abnormalities involves replacement of the deficient hormones. Replacement therapy has been successful in reversing the signs and symptoms of growth hormone, thyroid hormone, sex hormone, and corticosteroid deficiencies (Tan *et al.*, 1967; Richard *et al.*, 1976, Perry-Keene *et al.*, 1976). Unfortunately, Shalet has shown that growth hormone abnormalities following therapy may progress with time, thus making spontaneous recovery unlikely (Shalet *et al.*, 1977).

The effect of antineoplastic therapy upon neuropsychologic functions and intelligence is much more difficult to define than the encephalopathic or neuroendocrine abnormalities described above. The major reasons for this impression are the long latent period (especially in children) required from the time of therapy until clinically recognizable abnormalities are identified, and the difficulty in determining which factor(s) are primarily responsible for the observed neuropsychologic dysfunction; therapy, underlying malignancy, or the emotional stress associated with prolonged illness. It is not surprising therefore that several groups have reached different conclusions concerning the occurrence of these abnormalities.

B. Thyroid–Parathyroid

Hypothyroidism is the most common late complication of local radiotherapy involving the thyroid gland (Adler *et al.*, 1976; Markson and Flatman, 1965; Rosenthal and Goldfine, 1976). The incidence of hypothyroidism among patients with Hodgkin's disease following neck irradiation varies from 5 to 25% (Slanina *et al.*, 1977; Schimpff *et al.*, 1980; Nelson, 1978; Poussin-Rosillo *et al.*, 1978).

Similar incidence figures have been reported for patients with non-Hodgkin's lymphoma, laryngeal carcinoma, and other head and neck tumors following radiotherapy (Glatstein *et al.*, 1971; Shafer *et al.*, 1975; Fuks *et al.*, 1976). However, impaired thyroid function can be demonstrated in 60–90% of these patients using biochemical parameters such as the response to thyrotropin-releasing hormone or baseline TSH levels (Shalet *et al.*, 1977; Schimpff *et al.*, 1980).

Thyroid dysfunction following radiotherapy has been reported over a wide range of radiation doses (2500–7000 rads) (Markson and Flatman, 1965; Shalet *et al.*, 1977; Shafer *et al.*, 1975; Fuks *et al.*, 1976). Fewer abnormalities are produced with lower radiotherapy doses or with only partial exposure of the thyroid gland to radiation (Schimpff *et al.*, 1980; Glatstein *et al.*, 1971). Hemithyroidectomy following radiotherapy or X-ray procedures involving iodine-containing dyes (e.g., lymphangiography) prior to radiation can increase the risk of hypothyroidism (Shafer *et al.*, 1975; Fuks *et al.*, 1976).

Most thyroid dysfunction develops within the first 24 months following radiation (Glatstein *et al.*, 1971) but hypothyroidism can occur up to 6 years after radiotherapy (Markson and Flatman, 1965; Schimpff *et al.*, 1980; Murken and Duvall, 1972). The severity of this syndrome can vary from asymptomatic impairment of thyroid reserve to clinical hypothyroidism and even myxedema coma (Shalet, 1977; Formeister *et al.*, 1978). The etiology of these abnormalities appears to be radiation-induced atrophy and/or fibrosis of the thyroid gland (Glatstein *et al.*, 1971). However, Markson and Flatman (1965) have suggested an autoimmune mechanism involving antithyroidal antibodies as the basis of radiation induced hypothyroidism. Other investigators have failed to identify any autoantibodies in their patients with radiation-related hypothyroidism (Shafer *et al.*, 1975; Formeister *et al.*, 1978).

Radiation-induced thyroid dysfunction can be successfully and easily treated with hormonal replacement therapy. Hormonal therapy has been recommended for all patients with elevated TSH levels following radiotherapy in order to prevent overt hypothyroidism and to reduce the risk of radiation-induced thyroid carcinoma (Schimpff *et al.*, 1980).

Parathyroid abnormalities can also occur secondary to radiation therapy of the head and neck. In one series 30% of the patients operated on for primary hyperparathyroidism had a history of radiation to the head or neck for benign diseases in childhood (Prinz *et al.*, 1977). These disorders developed after an average of 30 years.

C. Gonadal

Primary tumors of the gonads are rare in the pediatric age group. However, testicular involvement in childhood leukemia and lymphoma has been reported as high as 30%. Isolated leukemic relapses of the testes occur in approximately 5% of patients (Finkelstein *et al.*, 1969; Stoffel *et al.*, 1975). Pharmacokinetic studies have indicated that the testes may act as a sanctuary for leukemic cells during systemic chemotherapy preventing the penetration of adequate levels of cytotoxic drugs. This situation would be analogous to that which occurs in the CNS, and therefore prophylactic antileukemic therapy directed at the testicles may be advisable (Nesbit *et al.*, 1977). Radiotherapy is the treatment of choice for leukemic relapses confined to one organ. Usually a dose of 1200 rads is sufficient to eliminate all evidence of microscopic disease (Stoffel *et al.*, 1975).

The late effects of radiotherapy on the gonads may manifest themselves as either reduced fertility or sterility. Lushbaugh and Casarett (1976) have found that testicular tolerance to radiation doses of 15 to 416 rads resulted in diminished or temporary infertility, while doses of 500 to 950 rads resulted in permanent sterility. These data are in contrast to the report of Rowley *et al.* (1974) who found recovery of testicular function several years after local radiotherapy up to 600 rads. Rowley demonstrated that recovery from radiation in the range of 200 to 300 rads takes approximately 30 months although evidence of sperm production may be visible as early as 1 year posttreatment. Patients receiving fractionated radiation are reported to be more susceptible to the sterilizing effects of radiotherapy. Speizer *et al.* (1973) noted complete azospermia 1 month after fractionated radiation of 250 rads delivered to the lower trunk for Hodgkin's disease. This depression in sperm production persisted for up to 40 months.

Radiotherapy directed at the ovaries can also result in infertility. In this case the age of the patient is very important in assessing the potential damage done by radiation exposure. While 600 rads has been reported to cause sterility in women over the age of 40, women below 40 can tolerate this dosage without permanent deficits (Lushbaugh and Ricks, 1972). Conflicting data have accumulated concerning the precise dose of radiation required to cause permanent sterility in both males and females (Rubin and Casarett, 1972; Lushbaugh and Casarett, 1976). However, it is clear that doses in excess of 600 rads, and especially if fractionated in their delivery, will cause significant infertility and may lead to permanent sterility. The situation in children is much less clear since fewer studies have been undertaken, but it seems safe to conclude that problems of infertility will also occur in these patients following local radiotherapy of the gonads. More to the point, patients of reproductive age, should be spared gonadal radiation whenever possible. In patients with Hodgkin's disease the recent practice of oophoropexy at the time of staging laporotomy has resulted in reduced exposure to radiation and the preservation of reproductive function (Le Floch *et al.*, 1976). The question of teratogenic effects from radiotherapy delivered to the gonads has been raised. In at least one study, a series of female patients who had received approximately 400 rads to their ovaries were followed through childbirth. Two of three of these patients were fertile and no abnormalities were noted among their offspring (Le Floch *et al.,* 1976). In summary, permanent sterility may result from radiation delivered to either the testes or the ovaries in doses as low as 200 rads, but late recovery of function has been noted. While these data have been accumulated predominantly in adult populations, it is probable that the gonads of prepubertal children will also be sensitive to radiotherapy but to a lesser degree.

The effect of chemotherapy upon the gonads has received recent attention, both in the treatment of neoplastic diseases and in therapy of steroid-resistant nephrotic syndrome treated with cyclophosphamide (Parra *et al.*, 1978; Etteldorf *et al.*, 1976; Kirkland *et al.*, 1976). The maturation and development of the gonads in children are reflected in the variable sensitivity of these organs to chemotherapy at different stages of their development. Prepubertal boys given the same dose of cyclophosphamide as pubertal boys have been reported to suffer much less toxicity (Parra *et al.*, 1978). Similarly, Sherins and DeVita (1973) have shown that while 9 of 13 pubertal boys treated for Hodgkin's disease with MOPP developed hormonal disturbances and gynecomastia, all six of his prepubertal patients treated in the same manner were normal. The other major factor involved in determining the degree of damage caused by systemic chemotherapy is the total drug dose. Etteldorf *et al.* (1976) reported that prepubertal boys treated with cyclophosphamide in total doses of 6.2 to 14.3 g had normal sperm counts and testicular histology while patients receiving 11.8 to 39.3 g were uniformly azoospermic and exhibited evidence of germinal aplasia within their testes. These results were confirmed by Lentz *et al.* (1977) who found that prepubertal boys who had received more than 365 mg/kg of cyclophosphamide were azoospermic while other patients receiving lower doses of this agent had either normal or only slightly diminished sperm counts. Additional studies on prepubertal boys treated with relatively low doses of cyclophosphamide for long periods of time have found essentially normal gonadal function. These studies have established that it is the total dose of cyclophosphamide not the duration of therapy which is important in determining whether testicular damage will occur (De Groot *et al.*, 1974; Pennisi *et al.*, 1975). The pathologic findings associated with this form of toxicity include normal Sertoli cells lining atrophic tubules and the total elimination of germinal cells. Spermatozoa are rare and peritubular fibrosis is common. Focal tubular necrosis has also been reported with cyclophosphamide therapy (Pennisi *et al.*, 1975; Fairley *et al.*, 1972; Etteldorf *et al.*, 1976). Gonadotropin levels are generally high in those patients suffering from gonadal damage secondary to chemotherapeutic agents and testosterone levels are low. However, these values may not accurately reflect the patient's fertility status (Pennisi *et al.*, 1975).

Chlorambucil has been associated with a dose-dependent gonadal toxicity leading to azoospermia and germinal cell aplasia (Richter *et al.*, 1970). Procarbazine has been implicated in producing an irreversible form of azoospermia when used in combination with other chemotherapeutic agents (Roeser *et al.*, 1978). In general, recovery from the testicular toxicity of combination chemotherapy is uncommon. Sherins and DeVita (1973) failed to detect any signs of recovery from the oligospermia of MOPP therapy up to 4 years after therapy. However, some exceptions to this generalization have been reported with chlorambucil (Cheviakoff *et al.*, 1973), cyclophosphamide (Buchanan *et al.*, 1975), and combination chemotherapy (Roeser *et al.*, 1978).

The effect of chemotherapy upon ovarian function has been studied less thoroughly. Several studies have reported that prepubertal girls treated with cyclophosphamide have had normal hormonal development, normal menses, and a number of successful pregnancies (Parra *et al.*, 1978; Etteldorf *et al.*, 1976; De Groot *et al.*, 1974; Lentz *et al.*, 1977; Arneil, 1972; Himelstein *et al.*, 1978). The experience with postpubertal women has been more disappointing. Premature ovarian failure characterized by amenorrhea and infertility has been reported in association with systemic chemotherapy in a number of studies (Uldall *et al.*, 1972; Koyama *et al.*, 1977; Warne *et al.*, 1973; Miller *et al.*, 1971). The use of cyclophosphamide in one of these studies has indicated that older women may be more susceptible to ovarian failure than their younger counterparts. In this study the onset of amenorrhea occurred after an average total dose of cyclophosphamide of 5.2 g for women in their 40s versus 20.4 g for women in their 30s (Koyama *et al.*, 1977). Conflicting reports have appeared concerning the reversibility of these abnormalities following therapy, and this question remains unanswered at present (Kumar *et al.*, 1972; Uldall *et al.*, 1972).

V. Skeletal Growth

Antineoplastic therapy may influence linear body growth at several levels. Local treatments such as surgical removal of a long bone or radiation therapy to the spinal column will inhibit normal skeletal growth (Probert *et al.*, 1973). Systemic chemotherapy can also delay linear growth during therapy. Psychosocial dwarfism is another example of the multiple levels at which the normal growth can be interrupted.

Pinkel (1971) reported that five of seven children receiving systemic chemotherapy exhibited growth retardation during treatment. After the completion of therapy three of these patients showed "catch-up" growth while growth retardation persisted in the remaining two patients. Alternatively, Sundermann and Pearson (1969) observed normal growth patterns in children receiving small doses of maintenance chemotherapy during periods of remission. We have also examined the growth records of a series of 56 pediatric patients treated for acute lymphocytic leukemia. The majority of these children suffered from growth retardation during their therapy. Virtually all of these children began to exhibit normal growth rates following therapy. However, none of the affected children demonstrated "catch-up" growth (Bode and Oliff, unpublished results). The use of systemic corticosteroids, a frequent component of pediatric chemotherapy protocols, has been associated with impaired growth (Brasel and Blizzard, 1974). Methotrexate, another common agent used for pediatric tumors, has also been shown to cause pathologic changes in normal bones including osteoporosis, pseudoscurvy, and fractures (Ragab *et al.*, 1970).

It has been recognized for many years that irradiation of immature epiphyses in children will result in growth arrest. Localized radiotherapy of this nature can produce direct toxicity to the bones encompassed within the radiation field, and/or it may cause indirect damage to the surrounding soft tissues resulting in fibrosis and deformity (Parker and Bery, 1976). In pediatric oncology patients following radiation therapy for Wilm's tumor, late skeletal changes were reported in 59 of 81 children (Riseborogh *et al.*, 1976). In this study the degree of deformity correlated directly with the amount of radiation used and inversely with the age of the child. The most commonly encountered pathologic features were growth arrest lines, end-plate irregularities, decreased vertebral body height, and failure of vertebral body development. Of the patients receiving more than 3000 rads irradiation for Wilm's tumor, 60 to 80% can be expected to develop severe osseous changes. Clinically these changes can present as scoliosis, kyphosis, or kyphoscoliosis (Donaldson and Wissinger, 1967; Katzmann *et al.*, 1969). These deformities frequently are severe enough to require corrective surgery to promote vertebral fusions.

VI. Psychosocial Development

Significant progress has been made in the treatment of a number of pediatric malignancies, and the "total care" concept of Farber has changed to a "total cure" concept for many patients (Sutow, 1980). The preceding text has dealt with the physical impairments which may result from the treatments used in combating cancer. The remainder of this article deals with the emotional and social problems which can arise and the possible means of intervention which can prevent or ameliorate these problems.

In general children are considered in terms of their future social and economic potential, but they are rarely dealt with as individual members of society. Adults frequently see children as a means of fulfilling their own social wishes. The affect of this attitude is to deny children a sense of social awareness and consciousness. This behavior leads to the well-intentioned but unfortunate tendency on the part of the parents and professionals to ignore the child's conscious participation in his situation. As an example, pediatric oncologists often spend more time with a child's parents than with the patient himself. This attitude is based on several erroneous premises. Foremost among these is the tendency of adults to shield their children from the unpleasant information at hand. This attempt on the part of parents and staff to assume the physical and psychological distress for the patient results in a nonfunctional situation for the child (Levine, 1977). In response to this situation children frequently regress. Children are continually developing and need to mature through problem solving. In pediatric cancer patients the need to continue this process is not overruled by the physical stresses the children are required to undergo. The combination of psychosocial regression in the child and a general attitude of guilt in the parents often leads to excessive dependency of the child on his parents (Hoffmann and Futterman, 1971). This dependency spurs the child's separation anxiety and helps create a mother–child symbiosis which often leads to, among other things, school phobia (Lansky *et al.,* 1975; Lansky and Carins, 1978).

Children's awareness of their disease can also disrupt their psychosocial development by generating sufficient anxiety to disrupt their emotional stability and their interpersonal relationships (Spinetta, 1977; Goggin, 1976). Frequent in-patient treatments and out-patient fatigue will tend to isolate the patient from his normal school and extracurricular activities. This isolation is both self imposed and initiated by others (Zwartjes, 1980). Stigmata of therapy such as alopeica and weight loss may tend to force the patient into isolation in order to prevent ridicule. General societal attitudes at present tend to see all forms of cancer as invariably fatal, and few people feel comfortable in dealing with death. Therefore many people who would normally interact with the patient (e.g., teachers and employers) tend to avoid interpersonal contact with cancer patients. This phenomena has been termed "psychological euthanasia" (Van Eys, 1977b). The patient will also alter his own sense of personal value by virtue of having a putatively terminal disease. The combination of increased dependency on parents and progressive isolation from other social contacts results in a severe inhibition of the child's normal psychological and social development.

Reduced educational performance is an outgrowth of the school phobia mentioned above as well as the reduced expectations of teachers, classmates, and parents. Absenteeism necessitated by therapy also contributes to this problem. The resulting educational deficits can further lower the patient's self-esteem. Thus a vicious cycle is established where anxiety and isolation lead to further separation from the normal social contacts and support mechanisms employed by children as they mature.

In summary pediatric cancer victims undergo a high degree of psychological stress. Recognition of the factors contributing to this stress is necessary in order to ameliorate the psychosocial disruption caused by the patient's disease and its therapy. Specifically, it is necessary to honestly inform the *patient,* his relatives, teachers, and peers about the therapeutic possibilities and consequences of the disease in question. In this manner physical cures need not be associated with severe impairment of the patient's psychosocial development. Professionals must also strive to learn more about the psychological and social implications of their therapies and attitudes.

VII. Concluding Remarks

More than 50% of all childhood cancer patients can now be expected to survive at least 3 years and many of these patients will become long-term survivors (Draper, 1980). We have tried to describe the multiplicity of long-term adverse effects from antineoplastic therapy which can significantly impair these patients' quality of life. Meadows *et al.* (1980) have recently reported on the incidence of late effects of therapy in childhood cancer, and found that 20% of patients surviving leukemia, 28% in Wilms tumor, and more than 50% of patients with soft tissue sarcomas exhibit one or another of these sequellae. These numbers indicate the magnitude of this problem. Medical science has won a major victory against cancer by demonstrating the curability of certain tumors. Now some attention is needed to the traditional values of "do no harm." No one advocates a retreat from these hard won therapeutic triumphs. But more selective treatment may be possible without decreasing the overall effectiveness of therapy.

Learning more about cancer and its treatment also includes learning more about the patient and his social environment. As we begin to appreciate the psychosocial effects of cancer and its treatment, we should invest in the prevention and treatment of these complications as well. This includes a nearly forgotten feature of medicine: to spend time with the patient and listen.

References

Adams, G. E., Fowler, J. F., and Wartman, P. (1978). *Br. J. Cancer* **37,** Suppl. 13, 321.

Adler, R. A., Corrigan, D. F., and Wartkofsky, L. (1976). *Bull. Johns Hopkins Hosp.* **138,** 180.

Aisner, J., Weiss, H.D., Chang, P., and Wiernik, P. H. (1974). *Cancer Chemother. Rep.* **58,** 927.

Albert, D. M., Wong, V. G., and Henderson, E. S. (1967). *Arch. Ophthalmol.* **78,** 709.
Alexander, P., Dean, C. J., Hamilton, L. D. G., Lett, J. T., and Parkins, G. (1965). "Cellular Radiation Biology." Williams & Wilkins, Baltimore.
Allen, J. C. (1978). *J. Pediatr.* **93,** 903.
Allen, J. C., and Rosen, G. (1978). *Ann. Neurol.* **3,** 441.
Altman, A. Y., and Schwartz, A. D. (eds.) (1978). "Malignant Diseases of Infancy, Childhood and Adolescence." Saunders, Philadelphia.
Altman, K. T., Genada, S., and Gerber, G. B. (1970). "Radiation Biochemistry," Vol. I. Academic Press, New York.
Anderson, E. E., Cobb, O. E., and Glenn, J. F. (1967). *J. Urol.* **97,** 857.
Ariel, I. M. (1961). *Am. J. Surg.* **102,** 647.
Arneil, G. C. (1972). *Lancet* **2,** 1959.
Aur, R. J., Verzosa, M. S., Hustu, H. O., Simone, J., and Barker, L. (1975). *Assoc. Cancer Res.* **16,** 92.
Back, E. H. (1969). *Lancet* **2,** 1005.
Bagshaw, K. D., Magrath, I. T., and Golding, P. R. (1969). *Lancet* **2,** 1258.
Bamford, F. V., Morris-Jones, P., Pearson, D., Ribiero, G. G., Shalet, S. M., and Beardwell, C. G. (1976). *Cancer* **37,** 1149.
Band, P. R., Holland, J. F., Bernard, J., Weil, M., Walker, M., and Rall, D. (1973). *Cancer* **32,** 744.
Barendson, G. W., and Janse, H. C. (1978). *Int. J. Radiat. Oncol. Phys.* **4,** 95.
Baum, E. S., Koch, H. F., Corby, D. G., and Plunket, D. C. (1971). *Lancet* **1,** 649.
Bender, R. D., Bleyer, W. A., Frisby, S. A., and Oliviero, V. T. (1975). *Cancer Res.* **35,** 1305.
Berger, P. S., and Bataini, J. P. (1977). *Cancer* **40,** 152.
Bethlenfalvay, N. C., and Bergin, J. J. (1972). *Cancer* **29,** 366.
Beuer, A. C., Blank, N. K., and Schone, W. C. (1978). *Cancer* **41,** 2112.
Billmeier, G. J., and Holton, C. P. (1969). *J. Pediatr.* **75,** 892.
Bladin, P. F., and Royle, J. (1977). *J. Clin. Exp. Neurol.* **14,** 8.
Bland, J. E., Windmiller, J., Whitaker, J., and Clark, K. (1961). *Cancer* **14,** 1115.
Bleyer, W. A. (1977a). *Natl. Cancer Inst. Monogr.* **46,** 171.
Bleyer, W. A. (1977b). *Cancer Treat. Rev.* **4,** 67.
Bleyer, W. A., Drake, J. C., and Chabner, B. A. (1973). *N. Engl. J. Med.* **289,** 770.
Bloom, H. J. R. (1978). *Prog. Clin. Biol. Res.* **25,** 55.
Bode, U., Oliff, A., Bercu, B., DiChiro, G., and Poplack, D. G. (1979). *Am. J. Hematol. Oncol.* **2,** 21.
Bode, U., Seif, S. F., and Levine, A. S. (1980a). *Med. Pediatr. Oncol.* **8,** 295.
Bode, U., Magrath, I. T., Bleyer, W. A., Poplack, D. G., and Glaubiger, D. (1980b). *Cancer Res.* **40,** 2184.
Bohannon, R. A., Miller, D. G., and Diamond, H. D. (1963). *Cancer Res.* **23,** 613.
Bradley, W. G., Lassman, L. P., Pearch, G. W., and Walton, J. N. (1970). *J. Neurol. Sci.* **10,** 107.
Brady, L. W. (1980). (ed.) "Radiation Sensitizers." Masson, New York.
Brasel, J. A., and Blizzard, R. M. (1974). *In* "Textbook of Endocrinology" (R. H. Williams, ed.). Saunders, Philadelphia.
Brenner, H. J., and Har-Kedar, I. (1977). *In* "Radiobiological Research and Radiotherapy." Intern Atomic Energy Agency, Vienna.
Bresnan, M. J., Gilles, F. H., Lorenzo, F. H., Watters, G. V., and Barlow, C. F. (1972). *Trans. Am. Neurol. Assoc.* **97,** 204.
Brook, J., and Schreiber, W. (1971). *Cancer Chemother. Rep.* **55,** 591.

Brunner, K. W., and Young, C. W. (1965). *Ann. Int. Med.* **63,** 69.
Buchanan, J. D., Fairley, K. F., and Barrie, J. U. (1975). *Lancet* **2,** 156.
Capizzi, R. L. (1975). *Cancer Chemother. Rep.* **1,** 37.
Carmichael, S. M., Eagleton, L., Ayers, C. R., and Mohler, D. (1970). *Arch. Intern. Med.* **126,** 290.
Carter, S. K. (1975). *Front. Radiat. Ther. Oncol.* **9,** 13.
Casey, E. B., Jellife, A. M., LeQuesne, P. M., and Millet, Y. L. (1973). *Brain* **96,** 69.
Chabner, B. A., Sponzo, R., Hubbard, S., Canellos, G. P., Young, R. C., Schein, P. S., and DeVita, V. T. (1973). *Cancer Chemother. Rep.* **57,** 361.
Chabner, B. A., Myers, C. E., Coleman, C. N., and Johns, D. G. (1975). *N. Engl. J. Med.* **292,** 1107, 1159.
Cheng, V. S. T., and Schultz, M. S. (1975). *Cancer* **35,** 1537.
Cheviakoff, S., Calamera, J. S., Morgenfeld, M., and Mancini, R. E. (1973). *J. Reprod. Fertil.* **57,** 361.
Clemente, C. D., and Holst, E. A. (1954). *Arch. Neurol. Phychiat.* **71,** 66.
Concord Trial (1971). *Br. Med. J.* **4,** 189.
Conomy, J. P., and Kellermeyer, R. W. (1975). *Cancer* **36,** 1702.
Court-Brown, W. M., Brickton, K. E., and McLean, A. S. (1965). *Lancet* **1,** 1239.
Cutting, H. O. (1971). *Am. J. Med.* **51,** 269.
D'Angio, G. J. (1969). *Front. Radiat. Ther. Oncol.* **4,** 174.
Davis, R. L. (1979). *Front. Radiat. Ther. Oncol.* **13,** 58.
DeConti, R. C. (1971). *J. Am. Med. Assoc.* **215,** 927.
DeFronzo, R. A., Colvin, O. M., Braine, H., Robertson, G. L., and Davis, P. J. (1973). *Cancer* **33,** 483.
DeGroot, G. W., Faiman, C., and Winter, J. S. D. (1974). *J. Pediatr.* **84,** 123.
Dickinson, W. P., Berry, D. H., Dickinson, K., Irvin, M., Schedewie, H., Fiser, R. H., and Elders, M. J. (1978). *J. Pediatr.* **92,** 754.
Donaldson, W. F., and Wissinger, H. A. (1967). *Proc. Am. Orthop. Assoc. Bone Joint Surg.* **49 A,** 1469.
Draper, G. J. (1980). *In* "Status of the Curability of Childhood Cancers" (J. van Eys, and M. P. Sullivan, eds.). Raven, New York.
Duttera, M. J., Bleyer, W. A., Pomeroy, T. C., Leventhal, C. M., and Leventhal, B. G. (1973). *Lancet* **2,** 703.
Dynes, J. B., and Smedel, J. I. (1960). *Am. J. Roentgenol.* **83,** 78.
Egorin, M., Kaplan, R., Salomon, M., Colvin, N., Wiernik, P., and Bachur, N. (1981). *Proc. Am. Assoc. Cancer Res.* **72,** 210.
Eiser, C. (1978). *Arch. Dis. Child* **53,** 391.
Eiser, C., and Landsdown, R. (1977). *Arch. Dis. Child* **52,** 525.
Elkind, M. M., and Sakamoto, K. (1969). *Front. Radiat. Ther. Oncol.* **4,** 53.
Ernst, P., and Killmann, S. (1971). *Blood* **38,** 689.
Etteldorf, J. N., West, C. D., Pitcock, J. A., and Williams, D. L. (1976). *J. Pediatr.* **88,** 206.
Fairley, K. F., Barrie, J. U., and Johnson, W. (1972). *Lancet* **1,** 568.
Falkson, G., deVilliers, P. C., and Falkson, H. C. (1965). *Cancer Chemother. Rep.* **46,** 7.
Fine, R. N., Clarke, R. R., and Shore, N. A. (1966). *Am. J. Dis. Child* **112,** 256.
Finkelstein, J. Z., Dyment, P. G., and Hammond, G. D. (1969). *Pediatrics* **43,** 1042.
Flament-Durand, J., Ketelbant-Balasse, P., Maurus, R., Regier, R., and Spehl, M. (1975). *Cancer* **35,** 319.
Formeister, J. F., Sako, K., Razack, M. S., and Aungst, C. W. (1978). *J. Surg. Oncol.* **10,** 493.
Freeman, J. E., Johnson, P. G., and Voke, J. M. (1973). *Br. Med. J.* **4,** 523.

Frei, E., III, Franzino, A., Schnider, B. I., Costa, G., Golsky, J., Brindley, C. O., Hosley, H., Holland, J. F., Gold, G. L., and Jonsson, U. (1961). *Cancer Chemother. Rep.* **12,** 125.
Frei, E., III, Jaffe, N., Tattersall, M. H. N., Pitman, S., and Parker, L. (1975). *N. Engl. J. Med.* **292,** 846.
Fuks, Z., Glatstein, E., Marsa, G. W., Gabshaw, M. A., and Kaplan, H. S. (1976). *Cancer* **35,** 1152.
Fusner, J. E., Poplack, D. G., Pizzo, P. A., and DiChiro, G. (1977). *J. Pediatr.* **91,** 77.
Gagliano, R., and Costani, J. (1976). *Cancer* **37,** 1663.
Geiser, C. F., Bishop, Y., and Frei, E., III (1974). *Cancer Res.* **15,** 77.
Glatstein, E., McHardy-Young, S., Brast, N., Eltringham, J. R., and Kriss, J. P. (1971). *J. Clin. Endocrinol. Metab.* **32,** 833.
Godwin-Austen, R. B., Howell, D. A., and Worthington, B. (1975). *Brain* **98,** 557.
Goggin, E. L., Lansky, S. B., and Hassanein, K. J. (1976). *J. Am. Child Psych.* **15,** 314.
Goldie, J. H., Price, L. A., and Harrap, K. R. (1972). *Eur. J. Cancer* **8,** 409.
Gottlieb, J. A., and Luce, J. K. (1971). *Lancet* **1,** 138.
Gottlieb, R. J., and Buttner, J. (1971). *Cancer* **28,** 674.
Gottschalk, P. G., Dyck, P. J., and Kiely, J. M. (1968). *Neurology* **18,** 875.
Gray, L. H. (1961). *Am. J. Roentgenol. Rad. Ther. Nucl. Med.* **85,** 803.
Green, A. A., and Naiman, J. L. (1968). *Am. J. Dis. Child* **116,** 190.
Greenhouse, A. H., Neuberger, K. T., and Bowerman, D. L. (1964). *Arch. Neurol.* **11,** 618.
Griem, M. L., and Malkinson, F. D. (1969). *Front. Radiat. Ther. Oncol.* **4,** 24.
Griffin, T. W., Rasey, J. S., and Bleyer, W. A. (1977). *Cancer* **40,** 1109.
Haggard, M. E., Chairman, J., Fernbach, D. J., Holcomb, T. M., Sutow, W. W., Vietti, T. J., and Windmiller, J. (1968). *Cancer* **22,** 438.
Hahn, C. M. (1974). *Cancer Res.* **34,** 3117.
Hannawalt, P., Friedberg, E., and Fox, F. (eds.) (1978). "DNA Repair Mechanisms." Academic Press, New York.
Hancock, B. W., and Naysmith, A. (1975). *Br. Med. J.* **3,** 207.
Hardisty, R. M., McElwain, T. J., and Darby, C. W. (1969). *Br. Med. J.* **2,** 662.
Haskell, C. M., Canellos, G. P., Leventhal, B. G., Carbone, P. P., Sherpick, A. A., and Hansen, H. H. (1969). *Cancer Res.* **29,** 974.
Hayward, R. H. (1972). *Surg. Clin. North Am.* **52,** 359.
Hendin, B., DeVivo, D. C., Torack, R., Lell, M. E., Ragab, A. H., and Vietti, T. J. (1974). *Cancer* **33,** 468.
Hersh, S. P. (1978). *In* "Processing of the National Conference of Human Values and Causes," p. 20. American Cancer Society.
Hertz, R., Lipsett, M. B., and Moy, R. H. (1960). *Cancer Res.* **20,** 1050.
Himelstein-Braw, R., Peters, H., and Faber, M. (1978). *Br. J. Cancer* **38,** 82.
Hoffmann, I., and Futterman, E. H. (1971). *Comp. Psychiat.* **12,** 67.
Holland, J. F., Scharlau, C., Gailani, S., Krant, M. J., Olson, K. B., Horton, J., Shnider, B. J., Lynch, J. J., Owens, A., Carbone, P. P., Colsky, J., Grob, D., Miller, S. P., and Hall, T. C. (1973). *Cancer Res.* **33,** 1258.
Holland, J. F. (1981). *In* "Cancer Medicine" (J. F. Holland and E. Frei III, eds.). Lea & Febiger, Philadelphia
Hustu, H. O., Aur, R. J., Verzosa, M. S., Simone, J. V., and Pinkel, D. (1973). *Cancer* **32,** 585.
Irwin, L. (1977). *Natl. Cancer Inst. Monograph* **46,** 253.
Itabashi, H. H., Bebin, J., and DeJong, R. N. (1957). *Neurology* **7,** 844.
Jenkin, R. D. (1969). *Can. Med. Assoc. J.* **100,** 51.

Johnson, R. L., Bernstein, I. D., Hartimann, J. R., and Chard, R. L. (1973). *J. Pediatr.* **82,** 699.
Journey, L. J., Burdman, J., and Whaley, A. (1969). *J. Natl. Cancer Inst.* **43,** 603.
Kagan, A. R., Steckel, R. J., Cancilla, P., Juillard, G., and Patin, T. (1976). *Int. J. Radiat. Oncol. Biol. Phys.* **1,** 729.
Kay, H. E. M., Knapton, P. J., O'Sullivan, J. P., Wells, D. G., Harris, R. F., Innes, E. M., Stuart, J., Schwartz, F. C. M., and Thompson, E. N. (1972). *Arch. Dis. Child.* **47,** 344.
Katzman, H., Waugh, T., and Berdon, W. (1969). *J. Bone Joint Surg.* **51 A,** 825.
Kirkland, R. T., Bongiovanni, A. M., Cornfeld, G., McCormich, J. B., Parks, J. S., and Tenore, A. (1976). *J. Pediatr.* **89,** 941.
Koenig, H., and Patel, A. (1970). *Neurology* **20,** 416.
Koyama, H., Wada, T., Nishizawa, Y., Iwanaga, T., Aoki, Y., Teresawa, T., Kosaki, G., Tamamoto, T., and Wade, A. (1977). *Cancer* **39,** 1403.
Kramer, S., Southard, M. E., and Mansfield, C. M. (1972). *Front. Radiat. Ther. Oncol.* **6,** 322.
Kumar, R., McEvoy, J., and McGeown, M. G. (1972). *Lancet* **1,** 1212.
Lampert, P. W., and Davis, R. L. (1964). *Neurology* **14.** 912.
Land, V. J., Sutow, W. W., Fernbach, D. J., Lane, D. M., and Williams, T. E. (1972). *Cancer* **30,** 339.
Lansky, S. B., and Carius, N. U. (1978). *In* "Proceeding National Conference on Human Values and Causes," p. 156. American Cancer Society.
Lansky, S. B., Lowman, J. T., Vats, T., and Gyulay, J. (1975). *Am. J. Dis. Child.* **129,** 42.
Larkins, R. G., and Martin, F. I. R. (1973). *Br. Med. J.* **1,** 152.
Lawrence, W. J., Kuehn, P., Masle, E. T., and Miller, D. G. (1961). *J. Surg. Res.* **1,** 142.
Le Floch, O., Donaldson, S. S., and Kaplan, H. S. (1976). *Cancer* **38,** 2263.
Lentz, R. D., Bergstein, J., Steffes, M. W., Brown, D. R., Prem, K., Michael, A. F., and Verneir, R. L. (1977). *J. Pediatr.* **91,** 385.
Lett, J. T., Keng, P. C., and Sun, C. (1978). *In* "DNA Repair Mechanisms" (P. C. Hanawalt, P. C. Friedberg, and C. F. Fox, eds.), p. 481. Academic Press, New York.
Levine, A. S. (1977). *In* "Proceedings, of American Cancer Society Second National Conference on Human Values and Cancer," p. 29. Chicago American Cancer Society.
Littman, P., Rosenstock, J. G., and Bailey, C. (1978). *Med. Pediatr. Oncol.* **5,** 145.
Little, J. B. (1968). *N. Engl. J. Med.* **278,** 308.
Liu, H. M., Maurer, H. S., Vongrivivut, S., and Conway, T. J. (1978). *Human Pathol.* **9,** 635.
Llena, J. F., Cespedes, G., Hirano, A., Zimmermann, H. M., Feiring, E. H., and Fine, D. (1976). *Arch. Pathol.* **100,** 531.
Locksmith, J. P., and Powers, W. E. (1968). *Am. J. Roentgenol.* **102,** 916.
Long, D. M. (1970). *J. Neurosurg.* **32,** 127.
Luddy, R. E., and Gilman, P. A. (1973). *J. Pediatr.* **83,** 988.
Lushbaugh, C. C., and Cassarett, G. W. (1976). *Cancer* **37,** 1111.
Lushbaugh, C. C., and Ricks, C. C. (1972). *Front. Radiat. Ther. Oncol.* **6,** 229.
McIntosh, S., Klatskin, E. H., O'Brien, R. T., Aspnes, G. T., Kammerer, B. L., Snead, C., Kalavsky, S. M., and Pearson, H. A. (1976). *Cancer* **37,** 853.
McIntosh, S., Fischer, D. B., Rothman, S. G., Rosenfield, N., Lobel, J. S., and O'Brien, R. T. (1977). *J. Pediatr.* **91,** 909.
McLeod, J. G., and Penny, R. (1969). *J. Neurol. Neurosurg. Psychiatr.* **32,** 297.
Maas, A. I. R. (1977). *J. Neurol. Neurosurg. Psychiat.* **40,** 655, 666.
Mahaley, M. S., Huneycutt, H., and Boone, H. (1961). *Cancer Chemother. Rep.* **11,** 29.

Mann, A. M., and Hutchinson, J. L. (1967). *Can. Med. Assoc. J.* **97,** 1350.

Margileth, D. A., Poplack, D. G., Pizzo, P. A., and Leventhal, B. G. (1977). *Cancer* **39,** 58.

Markson, J. L., and Flatman, G. E. (1965). *Br. Med. J.* **1,** 1228.

Martins, J. B., Reichlin, S., and Brown, G. M. (1977). "Clinical Neuroendocrinology," p. 340. David, Philadelphia.

Mathe, G., Schweisguth, O., Schneider, M., Amiel, J. L., Berunen, L., Brule, G., Cattan, A., and Schwarzengerg, L. (1963). *Lancet* **2,** 1077.

Meadows, A. T., and Evans, A. E. (1976). *Cancer* **37,** 1079.

Meadows, A. T., Krejmas, N. L., and Belasco, J. B. (1980). *In* "Status of the Curability of Childhood Cancers" (J. van Eys, and M. P. Sullivan, eds.), p. 263. Raven, New York.

Mikhael, M. A. (1978). *J. Comput. Assist. Tomogr.* **2,** 71.

Miller, J. J., III, Williams, G. F., and Leissring, J. G. (1971). *Am. J. Med.* **50,** 530.

Moress, G. R., D'Agostino, A. M., and Jarcho, L. W. (1967). *Arch. Neurol.* **16,** 377.

Moure, J. M. B., Whitecar, J. P., and Bodey, G. P. (1970). *Arch. Neurol.* **23,** 365.

Mubashir, B. A., and Bart, J. B. (1972). *N. Engl. J. Med.* **287,** 517.

Mueller, S., Bell, W., and Seibert, J. (1976). *J. Pediatr.* **88,** 650.

Muhlendahl, K. E., Gadner, H., Riehm, H., Helge, H., Weber, B., and Muller-Hess, R. (1976). *Helv. Pediatr. Acta* **31,** 463.

Murken, R. E., and Duvall, A. J. V. (1972). *Laryngoscope* **82,** 1306.

Myers, C. E., McGuire, W., and Young, R. (1976). *Cancer Treat. Rep.* **60,** 961.

Naiman, J. L., Rupprecht, L. M., Tanyeri, G., and Philippidis, P. (1970). *Lancet* **1,** 571.

Nelson, D. F., Reddy, K. V., O'Mara, R. E., and Rubin, P. (1978). *Cancer* **42,** 2553.

Nesbit, M. E., Ortega, J., and Donaldson, M. (1977). *Am. Soc. Clin. Oncol.* **13,** 201.

Norrell, H. N., Wilson, C. B., Slagel, D. E., and Clark, D. B. (1974). *Cancer* **33,** 923.

Ochs, J. J., Berger, P., Breder, M. L., Sinks, L. F., Kinkel, W., and Freeman, A. I. (1980). *Cancer* **45,** 2274.

Oettgen, H, F., Stephenson, P. A., Schwartz, M. K., Leeper, L. D., Talall, L., Tan, C. C., Clarkson, B. D., Golbey, R. B., Krakoff, H., Karnofsky, D. A., Murphy, M. C., and Burchenal, J. H. (1970). *Cancer* **25,** 253.

Ohnuma, T., Holland, J. F., Freeman, A., and Sinks, L. F. (1970). *Cancer Res.* **30,** 2297.

Oliff, A., Bleyer, W. A., and Poplack, D. G. (1978). *Lancet* **2,** 13.

Oliff, A., Bode, U., Vercu, B., DiChiro, G., Graves, V., and Poplack, D. G. (1979). *Med. Pediatr. Oncol.* **7,** 141.

Oliviero, V. T., Denham, C., DeVita, V. T., and Kelly, M. (1964). *Cancer Chemother. Rep.* **42,** 1.

Palmer, J. J. (1972). *Brain* **95,** 109.

Parker, R. G., and Bery H. C. (1976). *Cancer* **37,** 1162.

Parra, A., Santose, D., Cervantes, G., Sojo, I., Carranco, A., and Cortes-Gallegos, V. (1978). *J. Pediatr.* **92,** 117.

Pasquinucci, G., Pardini, R., and Fedi, F. (1970). *Lancet* **1,** 309.

Pennisi, A. J., Grushkin, G. M., and Lieberman, E. (1975). *Am. J. Dis. Child.* **129,** 315.

Perez, C. A. (1977). *In* "Clinical Pediatrics Oncology" (W. Sutow, T. Vietti, and D. Fernback, eds.), p. 139. Mosby, St. Louis.

Perry-Keene, D. A., Connelly, J. F., Young, R. A., Wettenhall, H. N. B., and Martin, F. I. R. (1976). *Clin. Endocrinol.* **5,** 373.

Peylan-Ramu, N., Poplack, D. G., Blei, C. L., Herdt, J. R., Vermess, M., and DiChiro, G. (1977). *J. Comput. Assist. Tumogr.* **1,** 216.

Peylan-Ramu, N., Poplack, D. G., Pizzo, P. A., Adornato, B. T., and DiChiro, G. (1978). *N. Engl. J. Med.* **298,** 6.

Phillips, T., Benals, S., and Ross, G. (1972). *Front. Radiat. Ther. Oncol.* **6,** 21.

Phillips, T. L., and Buschke, F. (1969). *Am. J. Roentgenol.* **105,** 659.

Pinkel, D. (1971). *J. Am. Med. Assoc.* **216,** 648.
Pizzo, P. A., Bleyer, W. A., Poplack, D. G., and Leventhal, G. G. (1976). *J. Pediatr.* **88,** 131.
Pizzo, P. A., Poplack, D. G., Bleyer, W. A. (1979). *Am. J. Hematol. Oncol.* **1,** 127.
Poussin-Rosillo, H., Nisoe, L. Z., and Lee, B. J. (1978). *Cancer* **42,** 437.
Powers, W. E., and Tolmach, L. J. (1963). *Nature (London)* **197,** 710.
Pratt, R. A., DiChiro, G., and Weed, J. C., Jr. (1977). *Surg. Neurol.* **77,** 117.
Price, R. A., and Jamieson, P. A. (1975). *Cancer* **35,** 306.
Primack, A. (1971). *J. Natl. Cancer Inst.* **47,** 223.
Prinz, R. A., Paloyan, E., Lawrence, A. M., Pickelman, J. R., Braithwaite, S., and Brocks, N. H. (1977). *Surgery* **82,** 296.
Probert, J. C., Parker, B. R., and Kaplan, H. S. (1973). *Cancer* **32,** 634.
Ragab, A. H., Frech, R. S., and Vietti, T. J. (1970). *Cancer* **25,** 580.
Reagon, T. J., Thomas, J. E., and Colby, M. Y. (1968). *J. Am. Med. Assoc.* **203,** 128.
Richard, G. E., Wara, W. M., Grumbach, M. M., Kaplan, S. L., Sheline, G. E., and Conte, F. A. (1976). *J. Pediatr.* **89,** 553.
Richter, P., Calamara, J. C., Morgenfeld, M. C., Kierszenbaum, A. L., Lavieri, J. C., and Mancini, R. E. (1970). *Cancer* **25,** 1026.
Riehl, J. L., and Brown, W. J. (1964). *Neurology* **14,** 254.
Risenborough, E. J., Grasias, S. L., Burton, R. I., and Jaffe, N. (1976). *J. Bone Joint Surg.* **58 A,** 526.
Robertson, G. L., Bhoopalam, N., and Zelkowitz, L. J. (1973). *Arch. Intern. Med.* **132,** 717.
Robinson, J. E., and Wizenberg, M. J. (1974). *Acta Radiol.* **13,** 241.
Roeser, H. P.. Stocks, A. E., and Smith, A. J. (1978). *Aust. N. Z. J. Med.* **8,** 250.
Rosenthal, M. B., and Goldfine, I. D. (1976). *J. Am. Med. Assoc.* **236,** 1591.
Rowley, M. M., Leach, D. R., Warner, G. A., and Heller, C. G. (1974). *Radiat. Res.* **59,** 665.
Rubin, P., and Casarett, G. W. (1972). *Front. Radiat. Ther. Oncol.* **6,** 1.
Rubinstein, L. J., Herman, M. M., Long, T. F., and Wilbur, J. R. (1975). *Cancer* **35,** 291.
Saiki, J. H., Thompson, S., Smith, F., and Atkinson, R. (1972). *Cancer* **29,** 370.
Samaan, N. A., Bakdash, M. M., Gaderao, J. B., Canfir, A., Jesse, R. H., and Ballantyn, A. J. (1975). *Ann. Intern. Med.* **83,** 771.
Samuels, M. C., Leary, W. B., and Alexauian, R. (1967). *Cancer* **20,** 1187.
Sanderson, P. A., Kuwabara, T., and Cogan, D. (1976). *Am. J. Ophthalmol.* **81,** 146.
Schiliro, G., Russo, Sciotto, A., Distefano, G., and Vigo, R. (1976). *Lancet* **2,** 1031.
Schimpff, S. C., Diggs, C. H., Wisell, J. G., Salvatore, P. C., and Wiernik, P. H. (1980). *Ann. Intern. Med.* **92,** 91.
Schochet, S. S., Jr., Lampert, P. W., and Earle, K. M. (1968). *J. Neuropathol. Exp. Neurol.* **27,** 645.
Shafer, R. B., Nuttall, F. Q., Pollack, K., and Kuisk, H. (1975). *Arch. Intern. Med.* **135,** 843.
Shalet, S. M., Beardwell, C. G., Pearson, D., and Morris-Jones, P. H. (1976). *Clin. Endocrinol.* **5,** 287.
Shalet, S. M., Beardwell, C. G., MacFarlane, T. A., Morris-Jones, P. H., and Pearson, D. (1977). *Acta Endocrinol.* **84,** 673.
Shalet, S. M., Price, D. A., Beardwell, C. G., Morris-Jones, P. H., and Pearson, D. (1979). *J. Pediatr.* **94,** 719.
Shapiro, W. R., Young, D. F., and Mehta, B. M. (1973a). *N. Engl. J. Med.* **293,** 161.
Shapiro, W. R., Chernik, N. L., and Posner, J. B. (1973b). *Arch. Neurol.* **28,** 96.
Shelanski, M. L., and Wisniewski, H. (1969). *Arch. Neurol.* **20,** 199.
Sheline, G. E. (1975). *Cancer* **35,** 957.
Sherins, R. J., and DeVita, V. T., Jr. (1973). *Ann. Intern. Med.* **79,** 216.

Sicher, K., and Backhouse, T. W. (1965). *Br. Med. J.* **1,** 858.
Sieber, S. M., and Adamson, R. H. (1975). *Adv. Cancer Res.* **22,** 57.
Silverberg, G. D., Britt, R. H., and Joffinet, D. R. (1978). *Cancer* **41,** 130.
Simila, S., Heikkinen, E., and Blanco, G. (1977). *Lancet* **1,** 1000.
Sinclair, W. K. (1968). *Radiat. Res.* **33,** 620.
Skipper, H. E., Sclabel, F. M., and Wilcox, W. S. (1964). *Cancer Chemother. Rep.* **35,** 1.
Slanina, J., Mussoff, K., Rahner, T., and Stiasny, R. (1977). *Int. J. Radiat. Oncol. Biol. Phys.* **2,** 1.
Smyth, J. F. (1976). *In* "Biological Characterization of Human Tumors," (W. Davis and E. Galtoni, eds.), p. 52. Excerpta Medica, Amsterdam.
Solheim, O. P. (1971). *Acta Radiol.* **10,** 474.
Speizer, B., Rubin, P., and Casarett, G. (1973). *Cancer* **32,** 692.
Spinetta, J. J. (1977). *J. Pediatr. Psych.* **2,** 49.
Stoffel, T. J., Nesbit, M. E., and Levitt, S. H. (1975). *Cancer* **35,** 1203.
Stolinsky, D. C., Solomon, J., Pugh, R. P., Stevans, A. R., Jacobs, E. M., Irwin, L. E., Wood, D. A., Steinfeld, J. L., and Bateman, J. R. (1970). *Cancer* **26,** 984.
Sullivan, M. P., Vietti, T. J., Fernbach, D. J., Griffith, K. M., Hardy, T. B., and Watkins, W. L. (1969). *Blood* **34,** 301.
Sunderman, C. R., and Pearson, H. A. (1969). *J. Pediatr.* **75,** 1058.
Sutow, W. W. (eds.) (1980). "Malignant Solid Tumors in Children, A Review." Raven, New York.
Swift, P. G. S., Kearney, P. J., Salton, R. G., Bullimore, J. A., Mott, M. G., and Savage, D. C. L. (1978). *Arch. Dis. Child.* **531,** 890.
Tan, C., Tasaka, H., Yu, K. P., Murphi, M. L., and Karnofsky, D. A. (1967). *Cancer* **20,** 333.
Tattersall, M. H., Parker, L. M., Pitman, S. W., and Frei, E., III (1975). *Cancer Chemother. Rep.* **6,** 25.
Terasima, T., and Tolmach, L. J. (1963). *J. Biophys.* **3,** 11.
Thompson, S. W., Saiki, J., and Kornfeld, M. (1971). *Neurology* **21,** 454.
Tobin, W., and Sandler, S. S. (1968). *Cancer Chemother. Rep.* **52,** 519.
Tolmach, L. J. (1961). *Ann. N.Y. Acad. Sci.* **95,** 743.
Uldall, P. R., Kerr, D. N. S., and Tacchi, D. (1972). *Lancet* **1,** 693.
Ushio, Y., Chernik, N. L., Posner, J. B., and Shapiro, W. R. (1977). *J. Neuropathol. Exp. Neurol.* **36,** 228.
Uy, Q. L., Moen, T. H., Johns, R̂. J., and Owens, A. H. (1967). *Bull. Johns Hopkins Hosp.* **121,** 349.
van Eys, J. J. (1977). *J. Sch. Health* **47,** 165.
van Eys, J. J. (1977). *In* "Clinical Pediatric Oncology" (W. W. Sutow, D. J. Fernbach, and T. Y. Vietti, eds.), p. 487. Mosby, St. Louis.
van Eys, J. J., and Sullivan, M. P. (eds.) (1980). "Status of the Curability of Childhood Cancers." Raven, New York.
Verity, G. L. (1968). *Radiology* **91,** 1221.
Verzosa, M. S., Aur, R. J. A., Simone, J. V., Hustu, M. O., and Pinkel, D. P. (1976). *J. Radiat. Oncol. Biol. Phys.* **1,** 209.
Vietti, T. J., and Valeriole, F. A. (1976). *Ped. Clin. N.A.* **23,** 67.
von Hoff, D. D., Rozenzweig, M., Layard, M., and Muggia, F. M. (1977). *Am. J. Med.* **62,** 200.
Wakem, C. J., and Bennett, J. M. (1975). *Aust. N. Z. J. Med.* **5,** 266.
Walker, M. D., Dalgard, D. W., and Hururtz, B. S. (1969). *Proc. Am. Assoc. Cancer Res.* **10,** 97.

Warne, G. L., Fairley, K. F., Hobbs, J. B., and Martin, F. I. R. (1973). *N. Engl. J. Med.* **189,** 1159.
Weiden, P. L., and Wright, S. E. (1972). *N. Engl. J. Med.* **286,** 1369.
Weiss, H. D., Walker, M. D., and Wiernik, P. H. (1974). *N. Engl. J. Med.* **291,** 75, 126.
Wheeler, K. T., and Lett, J. T. (1974). *Proc. Natl. Acad. Sci. U.S.A.* **71,** 1862.
Whittaker, J. A., Parry, D. H., Bunch, C., and Weatherall, J. (1973). *Br. Med. J.* **4,** 335.
Willoughby, M. L. N. (1976). *Br. Med. J.* **1,** 864.
Wilson, C. B., and Norrell, H. A., Jr. (1969). *Cancer* **23,** 1038.
Wolff, L., Zighelboim, G., and Sale, R. P. (1979). *Cancer* **43,** 83.
Wolfson, S., and Olney, M. B. (1957). *J. Am. Med. Assoc.* **165,** 239.
Wright, T. L., and Bresnan, M. J. (1976). *Neurology* **26,** 540.
Young, D. F., Shapiro, W. R., and Mehta, B. (1974). *Proc. Am. Assoc. Cancer Res.* **15,** 140.
Zubrod, C. G. (1970). *Pediatrics* **45,** 555.
Zwartjes, W. J. (1980). *In* "Status of the Curability of Childhood Cancers" (J. van Eys and M. P. Sullivan, eds.), p. 277. Raven, New York.

Biological Properties of ICRF-159 and Related Bis(dioxopiperazine) Compounds

EUGENE H. HERMAN,* DONALD T. WITIAK,† KURT HELLMANN,‡ AND VAMAN S. WARAVDEKAR§

* *Division of Drug Biology, Food and Drug Administration, Washington, D.C.*
† *Division of Medicinal Chemistry, College of Pharmacy, Ohio State University Columbus, Ohio*
‡ *Imperial Cancer Research Fund, Lincoln's Inn Fields, London, England*
and
§ *Office of the Director, National Cancer Institute, National Institutes of Health Bethesda, Maryland*

I. Historical . . . 249
II. Chemistry and Structure–Activity Relationships . . . 250
III. Biological Characteristics . . . 260
A. Cytotoxicity . . . 260
B. Cell Cycle Specificity . . . 264
C. Antimetastatic Activity . . . 266
IV. Radiosensitization . . . 268
V. Pharmacology . . . 269
VI. Toxicology . . . 270
A. Preclinical ICRF-159 . . . 270
B. Clinical ICRF-159 . . . 271
C. Preclinical ICRF-187 . . . 272
D. Clinical ICRF-187 . . . 274
VII. Clinical . . . 274
VIII. Interactions of ICRF Compounds with Other Agents . . . 278
IX. Prospective Views . . . 286
References . . . 286
Note Added in Proof . . . 290

I. Historical

The bis(dioxopiperazines) were first synthesized in the late 1950s by Geigy chemists (U.K. patent 961065) with the objective that they might be useful as textile leveling agents or possibly as pharmaceuticals, however, no clear indication for their use was given. These compounds were later synthesized by Creighton (1970, 1971) as potential intracellular activated chelating agents and were shown to elicit antitumor activity against sarcoma 180 and leukemia L1210 (Creighton *et al.*, 1969) and inhibit [^{3}H]thymidine incorporation into the cellular DNA of mouse fibroblasts (Creighton *et al.*, 1969).

ISBN 0-12-032919-0

Although no firm evidence has yet been presented regarding the intra- or extracellular chelating action of these compounds it appears that the antitumor action is probably independent of this activity. The initial antitumor observations made with ICRF-154 and ICRF-159 led subsequently to a systematic study of a family of bis(dioxopiperazines) at the Imperial Cancer Research Fund (ICRF) laboratories in London.

Clinical studies with ICRF-154 (NSC 129942) were soon initiated but in a Phase I/II study in patients with either acute leukemia or malignant melanoma it was found to be totally devoid of activity (Hellmann *et al.*, 1969). Chemical exploration of the bis(dioxopiperazine) series led to the conclusion that the antimitotic activity resided in a very closely defined structure, one of which was ICRF-159; (NSC 129943, ICI 59118) the official name given to this compound by the British Pharmacopoeia Commission is razoxane.

ICRF-159 in contrast to ICRF-154 appeared to be well absorbed and showed some activity. It produced remissions in children with acute leukemia and non-Hodgkin's disease (Hellmann *et al.*, 1969; Mathé *et al.*, 1970; Krepler and Pawlowsky, 1975) and it did so with few side effects.

These studies were accompanied by toxicology (Gralla *et al.*, 1974) and pharmacokinetic investigations (Creaven *et al.*, 1974, 1975; Sadee *et al.*, 1975). A number of Phase I and II studies were set up in the United States, some of which are still in progress.

Clinical trials of ICRF-159 in the United Kingdom were sporadic at first followed later by several major studies; however, only two of these studies used the drug as a single agent. In one trial razoxane was used as adjuvant treatment in resectable colorectal cancer (Gilbert *et al.*, 1981) and as single agent treatment in acute and chronic leukemia (Bakowski *et al.*, 1979). In addition there has been a study to determine possible activity in psoriasis (Atherton *et al.*, 1980). Studies at the Mayo Clinic and elsewhere have found no activity in melanoma (Ahmann *et al.*, 1978), breast cancer (Ahmann *et al.*, 1977), non-oat cell carcinoma of the bronchus (Eagan *et al.*, 1976), or cancer of the prostate (Kvols *et al.*, 1977).

In combination with radiotherapy it has significantly prolonged the recurrence free interval of soft tissue sarcomas (Ryall *et al.*, 1974).

II. Chemistry and Structure–Actvity Relationships

Ethylenediaminetetraacetic acid (EDTA **1**) failed to demonstrate any significant antitumor activity (Leiter *et al.*, 1959), however a few compounds synthesized in a series of bis(dioxopiperazines) did exert cytotoxic activity (Creighton *et al.*, 1969; Creighton, 1970). Ethyl (**2**) and methyl (**3**) esters of EDTA were inactive and reaction between the EDTA and formamide in an attempt to prepare the tetraamide (**4**) generally yielded diimides (**5**) via loss of ammonia. Initial screening results with the bis(dioxopiperazine) of EDTA (ICRF-154; **5**) were encouraging and prompted synthesis of other derivatives. Early investigations revealed that antitumor activity was retained by insertion of methyl (ICRF-159; **6**) but not by ethyl substitution (ICRF-192; **7**) of the central ethylene chain. Racemic ICRF-159 and both its optical isomers, the + enantiomorph of which is known as ICRF-187, exhibited significant antitumor activity as did meso isomer **8** (ICRF-193). Meso **8** was much more toxic possibly reflecting increased lipophilicity owing to insertion of methyl functions. However, inhibition of [^{3}H]thymidine incorporation was lost in the *dl*-diastereoisomer of **8** (namely **13**). Other *dl*-erythro (**9–12**) and *dl*-threo (**14**)

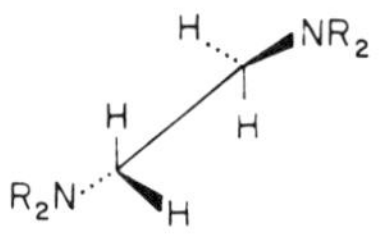

1, R = CH_2CO_2H
2, R = CH_2CO_2Et
3, R = CH_2CO_2Me
4, R = CH_2CONH_2

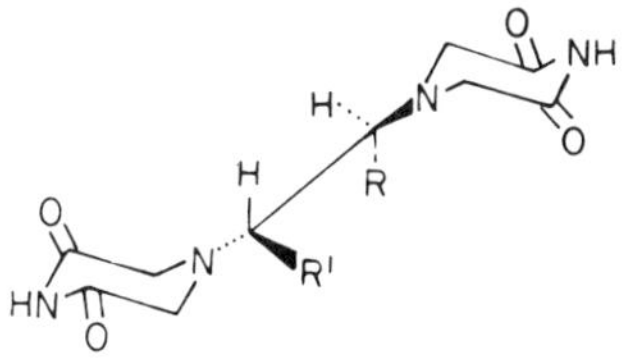

5, R = R' = H (ICRF-154)
6, R = H, R' = Me (ICRF-159; ICRF-187 = + enantiomer)
7, R = H, R' = Et (ICRF-192)

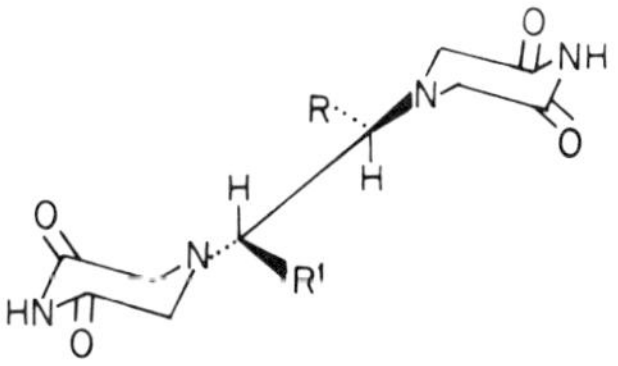

8, R = R' = Me (ICRF-193)
9, R = Me, R' = n-Pr
10, R = Me, R' = i-Pr
11, R = Me, R' = CH_2OMe
12, R = Et, R' = n-Pr

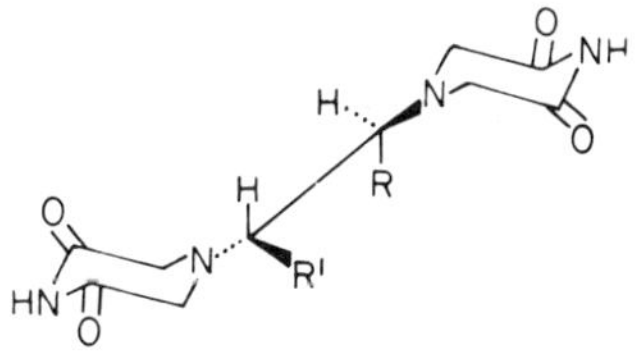

13, R = R' = Me (dl)
14, R = Me, R' = CH_2OMe

analogs of increased lipophilicity have considerably decreased activity in this regard (Creighton, 1970, 1974). Creighton *et al.* (1969) also observed that the hydrolysis product of ICRF-154 (**5**), namely, *N*,*N'*-dicarboxamidomethyl-*N*,*N'*-dicarboxymethyl-1,2-diaminoethane (**15**), also was inactive.

In cell culture [^{14}C]ICRF-159 (**6**) uptake has been compared with the corresponding ^{14}C-labeled 1,2-propylenediaminetetraacetic acid (**16**) and inactive 1,3-isomer (**17**) (Livingston *et al.*, 1972). [^{14}C]ICRF-159 was taken up rapidly by mouse embryo fibroblast cells, but the net amount of label within or attached to the cells decreased after 1.5 hours. This was followed by a rise after 5 hours. The highly polar tetraacid (**16**) was absorbed very slowly, but after 24 hours the concentration in cells was greater than the concentration found for ICRF-159. Incubation of [^{14}C]ICRF-159 with whole calf thymus histone for 2 hours at 37°C followed by gel filtration showed a significant association of the label with histones. Since the inactive isomer (**17**) did not associate with histone under these conditions, it was proposed (Livingston *et al.*, 1972) that specific binding of [^{14}C]ICRF-159 to histones might result in interference with DNA transcription and subsequent inhibition of DNA synthesis (Creighton and Birnie, 1970).

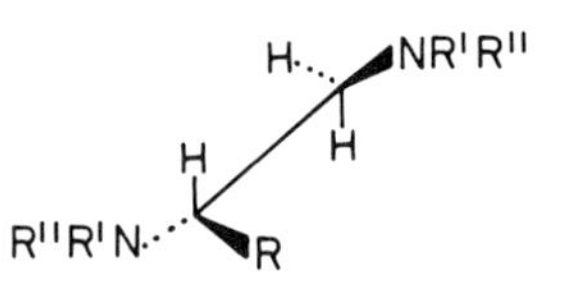

15, R = H, R' = CH_2CONH_2, R'' = CH_2CO_2H **17**

16, R = Me, R' = R'' = CH_2CO_2H

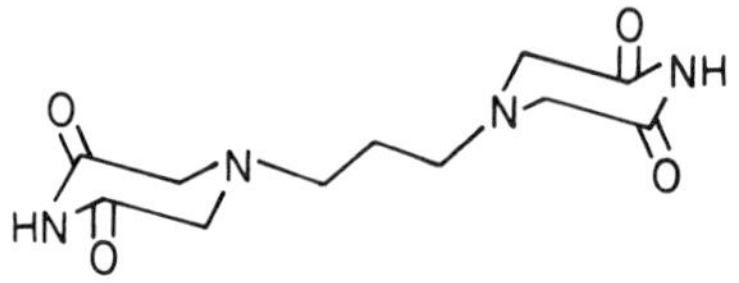

Several reviews (Wasserman *et al.*, 1973; Hellmann, 1972b; Sartorelli and Johns, 1975; Bakowski, 1976; Bellet *et al.*, 1977) concerning ICRF-159 have appeared and attest to the interest generated by the compounds. ICRF-193 proved to be too toxic in preclinical trials (Creighton *et al.*, 1969) and ICRF-154 given orally lacked biological activities in man (Hellmann *et al.*, 1969). Analogs of ICRF-154 (**5**) and 159 (**6**) are administered dissolved in oil or in suspension with carboxymethylcellulose. Racemic ICRF-159 has a solubility of only 3 mg/ml in water at 25°C (Repta *et al.*, 1976). Use of cosolvents, complexation, chemically derived prodrugs, or crystalline modification to overcome low water solubility problems in clinical tests requiring concentrations of 25 mg/ml were unsuccessful. However, the resolved enantiomers (+)*S* and (−)*R* of ICRF-159 individually possessed significantly greater water solubility when compared to racemic material. Interestingly, using the single crystal X-ray diffraction analysis, Camerman and Camerman (1981) have shown that the racemic compound (ICRF-159) in the crystalline state has the eclipsed conformation whereas the resolved material (ICRF-187) has the anticonformation. The number and degrees of intermolecular attraction in the racemate crystal structure are far greater than in the crystal structure of the enantiomer thereby accounting for differences in solubility between the two crystal forms. Whereas solubility differences between ICRF-159 and 187 are beneficial for drug formulation, antitumor activity for each enantiomer is equivalent to that of the racemate. However, because of solubility advantages ICRF-187 has been preferred in most recent investigations. Comparative analysis also revealed no differences in stability, uptake, metabolism, or binding which could explain why ICRF-159 (**6**) and 154 (**5**) are cytotoxic, but ICRF-192 (**7**) is not (Dawson, 1975).

In mouse embryo fibroblast cultures incubation for 22 hours with 5 μg/ml of ICRF-159 inhibited incorporation of pyrimidine into DNA by 62–69%, whereas syntheses of RNA and protein were inhibited by only 22–30 and 18%, respectively. Incubation of cell cultures with ICRF-193 (0.13 μg/ml) for 22 hours similarly inhibited DNA synthesis by 64–68%, whereas synthesis of RNA and protein was affected to a much smaller degree (34 and 16% inhibition, respectively). Neither cell death nor a detergent action could be invoked to explain inhibition of DNA synthesis by these analogs (Creighton and Birnie, 1970).

In addition to their possible role as chelating agents following metabolic degradation, Creighton and Birnie (1970) have suggested that the imide rings of the bis(dioxopiperazines) may function as acylating groups undergoing reaction *in vivo* with various amines, thiols, and phosphates. Although such compounds may act as bifunctional acylating agents on DNA the relative stability of imides would speak against this possibility. Clearly, further work is required to determine chemical mechanisms by which these compounds exert their effect. Nonetheless, structural requirements for antitumor activity in this area seem to be relatively specific. Replacement of the dioxopiperazine rings with other heterocyclic functions (**18–23**) led to inactive compounds. Activity also seems to be limited to those compounds in which the sum of the carbons in the central chain was not more than 5. Thus, the *trans*-cyclohexane bis(dioxopiperazine) exhibited little or no activity (Creighton, 1970).

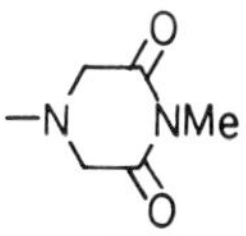

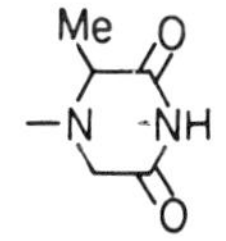

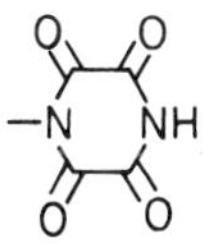

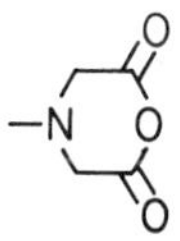

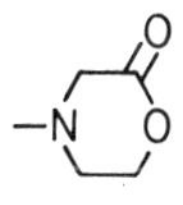

Witiak *et al.* (1977) suggested that *trans*- and *cis*-cyclopropyl analogs (**24** and **25**) could represent ideal molecules for assessing stereochemical requirements for biological activity since the molecular weights of the acyclic (**6**) and cyclic (**24** and **25**) compounds differ by only 2 hydrogen atoms. Possibly, lipophilicity differences between acyclic and cyclic analogs would not differ markedly and differences in activity might better reflect

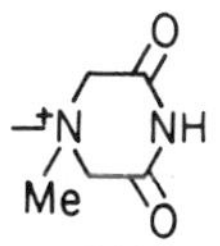

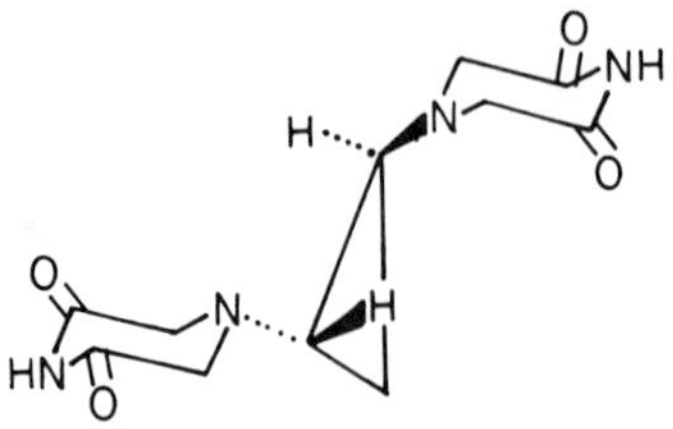

24

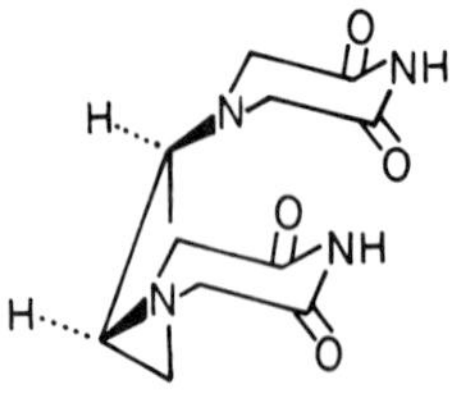

25

differences in molecular geometry. However, solubility differences between *cis*- and *trans*-cyclopropane dioxopiperazines have also been observed (Zwilling *et al.*, 1981) and these, in addition to geometric differences, may be responsible for the observed differences in biological activities.

Creighton (1970) previously had shown that meso isomer **8,** expected to be most stable in the anticonformation, was more potent than ICRF-159 in blocking $[^3H]$thymidine incorporation into the DNA of mouse embryo fibroblasts. Its diastereomer **13** was inactive. Cyclobutyl analog *trans*-26, which is stereochemically related to *dl*-**13** (when the dioxopiperazine functions are in the anticonformation), was considerably less potent than either ICRF-159 (**6**) or meso-**8** when assessed for its ability to block $[^3H]$thymidine incorporation into mouse embryo fibroblasts (Creighton, 1970). Evaluation of *cis*-cyclobutyl analogs has not been reported since attempted preparation of the precursor *cis*-diamine by Curtius rearrangement afforded a violent explosion (Witiak *et al.*, 1981). Landgrebe (1981) experienced a similar explosion during attempted synthesis of the *cis*-cyclopropane-1,2-diamine precursor to **25** by Curtius rearrangement of the bis(acid azide).

The relatively nontoxic nature of *trans*-cyclopropyl bis(dioxopiperazine) (**24**) in V-79A fibroblasts in tissue culture is in accord with the reported decrease in activity for the *trans*-cyclobutyldioxopiperazine in the sarcoma 180, leukemia L1210, and $[^3H]$thymidine assays (Creighton, 1970). The decrease in activity observed for analogs **24** and **26** (Witiak *et al.*, 1977) has been suggested to be a reflection of their structural relationships to inactive *dl*-**13** (Creighton, 1970). However, cis analog **25** was not assessed in the V-79A system. For cytotoxicity, the order of increasing potency ($24 < 16 < 27 < 28 < 6$) did not follow the exact order of increasing mutagenicity ($24 < 16 < 28 < 6 < 27$). However those compounds which were among the most mutagenic were also among the most cytotoxic. Owing to marked differences in chemical properties between imides (**6** and **24**) and tetraacids (**16** and **28**), Witiak *et al.* (1977) suggested that their modes of actions are also likely to differ. The rigid trans geometry for **24** rendered the compound less toxic and mutagenic in these tests than its acyclic analog ICRF-159 (**6**). Interestingly, for the strongly chelating tetraacid precursors to the bis(dioxopiperazines), the rigid trans geometry of **28** rendered the compound more toxic at all concentrations and generally more mutagenic than acyclic analog **16.** That tetraester **27** is more mutagenic than tetraacid **28** may be a reflection of enhanced cellular uptake of this non-zwitterionic compound. However, Witiak *et al.* (1977) suggested that if sequestering cations in the medium were responsible for the cytotoxic effects, both **16** and **28** would be expected to be equally active; if asymmetric "error-free postreplication gap filling" enzymes were involved one might anticipate a difference in activity between **16** and **28** and such differences in mutagenicity were observed.

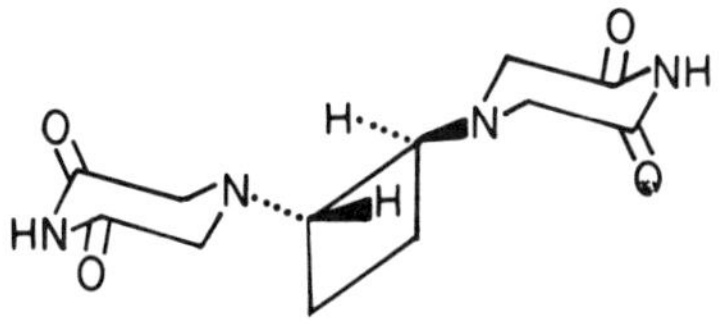

26

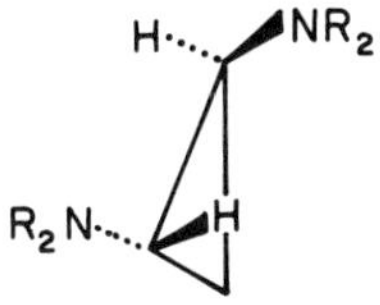

27, R=CH_2CO_2Me (HCl salt)
28, R=CH_2CO_2H

At rather high concentrations ($10^{-3}\,M$) cyclopropyl tetraacid **28,** one of the most cytotoxic and mutagenic agents studied, was the most effective blocker of scheduled DNA synthesis, but a weak inducer of unscheduled DNA synthesis. Possibly, the differential action of **28** at higher concentrations reflects inhibition of asymmetric enzymes involved in both scheduled and unscheduled DNA synthesis, thus permitting DNA damage, caused by the compound, to enter DNA replication with subsequent activation of "error-prone" postreplication repair processes. All other analogs (**6, 24,** and **16**) examined showed a decreased ability to inhibit scheduled DNA synthesis and induce unscheduled DNA synthesis as a function of dose. Again, the considerably decreased effect of cyclopropyl bis(dioxopiperazine) when compared to ICRF-159 (**6**) likely reflects its unfavorable rigid trans geometry. Acyclic tetraacid (**16**) exhibited only marginal effects on scheduled DNA synthesis, an observation consistent with the lack of cytotoxicity reported for acyclic tetraacids.

In addition to their activity in mammalian tissue culture assays bis(dioxopiperazines) such as ICRF-187 are active in reducing daunorubicin toxicity (Herman *et al.,* 1974, 1979). Although ICRF analogs 192 (**7**) and 200 (**29**) also provided some protection against daunorubicin-induced toxicity, analogs 154 (**6**), 158 (**30**), 193 (**8**), and 202 (**31**) were devoid of such properties. Additionally, none of the cyclopropyl bis(dioxopiper-

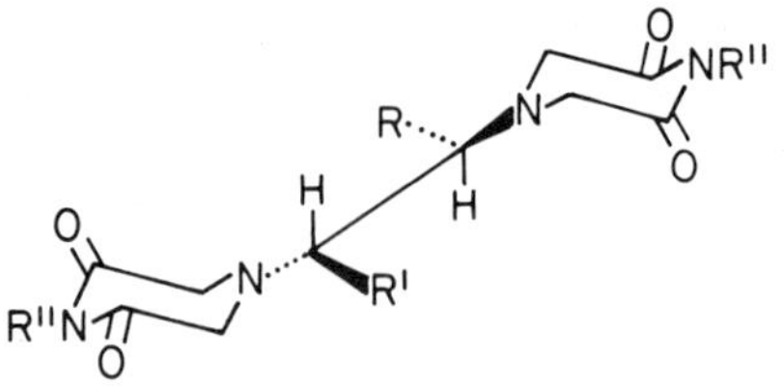

29, R = R'' = Me, R' = H (ICRF-200)

30, R = R' = H, R'' = Me (ICRF-158)

31, R = Me, R' = Et, R'' = H (ICRF-202)

azines) or their synthetic intermediates were active in this assay at equivalent doses.

Since structural influences on pharmacokinetic parameters may reflect differences in the ability of a given compound to protect against daunorubicin-induced toxicity, direct extrapolation of these results to intrinsic protection cannot be done at this time. For a more detailed discussion of ICRF-187 effects on anthracycline-induced toxicity the reader is referred to Section VIII.

The observation that ICRF-159 (**6**) inhibits metastasis in the Lewis lung tumor (3LL) animal model without impeding the growth of the primary implant (Hellmann and Burrage, 1969; Salsbury *et al.,* 1970; Burrage *et al.,* 1970; Hellmann, 1972a; LeServe, 1971; LeServe and Hellmann, 1972; James and Salsbury, 1974; Salsbury *et al.,* 1974; Hoover and Ketcham, 1975; Hellmann *et al.,* 1973, 1974) provided the impetus for Witiak *et al.* (1978) to investigate stereoselective effects on metastases by examining both the *cis-* and *trans-*cyclopropyl bis(dioxopiperazines) **25** and **24** in Syrian hamster lung adenocarcinoma (LG1002). Following intraperitoneal administration of ICRF-159 or the *cis-* and *trans*-cyclopropyl analogs at doses of 15 mg/kg, only the open chain and cis compound reduced metastatic growth whereas the trans compound stimulated the number of metastases in the lung. In this animal model, the trans isomer stimulated growth of the primary tumor whereas ICRF-159 (**6**) and *cis*-**25** had no effect on primary tumor growth. It was suggested that the potentiating effects of the trans isomer may be related to an effect on cell volume and glycosaminoglycan biosynthesis as proposed by Lazo *et al.* (1978), whereas the cis isomer may selectively cause normalization of developing blood vessels in the primary tumor and, thus, inhibit metastasis by angiometamorphic mechanisms (Salsbury *et al.,* 1970; James and Salsbury, 1974). The angiometamorphic effect is not unique to 3LL infected animals (LeServe and Hellmann, 1972; Stephens and Creighton, 1974; Atherton,

1975), but histological features suggested that the antimetastatic effects of ICRF-159 in an experimental transplanted murine squamous carcinoma did not depend upon morphological changes in vascularity (Peters, 1975). Furthermore, ICRF-159 did not reduce metastases in all tumor models (Pimm and Baldwin, 1975).

Lazo *et al.* (1978) observed the incubation of exponentially growing B16 melanoma cells with ICRF-159 significantly increased their *in vivo* colony forming efficiency. To explore further stereostructure activity relationships, as a prerequisite to mechanism studies, Zwilling *et al.* (1981) reexamined the activity of ICRF-159, *cis*- and *trans*-cyclopropyl analogs (**25** and **24**), and various tetraacids [EDTA (**1**), **16, 28, 32**] and tetraesters (**27,33**) using the syngeneic B16-F1 and F10 melanoma in C57BL/6 mice (Fidler and Nicolson, 1976). Stereoisomeric analogs **24** and **25** again exhibited opposing effects on the ability of the B16 melanoma to form lung colonies. When cultures of B16-F10 cell lines were pretreated for 24 hours with the trans analog at concentrations of 2 and 20 μM, an increase in lung colony formation was noted. Pretreatment with the cis isomer **25** reduced lung colony formation. The effect of 2 μM ICRF-159 (**6**) was similar to that of the cis isomer at that concentration. A concentration of 20 μM resulted in an increased number of lung colonies although the increase was not statistically significant. Results with regard to colony formation *in vitro* paralleled those obtained *in vivo* except with the cis isomer. While lung colony formation was inhibited by the cis isomer, colony formation *in vitro* was stimulated at 20 and 100 μM drug concentrations. Using the nonmetastasizing B16-F1 melanoma cell line, neither the cis nor trans isomer had an affect on lung colony formation. Treatment of tumor cells with ICRF-159 or related stereoisomeric analogs did not affect the viability of the tumor cells even after 3 days cocultivation.

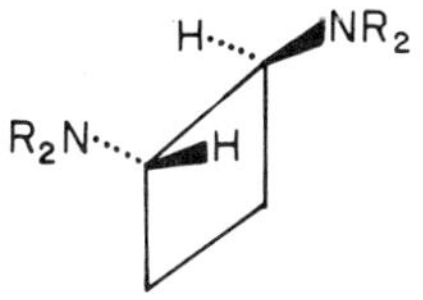

32, R = CH_2CO_2H

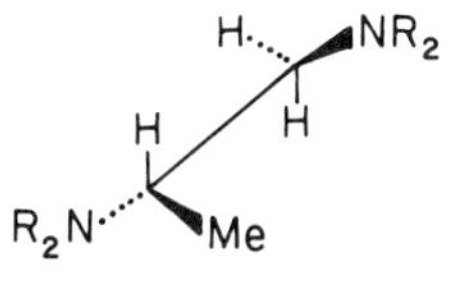

33, R = CH_2CO_2Me (2HCl)

In the B16-F1 melanoma model, injection of either the cis or trans isomers into tumor bearing animals resulted in an accelerated primary tumor growth. Palpable tumors were detected as early as 6 days after implantation and grew to a size of 100 to 250 mm^2 after 22 days. In contrast, tumors from animals injected with ICRF-159 did not appear until 17 days and were only 30 mm^2 in size after 22 days. Tumors from animals treated with saline or carboxymethylcellulose appeared from 12 to 15 days after implantation and reached 60 to 80 mm^2 by day 22. Little or no effect was observed for various synthetic intermediate zwitterionic acids (**16, 28, 32**) and tetraesters (**27, 33**), suggesting that bis(dioxopiperazine) functions play an important role in the stereoselective antimetastatic process. However, EDTA (**1**) treated tumor cells yielded significant decreases in lung colony formation at 2 and 100 *M* concentrations. Unpublished results from Adria Laboratories (Wolgemuth *et al.*, 1981) have shown that cis and trans analogs (**25** and **24**) or ICRF-159 inhibited lung colony formation (as assessed on day 17) when treated on days 1–9 following B16 melanoma tumor implantation. This action occurred at doses which had no effect on the primary tumor. However, when drug administration was begun 1 day prior to implantation, the trans isomer (**24**) enhanced primary tumor growth as well as lung metastasis whereas the cis analog had no effect on primary tumor growth and inhibited metastases.

The results of Zwilling *et al.* (1981) tend to indicate that ICRF-159 and the *cis*-cyclopropyl (**25**) isomer may inhibit metastases by a mechanism independent of an angiometamorphic effect because the tumor cells were pretreated with the drugs and no primary tumor was established. Although these stereoisomers proved to be noncytotoxic in tumor cells, they affected colony formation *in vitro*. This effect did not correlate with lung colony formation *in vivo*. Rather, colony formation *in vitro*, which was stimulated by both the cis and trans isomers, seemed to correlate best with the accelerated growth rates of the tumors in animals injected with these compounds (Zwilling *et al.*, 1981). Differences in reported stimulatory (Lazo *et al.*, 1978) and antimetastatic effects (Zwilling *et al.*, 1981) for ICRF-159 in the B16 model may reflect differences in protocol, use of EDTA, and percentage lung colony formation observed.

Target tricyclic analogs *trans*–anti-*trans*-**34** and *cis*–syn-*trans*-**35** having a "cisoid" relationship of dioxopiperazine rings similar to those found in *cis*-**25** were constructed in order to further assess stereostructure–activity relationships and provide analogs not having the undesirable solubility differences observed with the cyclopropane systems (Witiak *et al.*, 1981). Stereoisomers **34** and **35** are related to ICRF-154 (**5**) and differ only by 1 mole of hydrogen in molecular weight from this open chain structure. These compounds may be visualized as piperazine analogs of the ethylenediamine function in *cis*-**25** wherein the CH_2 of the cyclopropane ring is deleted and a C–C bond is formed between the C_2 and C_2^1 positions of the dioxopiperazine rings. Results with these tricyclic bis(dioxopiperazines) were compared with selected synthetic intermediates (**36, 37**, and **38**) on experimental metastasis using the B16-F10 melanoma model. Both **34** and tetraester **36** resulted in significantly decreased lung colony formation at all dose levels. Intermediate ester imide **37** exhibited no effect. When *trans*-**34** was compared to **35** and bicyclic analog **38** only **34** significantly inhibited metastases at all doses. Neither **35** nor **38** had any effect.

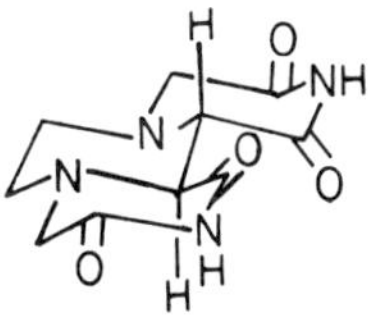

34 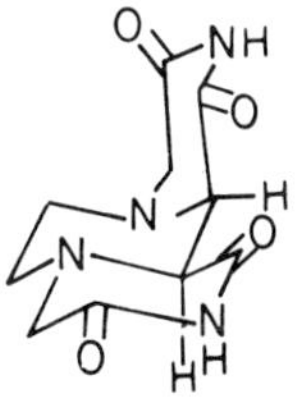 35

Witiak *et al.* (1981) rationalized that for bis(dioxopiperazines), antimetastatic activity seems to be independent of a preferred spacial orientation. Although the "cisoid" relationship of the bis(dioxopiperazine) rings found in **25** and **34** appears to be important for antimetastatic activity, the inactivity of **35,** also having "cisoid" bis(dioxopiperazine) rings, suggests that certain preferred conformations are required. Whereas ICRF-159 has a cis relationship of hetero rings in the crystalline state, the + isomer has a trans geometry indicating that differences in rotational energy between these two forms is small (Camerman and Camerman, 1981) and easily could be overcome during binding to macromolecules of biological consequence. It may well be that antimetastatic properties *in vitro* are a reflection of an eclipsed conformation similar to the juxtaposition of rings found in **25** and **34.** The stereoselective antimetastatic activity of **34** and **35** is of particular interest. These compounds have similar solubility properties and may serve as probes for mechanistic studies since their syntheses (3 to 4 steps) are relatively short in comparison to cyclopropane geometric isomers **24** and **25** which require 9 to 10 steps. The antimetastatic properties observed for analog **36** are unique since all other bis(dioxopiperazine) synthetic intermediates (Zwilling *et al.*, 1981) have no significant antimetastatic properties.

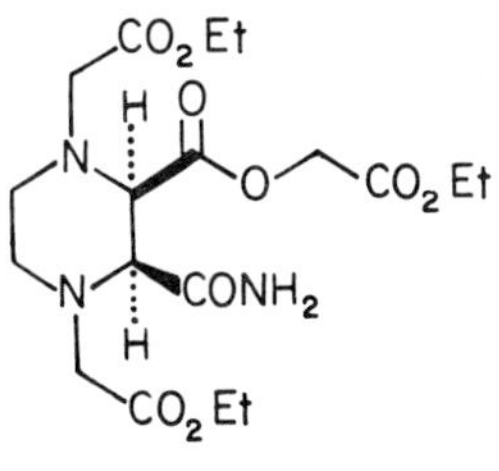

36 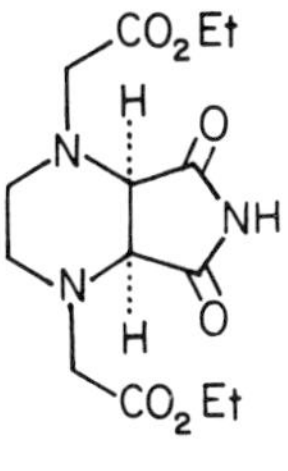 37 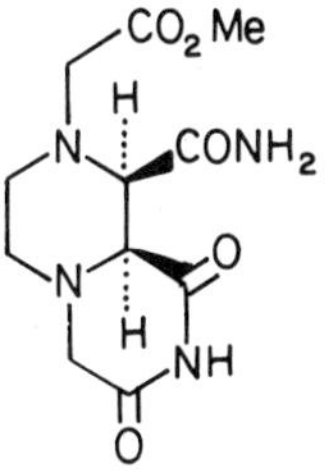 38

III. Biological Characteristics

A. Cytotoxicity

ICRF-159 inhibits cell division of most dividing cells *in vitro* and *in vivo*. *In vitro* it is active at approximately 1–5 μg/ml (Hellmann and Field, 1970), but *in vivo* effective doses show a good deal more variation (Creighton *et al.*, 1969). The *in vivo* tumor most sensitive to ICRF-159 is the solid sarcoma 180 with an ED_{90} of approximately 5 mg/kg. On the other hand some tumors such as the Lewis lung carcinoma are more resistant and the ED_{90} for this tumor is in the region of 30 mg/kg. Much depends on the scheduling of the dose since it is not the total daily dose but the number of doses given in 24 hours which influences activity. This effect is almost certainly connected with the fact that the drug is active only at one short period of the cell cycle and only a small proportion of cells is at the vulnerable phase during a single administration of the drug. Since the drug is also excreted rapidly (Field *et al.*, 1971) the delay in tumor growth which one dose, no matter how large, can produce is very small; on the other hand the delay which small doses, given repeatedly, can produce may be considerable.

Woodman *et al.* (1971) compared the effects of ICRF-159 and ICRF-154 against early and advanced leukemia L1210 and against leukemia P-388. The results showed that although both these compounds displayed activity against early and advanced leukemia L1210, ICRF-159 was more effective than ICRF-154.

Investigations on the influence of treatment schedules of ICRF-159 and ICRF-154 on leukemia P-388 revealed that a daily schedule or a day 1, 5, 9 schedule for these compounds produced higher increases in life span of leukemic mice than administration only on day 1. In the case of ICRF-159, the schedule of q3h/24h on days 1, 5, 9 was more effective in further extending the survival of the animals than if the total dose of the agent was given at one time on the same 3 days.

The effect of ICRF-159 was examined on several transplanted tumors (Table I).[1] AK lymphoma and leukemia L1210 resistant to BCNU (NSC 409962), cyclocytidine, vincristine or cytosine arabinoside (NSC 63878) were responsive to the action of ICRF-159 as were DC8F1 mammary carcinoma and Walker carcinosarcoma 256. In contrast, other tumors, such as xenografts of lung, breast and colon were not affected by the drug.

Several chemotherapeutic drugs including ICRF-159 have been employed against C1300 murine neuroblastoma as a model for the study of

[1] We are grateful to Drs. Venditti, Narayanan, Paull, Geran, Wolpert, and Schumacher of the Development Therapeutics Program, DCT, NCI for providing biological data on these ICRF compounds.

TABLE I

EFFECT OF ICRF-159 ON EXPERIMENTAL TUMORS

Tumor systems[a]	
Responsive[b]	Less or nonresponsive[c]
AK lymphoma	Colon 26
B16 melanoma	Colon 36
L1210 lymphoid leukemia	Colon 51
L1210 leukemia/cytosine arabinoside	C3H mammary adenocarcinoma
L1210 leukemia/BCNU	C3H mammary carcinoma
L1210 leukemia/cyclocytidine	Colon xenograft
P388 lymphocytic leukemia	Ependymoblastoma
P388 leukemia/vincristine	Lewis lung carcinoma
CD8F1 mammary carcinoma*	M5076 ovarian carcinoma
Walker carcinosarcoma 256*	Madison Lung
Sarcoma 180*	P388 leukemia/adriamycin
Ca 755*	Breast xenograft*
	Colon 38*
	Lung xenograft*

[a] Evaluation of median survival time (MST) or mean tumor weight (MTW*) for test over control in percent, i.e., T/C.

[b] Greater than minimal response, MST = T/C > 130%, MTW = T/C < 42%.

[c] Those with minimal or less than minimal response.

CNS disease in children (Finkelstein *et al.,* 1975). The results indicated that ICRF-159 did not cause the tumor to regress but prolonged the life span of the treated animals by 50 percent.

The effect of ICRF-187 (NSC 169780), the more water-soluble *d* isomer of ICRF-159, was examined against several transplantable tumors (Table II). A pronounced antitumor effect was achieved against leukemia L1210 and leukemia P-388, but less effect was observed with Lewis lung carcinoma, melanoma B16, mammary tumor, ependymoblastoma, and colon 38. The compound failed to show any effect on colon 26, lung and breast xenografts, and ovarian carcinoma.

The treatment schedule plays an important role in antitumor activity of ICRF-187 (Fig. 1). A dose of 16 mg/kg per injection every 3 hours on days 1, 5, and 9 increased the mean survival time (MST) from 9 to 27 days. Doses above 16 mg/kg were toxic and survival time was close to that of the untreated controls. Figure 1 also illustrates that by maintaining the same schedule of treatment but administrating the total dose at one time the survival time of leukemic mice was markedly reduced. It appears therefore that optimal antitumor activity is achieved when the dose of ICRF-187 is divided and given at frequent intervals in a day. The route of

TABLE II

EFFECT OF ICRF-187 (NSC-169780) ON SEVERAL TRANSPLANTED TUMORS

Tumor system	Effect[a]
Leukemia L1210	Responsive[b]
Leukemia P388	Responsive[b]
Lewis lung carcinoma	Minimal response
Melanoma B16	Minimal response
Mammary $CD8F_1$*	Minimal response
Ependymoblastoma	Minimal response
Colon 38	Minimal response
Colon 26	No response
Lung xenograft LX-1*	No response
Breast xenograft MS-1*	No response
Ovarian carcinoma M5076	No response

[a] Evaluation of median survival time (MST) or mean tumor weight (MTW*) for test over control in percent, i.e., T/C.

[b] Greater than minimal response, MST = T/C > 130%, MTW = T/C < 42%.

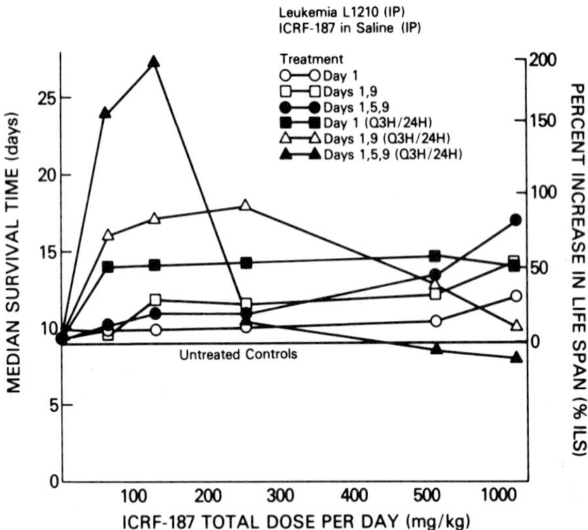

FIG. 1. Effect of various ICRF-187 treatment schedules on leukemia L1210 in mice. Leukemia L1210 ascites cells (10^5) inoculated intraperitoneally (ip) followed by ip administration of ICRF-187 on day 1; days 1 and 9; days 1, 5, and 9; day 1 every 3 hours for 24 hours; days 1 and 9 every 3 hours for 24 hours or days 1, 5, and 9 every 3 hours for 24 hours. Untreated controls were injected with saline and the median survival time (MST) was 9.2–9.3 days.

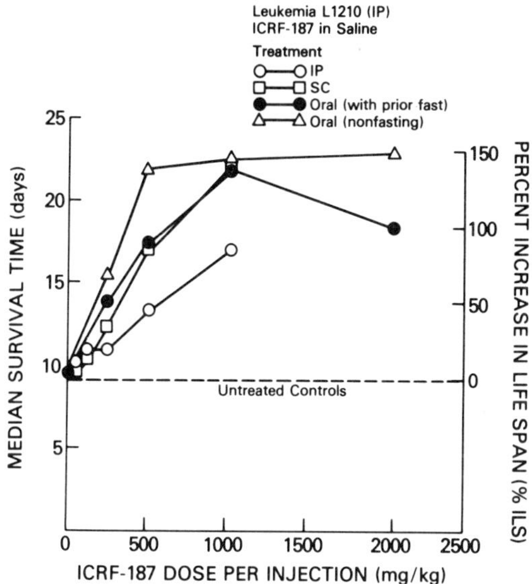

FIG. 2. Influence of route of administration on the action of ICRF-187 against leukemia L1210 in mice. Leukemia L1210 ascites cells (10^5) were inoculated ip and ICRF-187 was administered once on days 1, 5, and 9, subcutaneously (sc); ip; orally in fasted or nonfasted animals. The median survival time (MST) of untreated controls injected with saline only was 9.1–9.3 days.

administration can also influence the antitumor activity of ICRF-187 (Fig. 2). In this instance maximal increases in survival times of leukemic mice occurred at lower doses when the compound was given orally.

ICRF-159 has been utilized in conjunction with other agents against experimental leukemia. Treatment of early L1210 leukemia with combination of ICRF-159 and *cis*-diamminedichloroplatinum (*cis* platin) increased the survival time of treated mice by five to six times over that found when either drug was administered alone (Woodman, 1974). Even in the case of advanced systemic disease the increase in life span observed with the combination was about twice that found when *cis*-platin was given alone. In addition, the optimal combination dose of *cis*-platin was only one-half the amount necessary to produce comparable results when the agent was employed alone.

Experiments utilizing ICRF-159 plus daunorubicin in combination demonstrated alleviation of drug toxicity and enhancement of therapeutic responses (Woodman *et al.*, 1975). In leukemic mice combination treatment was more effective when the treatment schedule was daily from days 1–9 or on days 1, 5, and 9. The optimal combination dose (6 mg/kg daunorubicin plus 200 mg/kg of ICRF-159) increased the survival time over twice that observed when the optimal dose of either drug was given alone. Similarly treatment of normal mice with optimal therapeutic combination doses of ICRF-159 and daunorubicin resulted in no deaths from drug toxicity by the sixtieth day after treatment whereas the same dose of daunorubicin (6.0 mg/kg) when given alone was lethal. The reduction in toxicity is not absolute and there are conditions under which the opposite can occur. For example certain combinations of high doses and/or multiple injections of ICRF-159 and doxorubicin caused increased lethality in mice (Guiliani *et al.*, 1981).

The potential for therapeutic synergism led to a series of experiments in which several antitumor drugs were employed in combination with ICRF-159 against leukemia L1210 (Kline, 1974). The data in Table III summarize the efficacy of various combinations of antineoplastic drugs with ICRF-159 on leukemia L1210 when the treatment was started on days 1, 3, or 5 after transplantation of the tumor. Combination therapy was considered superior to single drug therapy if the percentage increase in life span (ILS) observed with the combination therapy was at least 50% higher than the percent ILS obtained with the more active single drug. Of the 15 drugs examined only 6 [daunorubicin, doxorubicin, camptothecin (NSC 100880), a quinolinium derivative (NSC 113089), *cis*-platin, and cytosine arabinoside] demonstrated enhanced antitumor activity with ICRF-159. The combination of other antitumor drugs with ICRF-159 produced an increase in life span of leukemic mice only slightly greater than that found when either drug was used separately. These increases were not of sufficient magnitude to be considered superior to single drug therapy.

B. Cell Cycle Specificity

In order to gain a closer insight into the biochemical mechanisms by which ICRF-159 might exert its inhibitory activity, human peripheral lymphocytes were stimulated into division by the mitogen phytohemagglutinin. To arrest cell cycle progression in metaphase, colcemid was then added at various times after administration of ICRF-159 so that the temporal relationship between ICRF-159 addition and metaphase arrest could be accurately gauged. By means of this reverse synchronization Sharpe *et al.* (1970) were able to pinpoint the phase specificity of the drug. Although initially this was thought to be the S phase as a result of experiments which claimed to show inhibition of DNA synthesis (Creighton and Birnie, 1970), it seems likely that the sensitive phase was not DNA synthesis, but late G_2 or possibly the interphase between G_2 and the beginning of prophase (Sharpe *et al.*, 1970). Subsequently this was

TABLE III

EFFECT OF ICRF-159 IN COMBINATION WITH OTHER DRUGS ON LEUKEMIA L1210[a,b]

ICRF-159 and other drugs	ICRF-159[c]	ICRF-159 and other drugs[c]	Increase in median life span (%)			Effect of combination therapy
			ICRF-159	Other drugs	ICRF-159 and other drugs	
Doxorubicin[a]	Q3H/1	Q3H/1	55	60	172(3)[d]	+[e]
Daunorubicin[a]	1,5,9	1,5,9	60	20	170(3)	+
Camptothecin[a]	1,5,9	1,5,9	155	112	565(5)	+
Quinolinium derivative[a] (NSC-113089)	3,7,11	3–11	80	125	180	+
cis-Diamminedichloroplatinum[b]	5,9,13	Q3H/5,9,13	61	67	161	+
Cytosine arabinoside[b]	5,9,13	5,7,9,11,13	68	100	158	+
Harringtonine[a]	1,5,9	1–9	70	40	110	–[f]
Coralyne[a]	1,5,9	1–9	70	25	95	–
Anguidin[a]	1,5,9	1–9	70	20	80	–
Chromomycin A_3[a]	1,5,9	1,5,9	70	20	75	–
Ellipticine[a]	1	1	75	40	60	–
5-Azacytidine[b]	1,5,9	1,5,9	139	117	139	–
5-HP[b]	5,9,13	5,9,13	78	100	133	–
Camptothecin[b]	5,9,13	5,9,13	60	55	90	–
Methotrexate[b]	5,9,13	5–13	44	83	111	–
Cyclophosphamide[b]	5,9,13	5,12,19	68	279	247	–

[a] Ascites leukemic cells (10^5) inoculated intraperitoneally.

[b] Ascites leukemic cells (10^6) inoculated subcutaneously.

[c] Days of treatment after tumor inoculation; Q3H/1 = injections every 3 hours for 24 hours on day 1.

[d] Numbers in parentheses indicate number of long-term survivors out of 8 mice.

[e] +, percentage increase in median life span either equal to or greater than 50% maximally effective single-drug therapy.

[f] –, percentage increase in median life span less than 50% maximally effective single-drug therapy.

confirmed by Taylor and Bleehen (1977) using flow cytometry. It was also confirmed by Hallowes *et al.* (1974) using tritiated thymidine incorporation and autoradiography. Further supporting evidence came from the studies of Greider *et al.* (1977), who showed that in contrast to most other anticancer drugs, ICRF-159 did not inhibit DNA synthesis, but instead it appeared to stimulate it. Protein and RNA synthesis were unaffected. All these effects were examined at doses which prevented cell division. Moreover Ward (1968) showed that it was not possible to fit the ICRF-159 molecule onto a model of DNA. It is clear therefore that the primary inhibition of cell division by ICRF-159 is not due to direct or indirect interference with DNA, RNA or protein synthesis or activity. Nondividing cells, i.e., those in plateau phase or in G_0 are unaffected by ICRF-159. This might account for the relative lack of toxicity the drug evokes in animals and in man since only those organ systems which contain dividing cells seem to be at risk. Undoubtedly the most critical of these tissues is the bone marrow, but even with this sensitive tissue where stem cells divide every 4 days, treatment that is timed well within this period, i.e., 2 or 3 consecutive days will not influence the production of white cells as much as treatment for 4 or more days. In a normal bone marrow, ICRF-159 does not usually affect red cells and platelets.

C. Antimetastatic Activity

Hellmann and Burrage (1969) described the activity of ICRF-159 in the Lewis lung carcinoma screen of selective antimetastatic compounds. Since this was a screen for compounds active against spontaneous metastases (Karrer *et al.*, 1967), ICRF-159 can be regarded as one of the first antimetastatic compounds. It had activity at doses which had no inhibitory effect on growth of the primary implant. The activity could be seen when the drug was given for only 7 days after the implantation of the tumor and even more strikingly when further treatment was given. It was less noticeable however when treatment was delayed until 2 weeks after implantation. The lungs in all these experiments were removed 3 weeks after the start of the experiment and all control animals had large numbers of metastases whereas the treated animals had very few or none.

Analysis of the mechanism of this antimetastatic action led Salsbury *et al.* (1974) to the conclusion that no tumor cells entered the circulation after treatment with ICRF-159 and that the problem therefore was not destruction of Lewis lung cells in the circulating blood or prevention of their implantation in the lungs. Histological examination of the peripheral areas of the primary tumors revealed a striking change in the anatomical and physiological characteristics of the tumor neovasculature. Whereas blood channels in the control tumor consisted mostly of irregular poorly endothelialized vascular sinusoids, many of which were lined by tumor cells and probably formed by blood streaming through the tumor mass, the ICRF-159 treated tumors had well endothelialized capillaries which were indistinguishable from those of normal tissues. Even more striking was the fact that the treated tumors had, in contrast to the control tumors, no or very few areas of hemorrhage. The treated tumors therefore appeared pale and strikingly different compared to the florid appearance of the control tumors. It was concluded that the action of ICRF-159 had been to normalize the developing neovasculature in such a way as to prevent the hemorrhages which carried the tumor cells into the circulation and that this angiometamorphic effect (as it was called) was responsible for the antimetastatic action of the drug in the Lewis lung carcinoma.

In a drug combination study for the treatment of Lewis lung carcinoma, Kline (1974) reported that cyclophosphamide administered on day 5 only after transplantation of tumor and ICRF-159 on days 5, 9, and 13 produced a 163% ILS in contrast to 87 and 9% ILS obtained with cyclophosphamide and ICRF-159 alone, respectively. This enhanced survival was thought to be due to the effectiveness of the former drug in inhibiting the primary tumor and metastases and the latter affecting essentially the metastatic growth.

Other investigators have found ICRF-159 to have an antimetastatic activity in a variety of tumors. Peters (1976) for example using the WHT carcinoma found the drug to have an antimetastatic action in that tumor and Pollard *et al.* (1981) using a prostate tumor in rats obtained similar results. Spreafico and Garattini (1974) confirmed the results of Hellmann and Burrage and extended them, but Pimm and Baldwin (1975) using a single dose of the drug found no effect on either the primary or secondary tumors of a rat epithelioma. Giuliani *et al.* (1981) found the compound had little activity on the virus MS tumor which metastasizes spontaneously. On the other hand experiments by Hellmann and Murkin (1978) on the B16 melanoma showed that ICRF-159, together with excision of the primary tumor at day 10 or 11, resulted in a considerable decrease in number of metastases.

Hellmann and LeServe (1974) investigated the effect of ICRF-159 on developing tumor blood vessels of the Walker tumor. Using X-ray microangiography they found that hemorrhages were much reduced in this tumor after ICRF-159. They also showed that in this system, the tortuous leaky tumor blood vessels were replaced by straight and apparently intact vessels. The functional state of these vessels also seemed to be affected by ICRF-159 treatment since injection of Pelikan ink revealed that, in contrast to the control vessels where Pelikan ink extravasated through the lumen of the vessels and was trapped between the basement membrane and the endothelium, no such trapping effect was seen in the blood vessels of the ICRF-159 treated tumors.

Salsbury *et al.* (1974) showed that ICRF-159 prevented not only Lewis lung carcinoma cell dissemination, but also that from the sarcoma S180. Normally this tumor does not appear to metastasize, but is clearly capable of hematogenous dissemination apparently by a similar process to that of the Lewis lung carcinoma, a process which may be profoundly altered by treatment with the drug. In the adenocarcinoma Ca755 however Salsbury *et al.* (1974) showed that the drug had little or no influence on dissemination; this may have been due to the fact that the tumor revealed no abnormal blood vessels.

Since no selective antimetastatic agent has been described among the clinically used anticancer drugs apart from ICRF-159, no clinical trials of any antimetastatic agent has yet been possible. A recent 4-year study of adjuvant ICRF-159 in resectable colorectal cancer however shows that the drug has a significant influence on the recurrence rate and on the distribution of metastases when they do appear (Gilbert *et al.*, 1981). Patients had fewer recurrences in the liver and more in areas which are not normally the sites of metastatic involvement, such as the brain and bones. Neither the statistics of such a shift in metastatic pattern nor the full clinical and biological significance of such a change have as yet been worked out.

IV. Radiosensitization

Some of the properties displayed by ICRF-159 seemed to suggest that the compound might potentiate the effects of radiation. These properties were first, the normalization of the developing tumor neovasculature in the Lewis lung carcinoma, which if it also applied to other tumors, make it seem likely that blood flow might be improved and oxygenation of hypoxic radioresistant areas of the tumor might thereby be increased. Second, because the compound blocked cell cycle progression at the end of G_2 or the interphase of G_2 and prophase, a point at which many cells become more sensitive to radiation, more cells would be held in a radiosensitive phase. Third, the demonstration that the compound in combination with a variety of other anticancer drugs would produce at least an additive effect with some and a synergistic effect with others.

Hellmann and Murkin (1974) therefore explored the interaction of ICRF-159 and radiation using the S180 sarcoma as a test system. They found the combination of ICRF-159 and radiation exerted more than an additive effect on the inhibition of tumor growth. At the same time using the white cell count as an indicator of simultaneous damage to normal bone marrow and lymphoid tissue they were unable to detect any additional myelosuppressive action other than that produced by the drug alone. Taylor and Bleehen (1977) using EMT6 tumor cells *in vitro* found that the drug produced radiosensitization of log phase cells, but not of plateau phase cells. Their studies indicated that the radiosensitization might be a direct effect and that nonproliferating cells were not at risk. Since most normal adult cells with the exception of those in bone marrow, gut, and gonads seldom proliferate no additional damage to normal tissues might be expected from the irradiation and ICRF-159 treatment of tumors located within normal tissues.

Peters (1976), using a mouse fibrosarcoma, also showed that ICRF-159 potentiated radiation. He went on to show that with this tumor the effect produced was unrelated to the degree of anoxia to which the tumor was exposed. It must be presumed therefore that the radiosensitization produced by ICRF-159 is not due to an increase of the effectiveness of radiation on hypoxic cells.

The radiosensitization effect of ICRF-159 was examined in several clinical trials. These are discussed in Section VII of this article.

V. Pharmacology

The pharmacology of ICRF-159 has been dealt with in only a limited number of studies. A consistent finding is that the compound disappears rapidly from the blood. The plasma half-life in the rat following intravenous administration of [^{14}C]ICRF-159 was found to be 30 minutes (Field *et al.*, 1971). In this study the agent was detected by a bioassay procedure which utilized cultured hamster cells. Utilizing this same species but with a GLC assay the plasma half-life was determined to be 40 to 45 minutes (Sadee *et al.*, 1975). The plasma half-life in the rabbit determined by a GLC–mass fragmentography technique was 85 minutes. In both rats and rabbits total ^{14}C levels were significantly higher than the parent ICRF-159 indicating rapid biotransformation to unknown metabolites. The plasma concentrations of ICRF-159 in both rats and rabbits following oral dosing were considerably lower than comparable intravenous doses of the compound. For example, 1 hour after an oral dose of 50 mg/kg in the rabbit the peak plasma concentration was 1.5 μg/ml; however when the same dose was administered intravenously the initial blood level was over 50 μg/ml and declined to 2 μg/ml by 2 hours.

The plasma concentration of ICRF-159 detected in humans after oral dosing was comparable to that detected in rats and rabbits (Sadee *et al.*, 1975). Two patients that received 3 g/m^2 ICRF-159 orally showed a peak plasma concentration of 3.8 μg/ml after 2 hours and a measurable level was still detected up to 12 hours after drug administration. A second study determined the bioavailability of orally administered ICRF-159 in 12 patients given [^{14}C]ICRF-159 at 3 different dose schedules, 10.5 g/m^2 as a single dose, 3.0 g/m^2 as a single weekly dose, and 3.0 g/m^2 divided into 1.0 g/m^2 given 6 hours apart 1 day a week for 6 weeks. The amount of radioactivity recovered in the urine of these patients, collected over a period of 96 hours, as percentage of the administered dose was 8.5 ± 3.0, 22.7 ± 10.7, and 52 ± 8.7%, respectively. The unrecovered radioactivity was largely accounted for in the feces. Using chromatographic separation techniques two metabolites were detected in the urine while none was found in the feces. These results indicate that a large oral dose of ICRF-159 is not well absorbed. The limited absorption following a single oral dose of ICRF-159 may be due to low solubility and/or restricted absorption through the gastrointestinal mucosa. In contrast moderate hematologic toxicity can occur when a smaller dose is subdivided and given at intervals over a 24-hour period. Thus it appears that the schedule dependent toxicity of ICRF-159 could at least be partly attributed to the limited bioavailability of the drug.

VI. Toxicology

A. Preclinical ICRF-159

The ICRF compounds were synthetized as less polar and potentially more biologically active derivatives of ethylenediaminetetraacetic acid (EDTA). EDTA exerts essentially no antitumor activity (Leiter *et al.*, 1959). Cytotoxicity is minimized because the highly polar nature of the molecule severely restricts intracellular uptake of EDTA (Foreman, 1960; Schroeder, 1960). The limited amounts of EDTA (2–4%) detected in the circulation do not concentrate in any tissue and consequently do not elicit any discernible systemic effects (Forman, 1960).

The bioavailability of ICRF-159 following oral administration is also limited (Sadee, 1975) but in this instance the amounts absorbed are sufficient to cause certain biological effects. The actions of both single and multiple oral doses of ICRF-159 were evaluated in the beagle dog (Gralla *et al.*, 1974). Toxic effects were found to be related to both the dose and frequency of drug administration. A single oral dose of 320 mg/kg or 5 consecutive daily 20 mg/kg doses of ICRF-159 caused little or no toxicity. A single 1000 mg/kg dose produced moderate but reversible hematopoietic and intestinal toxicity while a dose of 320 mg/kg given on 5 consecutive days was lethal. Other doses of ICRF-159 (40–160 mg/kg) given on this same 5 day regimen produced a toxicity pattern of increasing severity.

Clinical signs of intestinal toxicity such as anorexia, emesis, and diarrhea were coupled with histologic evidence of small intestine mucosal cell destruction. Bone marrow cytotoxicity resulted in leukopenia and reticulocytopenia. The cellular alterations in both organs were reversible. Orally administered ICRF-159 at doses of 40 mg/kg or more induced the same type of intestinal and bone marrow alterations in rhesus monkeys as was seen in the beagle dog. Anemia in addition to leukopenia was a consistent observation in these animals. Thus in both the rhesus monkey and the beagle dog ICRF-159 shares a cytotoxic profile similar to that of other antineoplastic agents. Some of these agents are also known to induce serious alterations in non-rapidly dividing organs such as heart, lung, or kidney. This type of activity apparently does not occur with ICRF-159 as tissue damage was limited to areas of rapidly dividing cells such as the bone marrow and the gastrointestinal tract (Gralla *et al.,* 1974).

B. Clinical ICRF-159

Initial phase I studies in patients were carried out with both single and multiple oral dose scheduling. The administration of single large doses (1.0 to 10.5 g/m^2) (25 to 263 mg/kg) resulted in variable mild leukopenia (Creaven and Taylor, 1973; Creaven *et al.,* 1974). Both the occurrence and severity of leukopenia was not dose related on this single dose regimen. Occasional occurrences of anemia, thrombocytopenia, nausea and vomiting, and alopecia were reported in these patients. ICRF-159 (3.0 g/m^2) was administered either as a single weekly dose or as a divided dose of 1 g/m^2 every 6 hours given 3 times a week. Administration of ICRF-159 in this manner for 6 consecutive weeks, resulted in consistent moderate to marked leukopenia. Previous exposure to chemotherapeutic drugs may enhance this effect as 2 patients who had prior extensive therapy experienced severe but reversible bone marrow suppression. These investigators concluded that a single-dose schedule of ICRF-159 was less toxic than administration of multiple doses.

In a second phase I trial, ICRF-159 was administered at oral doses ranging from 0.25 to 1.25 g/m^2/day in divided doses every 8 hours for 3 successive days (Bellet *et al.,* 1973). The dose-limiting toxicity again was leukopenia which occurred in all patients. The nadir of the leukopenia was 12 days and the white blood cell count returned to predrug levels within 8 days. Other toxic effects which occurred less frequently were mild and transient thrombocytopenia, nausea and vomiting, diarrhea, and alopecia. In these and in other clinical studies, the use of ICRF-159 has not been associated with cardiac, renal, hepatic, or pulmonary toxicity (Bellet *et al.,* 1973, 1977).

C. Preclinical ICRF-187

The limited aqueous solubility has limited the effective clinical use of ICRF-159. This problem was alleviated when it was found that ICRF-187, the *d*-isomer of ICRF-159, was more soluble in aqueous fluids and could be prepared in a solution for intravenous use (Repta *et al.*, 1976). The toxicity of single and multiple intravenous infusions of ICRF-187 was evaluated in beagle dogs (Levine *et al.*, 1980). In this study animals were treated with 250 to 2000 mg/kg as a single dose, with 15.6 to 250 mg/kg once daily for 5 consecutive days or 15.6 to 125 mg/kg for 5 consecutive days for 3 treatment periods with intervening 9-day rest periods.

The schedule of drug administration was found to be a primary factor in the degree of tissue alterations. A single infusion of 2000 mg/kg was lethal to 1 of 2 dogs while a similar situation occurred when a total dose of 1250 mg/kg was divided and given over a 5-day period. Hemorrhages in a number of organs and hemoconcentration were found in those animals which died from ICRF-187 administration. When an interval was allowed between each of 3 series of 5 consecutive daily doses a total dose of 1875 mg/kg could be given without lethality. The influence of schedule was also apparent on the effects exerted at the lower dose levels. The highest single ICRF-187 dose which caused little or no toxicity was found to be 250 mg/kg. However, 5 consecutive daily infusions of 15.6 mg/kg (78.0 mg/kg) produced slight to moderate changes in circulating blood cells and certain serum enzymes and microscopic lesions in lymphoid tissue.

As was noted with ICRF-159, the toxic effects of ICRF-187 are most pronounced on mitotically active tissues such as bone marrow, lymphoid tissue, and gastrointestinal mucosa. Bone marrow toxicity was evidenced by early neutrocytosis and delayed neutropenia, reduction in RBC and platelet counts, microscopic evidence of hypoplasia, and increased myeloid erythroid ratios. Repeated dose regimens had the greatest effect on circulating blood cells and anemia and neutropenia were most prominent after 3 series of 5 daily doses with 9-day rest periods between series. The drug also affected lymphocytes as demonstrated by a decrease in WBC count and morphologic evidence of lymphoid tissue necrosis.

Reductions in food consumption and weight loss were the clinical signs of gastrointestinal alterations following single or multiple ICRF-187 infusions. Gastrointestinal toxicity was also evidenced by emesis, bloody diarrhea, anorexia, and necrosis of the intestinal mucosa. The toxicity was most severe at lethal doses and was reduced or absent at lower doses.

The toxic effects of ICRF-187 on mitotically active tissue such as bone marrow, lymphoid tissue, and gastrointestinal mucosa were similar to those previously reported after ICRF-159 treatment (Gralla *et al.*, 1974;

Levine *et al.*, 1980). In addition, administration of ICRF-187 was also associated with evidence of liver and kidney toxicity. Total ICRF-187 doses of 2000 mg/kg (single) or 2500 mg/kg given on the 5 consecutive days schedule induced marked hepatotoxicity. Alterations in serum liver function tests were less severe when a cumulative dose of 1875 mg/kg was divided into 15 infusions with a 9-day rest period between each series of 5 consecutive daily doses. Hepatic dysfunction was indicated by increases in several clinical determinations such as SGOT, SGPT, BSP retention, prothrombin time, and bilirubin as well as morphologic evidence of swollen and vacuolated hepatocytes. The alterations in hepatic function persisted as evidenced by elevated liver function tests in a dog which survived for 45 days after a single 2000 mg/kg infusion of ICRF-187. Manifestations of hepatotoxicity following nonlethal doses of ICRF-187 were much less severe and in some instances amounted to only slight elevations of serum SGOT and SGPT levels.

Lethal doses of ICRF-187 are also associated with renal toxicity. Increases in serum BUN and creatinine levels and morphologic evidence of renal cellular damage were found in animals receiving the 2 highest single doses and the highest dose in the single 5-day study. The lesions were observed primarily in the proximal convoluted tubule and included vacuolization, degeneration, and necrosis of proximal tubule cells and proximal tubule lining cells. Similar alterations have been reported in clinical or experimental situations following intravenous administration of EDTA (Dubley *et al.*, 1967). For example, vacuolar changes were produced in the epithelium of the proximal tubule when $CaNa_2EDTA$ was given in high doses (300–500 mg/kg × 10 days) to rats (Doolan *et al.*, 1967). The degree of vacuolization appears to be similar whether the sodium, calcium, lead, or strontium salt of EDTA was utilized (Forman *et al.*, 1956). There was no evidence to indicate that the vacuoles or other alterations are the biochemical result of depletion of an essential metal from the proximal tubular cells (Doolan *et al.*, 1967). Although ICRF-187 treatment did not alter serum calcium, potassium, or sodium concentrations a selective depletion mechanism cannot be ruled out until renal metal concentrations have been determined following administration of the agent. Because ICRF-187 appears to exert a multiplicity of actions, there is a possibility that renal toxicity can occur independent of metal binding. In any case, the toxicity is dose dependent since at lower doses of ICRF-187 chemical or histologic evidence of renal alterations decreases or is absent. The toxic effects on the kidney and other tissues appear to be reversible since lesions which were present when animals were sacrificed within a day of the last infusion were not found when other animals receiving the same ICRF-187 dose were necropsied 45 days later.

D. Clinical ICRF-187

The results of a phase I study utilizing parenterally administered ICRF-187 have recently been reported (Von Hoff *et al.*, 1981). The amount of ICRF-187 administered ranged from 25 to 75 mg/kg (500 to 1500 mg/m^2) given for 3 consecutive days and repeated at 28-day intervals. Leukopenia and thrombocytopenia were found to be the major dose-limiting toxic effects. At the lowest dose, 25 mg/kg (500 mg/m^2), no decrease in either WBC or platelet counts was noted. Moderate to severe leukopenia and thrombocytopenia occurred when the doses were increased. The most severe hematopoietic toxicity occurred in patients who had prior nitrosourea treatment. In all patients the myelosuppression was not cumulative and recovery was complete by the twenty-first day of the treatment cycle. Nonmyelosuppressive toxic effects included mild elevations in SGOT and SGPT concentration. There was no indication that hepatotoxicity occurred to any significant degree and the serum enzyme concentrations returned to normal by the seventeenth day after drug administration. A further interesting observation was the detection of marked increases in the urinary clearances of iron and zinc after administration of ICRF-187. This finding may indicate the drug exerts chelating activity.

VII. Clinical

Like many new anticancer drugs, ICRF-159 received its first clinical examination against the acute leukemias. Hellmann *et al.* (1969) carried out a preliminary clinical assessment in 6 patients with acute leukemia and 3 with lymphosarcoma. In these studies a maximum dose of 40 mg/kg/day for 4 days caused a dramatic fall in circulating blast cells in 7 of the 9 patients. Partial bone marrow remission was obtained in one patient. No cross resistance was seen with other cytotoxic agents even where patients had received extensive prior chemotherapy. No toxic signs attributable to the drug were seen except in one patient who developed gastroenteritis and diffuse alopecia. Most of the patients with acute leukemia were children and in these the opportunity to use an oral drug was particularly appreciated.

Krepler and Pawlowsky (1975) reported similar results in their treatment of 20 children with relapsing acute leukemia. Despite the unfavorable selection of cases, 2 complete and 7 incomplete remissions of 1 to 6 months duration were obtained. More recently ICRF-159 has been used in combination with cytosine arabinoside in elderly patients with acute nonlymphoblastic leukemia and in these patients complete and partial remissions were obtained with very few side effects (Hellmann *et al.*, 1978).

This regimen was well tolerated and was subsequently extended to include children. In some of the children the disease continued, but the condition remained static for periods of up to 1 year.

ICRF-159 does not appear to be particularly active in adult leukemia with the exception of blast cell crisis of chronic myeloid leukemia (Bakowski *et al.*, 1979b). Bakowski *et al.* (1979a) have demonstrated that in this condition ICRF-159 can produce a response in 25% of the patients. ICRF-159 has also been found to be active in Hodgkin's and non-Hodgkin's lymphoma (Hellmann *et al.*, 1969; Mathe *et al.*, 1970; Krepler and Pawlowsky, 1975). In all of these conditions the drug treatment resulted in remissions even in heavily pretreated patients with an unfavorable histology. The remissions were for a reasonable length of time and confirmed earlier findings of Flannery *et al.* (1978) in non-Hodgkin's lymphoma. These authors had shown that patients who had failed both radio- and chemotherapy would still respond to this drug with good remissions, lasting in some cases over 1 year.

The rationale for the use of ICRF-159 in Kaposi's sarcoma was based on the findings of LeServe and Hellmann (1974) in regard to the normalization of the tumor neovasculature. Since Kaposi's sarcoma is a hemangiosarcoma it seemed reasonable to see if the drug would have any beneficial effect in this condition. Although there are sporadic reports of isolated cases of Kaposi's sarcoma in Europeans who have been treated with ICRF-159 and who have responded well, the experience of Olweny *et al.* (1980) in Uganda shows that the drug, as a single agent, is one of the most active anticancer drugs in this condition. It was given to patients who had relapsed on all standard drugs but despite these unfavorable circumstances still responded with minimal toxic side effects. The dosage used by Olweny *et al.* was 1 g/m^2 divided into three 8 hourly doses and given for 3 days every 3 weeks. It is not clear whether this was the optimal dosage, but since it was highly effective it is probable that the maximum tolerated dose in this instance was also the optimal dose. This may not be the case for other tumors.

An adjuvant study of ICRF-159 for resectable colorectal cancer used much lower doses, but on a continuous 5 days/week schedule (Gilbert *et al.*, 1981). A randomized controlled trial was set up in 1976. The latest interim analyses (November 1981) indicates that control and drug-treated patients with tumors in Dukes groups B and C show a statistically significant difference in recurrence free interval ($p < 0.01$) (Gilbert *et al.*, 1982). When the results were analyzed according to whether or not patients had received ICRF-159 as one of the drugs, the difference in recurrence free intervals was even more striking ($p < 0.004$). Overall differences in survival between the control and drug-treated groups however have not yet reached statistical significance ($p < 0.07$). In this study ICRF-159 was given at a dose of 125 mg twice daily for an indefinite period. This dosage was extremely well tolerated by 95% of patients and only an occasional patient suffered from either gastrointestinal disturbance or hair loss. However the white blood cell count was depressed in most patients, and about half experienced leukopenia (<3000 mm^3). An interesting feature of this study was the effect the drug appeared to have on the distribution of metastases when they occurred. Some drug-treated patients developed brain or bone metastases, sites where metastases are not normally found in colorectal cancer. Particularly noticeable was the diminution of the proportion with liver metastases in Dukes C patients. Liver metastases were found in 33% of the controls, but in only 12% of the group treated with the drug. The long-term significance of this is not yet certain but it could clearly have considerable repercussions on the vigor with which both the primary disease and its recurrence as well as the metastases are treated by surgeons in the future.

There are clinical trials in which ICRF-159 has been combined with radiotherapy. The first such study was a retrospective comparison of patients with a variety of soft tissue sarcomas treated either by radiation alone or with this drug and radiation (Ryall *et al.*, 1974). There were 14 patients treated with radiation alone and 19 with radiation plus the drug which were evaluable. These patients were not randomized to a particular treatment. Whether they received ICRF-159 in addition to radiation was decided by the clinician they chose. Some believed it was useful and gave it to all their patients and some remained to be convinced and gave it to none of theirs. Treatment policies in regard to radiation and general clinical care was largely identical. Log rank analysis of these two groups utilizing observations on regression and recurrence of the irradiated tumor showed that while there were no statistically significant differences in primary tumor response, the differences (64 vs 26%) in the incidence of time to recurrence were significant. There was no evidence from a careful scrutiny of the skin and deep tissues in the irradiated areas that the improved radiation response of the combined treatment had also resulted in greater normal tissue damage. Bates (1978), however, utilizing ICRF-159 and radiation combination in 12 patients with a variety of soft tissue sarcomas felt that normal skin and tissues had also been sensitized.

A total of nearly 100 cases of soft tissue sarcomas treated by irradiation and the drug have been described (Rhomberg, 1978; Bates, 1978; Ryall, 1978; Hellmann *et al.*, 1978a). Approximately 75% of these patients experienced tumor inhibition with combined treatment. A marked tumor regression was noted in 33% of the responding patients. In this study Rhomberg (1978) also reported that they obtained responses from other tumors not normally sensitive to irradiation such as melanomas when they were treated with the combined radiation and ICRF-159.

In another trial the effects of radiation and ICRF-159 and radiation alone were compared in patients with squamous cell carcinoma of the head and neck (Bakowski *et al.*, 1978). This study was performed double blind and the findings assessed by sequential analysis. The results indicated that patients responded more favorably to radiation alone. However, when all patients in the trial were analyzed there was essentially no difference between the ICRF-159 treated and the control group. It must be emphasized however that the dose of ICRF-159 employed in this trial was low (62.5 mg) because of fear of radiation sensitization reactions in the delicate membranes of the buccal cavity and the pharynx. When used as the sole agent in squamous cell carcinoma of the head and neck, ICRF-159 has a low order of antitumor activity (Shal *et al.*, 1982).

A trial of ICRF-159 and radiotherapy was evaluated in patients with carcinoma of the bronchus (Spittle *et al.*, 1979). The study was randomized and controlled using split dose radiotherapy. Patients were treated with 3000 rads in 10 fractions followed after 4 weeks rest by another 10 fractions of 300 rads each. In addition 125 mg of ICRF-159 was given twice daily on each of the radiation days. Patients received no further treatment after the end of these two radiotherapy/chemotherapy sessions. It appeared that there was some difference between the two groups chiefly in terms of survival but the differences did not reach statistical significance. A second trial was therefore initiated, in which the radiation was shortened to 5 fractions of 400 rads each for 1 week followed by 1 months rest and then a further 5 fractions of 400 rads giving a total dose of 4000 rads, either with or without the drug. This regimen was followed by maintenance chemotherapy or cyclophosphamide and ICRF-159 in all patients. Although the results at first seemed to indicate that survival differences might reach statistical significance, a recent final analysis showed that these differences had receded.

Using the standard United States dosage scheme (750–1000 mg/m^2 for 3 days every 3 weeks) the response of ICRF-159 has been examined in carcinoma of the breast (Ahmann *et al.*, 1977), prostate (Kvols *et al.*, 1977) and bronchus (non-oat cell) (Eagan *et al.*, 1976), and in melanoma (Ahmann *et al.*, 1978). No complete regressions were seen.

Finally the dramatic effect of ICRF-159 in psoriasis must be mentioned. In some 35 patients, Atherton *et al.* (1980) described the use of the drug in severe psoriasis, refractory to other treatment or where methotrexate had produced abnormalities of liver function. In nearly all these cases, the drug produced moderate to complete clearing of the skin with only minimal side effects.

VIII. Interactions of ICRF Compounds with Other Agents

ICRF compounds are capable of altering the actions of other agents. Some of the first evidence for this activity was obtained in studies with the antineoplastic drugs daunorubicin and doxorubicin. During exploratory investigations utilizing the isolated blood-perfused dog heart preparation both anthracyclines were found to cause an increase in coronary perfusion pressure (Herman *et al.*, 1972). After a number of attempts to ameliorate this toxicity it was found that if the hearts were pretreated with ethylenediaminetetraacetic acid (EDTA) or ICRF-159 prior to anthracycline administration, the changes in coronary perfusion pressure were negligible or absent. Additionally, it was noted that the increase in perfusion pressure occurred simultaneously with an increase in the appearance of aglycone metabolites. The formation of aglycone metabolites was reduced in those hearts pretreated with EDTA or ICRF-159. The mechanism for this protective activity was not determined.

Subsequent studies determined whether ICRF-159 would alter anthracycline toxicity in the intact animal. A single high dose of daunorubicin (50 mg/kg, iv) given to Syrian golden hamsters caused 100% lethality within 2 to 3 days but when this same dose was preceded by ICRF-159 (100 mg/kg, ip) half of the animals survived over 21 days (Herman *et al.*, 1974). Again less formation of aglycone metabolites occurred in the tissues of ICRF-159 pretreated hamsters than in hamsters pretreated with saline. The same large dose of daunorubicin (50 mg/kg) given to the rhesus monkey caused hyperglycemia and increased serum concentrations of CPK and SGOT suggesting that cardiac damage might have occurred. These alterations were absent or markedly attenuated by pretreatment with ICRF-159.

ICRF-187, the more water-soluble *d* isomer of ICRF-159, also attenuates high dose daunorubicin toxicity in Syrian golden hamsters (Herman *et al.*, 1979). By 3 weeks only 10% of the hamsters treated with daunorubicin alone (25 mg/kg) were alive while 80% of the animals pretreated with ICRF-187 (100 mg/kg) survived. Vitamin E pretreatment has been found to reduce acute doxorubicin toxicity in mice (Myers *et al.*, 1977). Other studies indicate that the protection observed initially is temporary and that by 60 days the death rate in both vitamin E treated and nontreated mice is identical (Gram *et al.*, 1978; Mimnaugh *et al.*, 1979). ICRF-187 pretreatment appears to afford both initial and long-term protection from daunorubicin toxicity since a significant number of animals receiving this agent survived over 4 months. This long-term survival is all the more impressive because the dose of daunorubicin was considerably higher than the dose of doxorubicin utilized in the vitamin E studies in mice.

The *in vivo* evidence clearly indicates that either ICRF-159 or ICRF-187 is capable of significantly reducing the toxic effects of a high dose of daunorubicin. The question of which tissues the ICRF compounds are protecting is of interest. Morphologic alterations in heart, liver, or kidney do not appear to be of sufficient magnitude to fully account for the ultimate lethality caused by high doses of daunorubicin (Herman *et al.*, 1979; Wang, *et al.*, 1981). Saline-pretreated hamsters stopped eating following daunorubicin administration and by the end of the second week had lost almost one-third of the total body weight. In contrast the weight loss in hamsters pretreated with ICRF-187 was reversible such that after 5 weeks the weight of these animals was above control levels. These observations tend to indicate that gastrointestinal toxicity may be responsible for high dose daunorubicin lethality. This possibility is further supported by the fact that marked histopathological changes have been found in the intestinal mucosa of mice receiving high doses of daunorubicin (Wang *et al.*, 1981). Intestinal alterations were minimized when mice were pretreated with ICRF-159 (Wang *et al.*, 1981). Thus the lethal effects of high doses of daunorubicin may be due to profound gastrointestinal alterations and ICRF compounds appear capable of attenuating anthracycline toxicity on this tissue.

The studies described above have utilized limited dosages and pretreatment times in order to demonstrate ICRF-159 or ICRF-187 reduction in daunorubicin toxicity. There have been attempts to vary certain factors in order to better define the scope of this protective activity. The degree of protective activity in mice can be altered when the timing of ICRF-159 treatment is varied in relation to the administration of daunorubicin (Wang *et al.*, 1981). These investigators found that the protective effect of ICRF-159 was greatest when given 24 hours before or at the same time as daunorubicin. Similar differences in protection with varying pretreatment times have been made in hamsters utilizing ICRF-187 (Herman *et al.*, 1982). In this study 90% of the hamsters given daunorubicin (25 mg/kg) alone died within 1 to 3 weeks while 45% of the animals pretreated with ICRF-187 (100 mg/kg) 48 hours prior to daunorubicin were alive at 8 weeks. However survival was only 20% when the pretreatment time was 24 hours. The highest numbers of animals surviving daunorubicin administration (50–80%) were found in those groups where ICRF-187 was given at time intervals between 3 hours before and 3 hours after daunorubicin administration. In contrast to the mice, no hamsters survived when the ICRF compound was given 12 or more hours after daunorubicin. The differences in the two studies could be due to the greater solubility of ICRF-187. However an additional factor may be related to the experimental design of the studies. The mouse study utilized a 3-week survival end-point while in the hamster study experiments were terminated after 8 weeks.

The amount of ICRF-159 in the mouse or ICRF-187 in the hamster at the time of daunorubicin administration was not determined in either of the above studies. Given the limited pharmacokinetic information available from other species the tissue concentrations of these compounds would be expected to be extremely small. It is therefore difficult to explain the fact that significant numbers of hamsters pretreated 48 hours or mice pretreated 24 hours prior to daunorubicin survived. It is possible that extremely small amounts of ICRF-159 or ICRF-187 in certain tissues would be sufficient to elicit protective activity. It is also possible that these compounds need not be present but they could modify some cellular mechanism such that the toxic effects of daunorubicin are reduced.

The course of daunorubicin toxicity was altered by ICRF-159 treatment doses of 50 mg/kg or more in mice (Wang *et al.*, 1981) and ICRF-187 treatment doses of 12.5 mg/kg or greater in hamsters (Herman *et al.*, 1982). In mice, all animals pretreated with 100 to 200 mg/kg ICRF-159 prior to administration of 10 mg/kg daunorubicin survived up to 21 days. There are limits to the beneficial actions of ICRF-159 in mice as the protective effects of these doses of ICRF-159 were reduced at daunorubicin doses of 20 to 30 mg/kg. The reduction in hamster toxicity during the first 2 weeks after 25 mg/kg daunorubicin was evidenced by the fact that ICRF-187 (12.5 to 100 mg/kg) treated animals lost less weight than those given daunorubicin alone. After 3 weeks only 10% of the nonpretreated hamsters were alive while 90 to 100% of the animals pretreated with the various doses of ICRF-187 survived. Even though survival rates were comparable there were some differences among the various treatment groups. Those animals given ICRF-187 (12.5 mg/kg) prior to daunorubicin experienced a progressive loss in weight such that body weight was reduced by one-third by the end of the fifth week. A pretreatment dose of 50 mg/kg ICRF-187 did not prevent the initial 8 to 9 g loss in body weight experienced during the first 1 to 2 weeks after daunorubicin but did prevent any further loss over the remainder of the experiment. Animals pretreated with 100 mg/kg ICRF-187 initially also lost weight. However, these were the only group of animals that actually weighed more after 5 weeks than they did prior to daunorubicin administration.

The bis(diketopiperazine) analogs such as ICRF-159 possess a number of biological properties some of which have been subjected to considerable structure–activity analysis (Creighton *et al.*, 1969, 1979; Witiak *et al.*,

1977). A similar evaluation of the structural requirements for the important action in reducing acute anthracycline toxicity has only recently been attempted (Herman *et al.*, 1982). In this study administration of a single dose of daunorubicin (25 mg/kg) was lethal to all hamsters by 4 weeks. In contrast 60% of animals pretreated with ICRF-187 (100 mg/kg) were alive after 8 weeks. Similar results were obtained with ICRF-186 the *l* isomer of ICRF-159, indicating that the protective activity is not stereospecific. Fifteen other ICRF analogs (Fig. 3) were also examined for potential protective activity. It was found that ICRF-192 and 200 were the only analogs to provide some protection against acute daunorubicin toxicity.

ICRF-200, while similar to ICRF-187 is racemic and due to *N*-methyl substitution does not have acidic ring functions. The number of animals (30%) alive after 8 weeks in groups given pretreatment doses of 50 or 200 mg/kg ICRF-200 indicates the degree of protection was considerably less than that obtained with ICRF-187. It is conceivable that *in vivo* demethylation of ICRF-200 could occur resulting in the formation of the racemic compound ICRF-159.

ICRF-192 has an ethyl function in place of the methyl found on the central chain of ICRF-187. Although a number of pretreatment doses were examined (6.25 to 100 mg/kg) the greatest number of 8 week survivors (30%) occurred in the group pretreated with 25 mg/kg. The amount of ICRF-192 available was limited and thus additional studies are needed to fully evaluate the protective activity of this compound.

Protection against daunorubicin lethality was negligible or absent when animals were pretreated with various doses of ICRF analogs 154, 158, 193, or 202. ICRF-154 may be envisioned as a central chain desmethyl analog of ICRF-187 with ICRF-158 being the *N*-methylimide derivative of ICRF-154. ICRF-193 and 202 represent butane and pentane side chains and thus are more lipophilic than ICRF-187. At the doses utilized neither ICRF-193 nor 202 provided protection against daunorubicin toxicity. Both compounds are considerably more cytotoxic than ICRF-187 (Creighton *et al.*, 1979). These two agents were also found to cause lethality in animals not treated with daunorubicin. The increase in cytotoxicity may be a reflection of the greater lipophilic properties of these compounds. Lower nontoxic doses of ICRF-193 or 202 need to be administered in order to confirm their inability to protect against daunorubicin toxicity.

At least 3 dose levels of the cyclopropane analogs **8–15** were given to hamsters prior to daunorubicin. A maximal survival rate of 20% was seen in the low dose groups of analog **13** (21.0 mg/kg) and **14** (21.25 mg/kg). Some inherent toxicity was noted with analogs **9** (88 mg/kg) and **12** (122 mg/kg) which by themselves caused 40 and 20% lethality in control animals. Thus it appears that the magnitude of the protective activity against

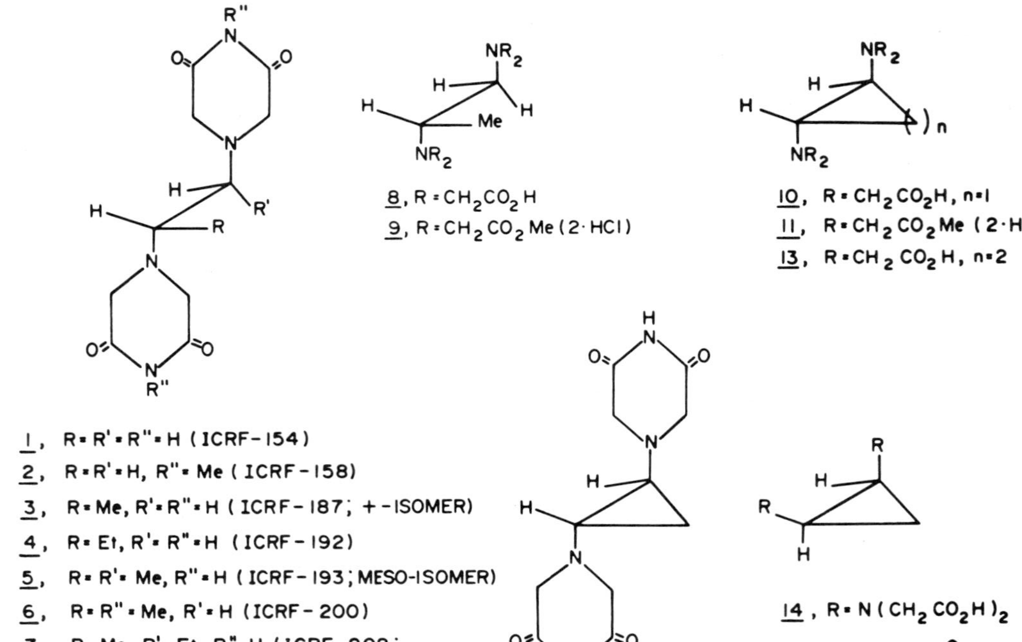

FIG. 3. Structures of ICRF-187 and related compounds examined for potential amelioration of acute daunorubicin toxicity in Syrian golden hamsters. Three to five different doses of each compound were given separately to each group of animals ip 1 hour prior to iv administration of daunorubicin (25 mg/kg).

daunorubicin toxicity can be altered by slight changes in the basic structure of ICRF-187.

Since ICRF-159 and 187 are nonpolar derivatives of EDTA, their presence might attenuate the toxic manifestations of daunorubicin by altering critical cation concentrations. For example an extracellular loss of calcium or magnesium might alter membrane permeability and thereby decrease the uptake of daunorubicin. It is doubtful that this does occur since mice treated with saline or ICRF-159 displayed identical tissue disposition and urinary excretion of daunorubicin (A.D. Little Progress Report, 1973). A decrease in intracellular cation levels might alter the interaction with DNA or interfere with the metabolic breakdown of the anthracyclines. There is no evidence to indicate that the presence of ICRF-159 modifies the DNA–daunorubicin interaction or the subsequent inhibition of nucleic acid turnover (A.D. Little Progress Report, 1973). A reduction in aglycone metabolites was observed in ICRF-159 treated isolated dog hearts given daunorubicin or doxorubicin (Herman *et al.*, 1972). Similarly the concentration of these metabolites in a number of tissues was less in ICRF-159 pretreated than in saline pretreated hamsters (Herman *et al.*, 1974). In contrast ICRF-159 pretreatment did not alter the metabolism of daunorubicin in mice or rats (A.D. Little Progress Report, 1973; Wang and Finch, 1980). These divergent findings tend to reduce the likelihood that an alteration in daunorubicin metabolism is responsible for ICRF-159 protection. Thus the exact mechanism for the protective action of ICRF-159 against acute anthracycline toxicity remains to be determined.

The reduction in acute anthracycline toxicity by ICRF compounds is of interest but questions have been raised as to the ultimate value of this observation. The cardiomyopathy which limits clinical use of the anthracyclines results from chronic administration of low doses of these agents (Tan *et al.*, 1967; Lefrak *et al.*, 1973, 1975). To determine whether ICRF-187 would attenuate chronic daunorubicin cardiac toxicity, rabbits were given 3.2 mg/kg daunorubicin (iv) alone or 30 minutes after 12.5 or 25.0 mg/kg of ICRF-187 (ip) at 3-week intervals (Herman *et al.*, 1981). The cardiac lesions seen 3 weeks after the fifth injection consisted mainly of vacuolization and myofibrillar loss. These alterations were observed in the hearts of all 12 rabbits given daunorubicin alone. The lesion severity in these 12 hearts ranged from 1 to 3 (average 1.8). In contrast no abnormalities were noted in the hearts of 4 of 12 rabbits pretreated with either 12.5 or 25.0 mg/kg ICRF-187. A second indication of protection concerned the frequency and extent of myocyte vacuolization. The 8 remaining hearts displayed minimal alterations ranging in severity from 0.5 to 1.0 (average 0.9). The difference in severity scores of cardiomyopathy between the ICRF treated and nontreated rabbits was highly significant ($p < 0.001$).

ICRF-159 has been shown to be consistently more effective in reducing acute high dose daunorubicin toxicity than doxorubicin toxicity (A.D. Little Progress Report, 1973; Woodman *et al.*, 1972; Giuliani *et al.*, 1981). Given these observations, a question arose as to whether ICRF-187 would also protect against chronic doxorubicin cardiotoxicity. This question was addressed in a study utilizing beagle dogs which were given 1.0 mg/kg doxorubicin (iv) alone or 30 minutes after 12.5 mg/kg ICRF-187 (ip) for 15 consecutive weeks (Herman and Ferrans, 1981). This regimen caused extensive intracellular vacuolization and myofibrillar loss. Five of six dogs receiving doxorubicin alone had a cardiac lesion score of 4+ (most severe). In contrast lesions were absent in the hearts from 4 of 6 animals given doxorubicin in combination with ICRF-187. Vacuolization and myofibrillar loss in the two other animals receiving ICRF-187 prior to doxorubicin was minimal. The difference in cardiomyopathy severity scores in the group given doxorubicin alone and the group given doxorubicin together with ICRF-187 again was highly significant ($p < 0.001$).

In many clinical protocols larger doses of doxorubicin are administered once every 3 weeks. The potential protective effect of ICRF-187 against such a dosage regimen was examined in a study utilizing miniature swine. In this study 2.4 mg/kg doxorubicin (iv) was given to miniature swine alone or 30 minutes after 12.5 mg/kg ICRF-187 (ip) at 3-week intervals (Herman and Ferrans, 1982). The experiment was terminated 3 weeks after the sixth injection. All 6 pigs (including 2 that died spontaneously) receiving doxorubicin alone developed myocardial lesions similar to those found in the other studies. These alterations were severe (3+) in the hearts from 4 of the 6 animals. No lesions were observed in 2 of 7 hearts from animals given doxorubicin in combination with ICRF-187; minimal changes (0.5 to 1+) were detected in the remaining hearts of this group. The differences between the cardiomyopathy scores in groups given daunorubicin with or without ICRF-187 were highly significant ($p < 0.001$). Thus with the study in miniature swine, the protective effect of ICRF-187 against chronic anthracycline cardiotoxicity has been demonstrated in 3 different species.

Neither ICRF-159 nor ICRF-187 appears to alter anthracycline actions in other tissues (Giuliani *et al.*, 1981; Wampler *et al.*, 1974; Woodman, 1974; Woodman *et al.*, 1972, 1975). For example, the alopecia in rabbits following daunorubicin and in dogs and miniature pigs following doxorubicin occurred despite treatment with ICRF-187. Likewise ICRF-187 does not interfere with daunorubicin myelosuppresion (Herman *et al.*, 1979). It should be noted that enhancement of anthracycline bone marrow toxicity did not occur at the doses of ICRF-187 utilized to reduce cardiotoxicity. These observations tend to indicate that anthracycline actions on the heart are mediated by a different mechanism than that on rapidly dividing tissues such as bone marrow.

The mechanism by which ICRF-187 reduces chronic anthracycline cardiac toxicity is not completely understood. Myers *et al.* (1982) have demonstrated that iron and doxorubicin can form a complex which when bound to erythrocyte ghost membranes can generate a locally destructive concentration of reactive oxygen species. The membrane damage is prevented when EDTA is added to the medium. Since ICRF-187 is a nonpolar derivative of EDTA, it could enter myocardial cells and exert protective effects by chelating divalent cations. This type of reaction between ICRF-187 and iron could be extremely important if the cardiotoxic action is mediated through the production of highly toxic oxygen containing radicals.

The question of whether ICRF-187 can alter a mechanism of tissue toxicity requiring iron for the formation of free radicals has been examined by El-Hage *et al.* (1981). These investigators found that pretreatment with either ICRF-187 or the free radical scavenger DMSO markedly attenuated the hyperglycemia and the destruction of pancreatic beta cells following alloxan administration in mice. When alloxan is given free radicals are generated through a series of reactions involving superoxide anion, hydrogen peroxide, and iron (Fisher and Hamburger, 1980). There is evidence that iron chelating substances such as diethylenetriaminepentaacetic acid (DETAPAC) can prevent the generation of hydroxyl radicals (Buettner *et al.*, 1978), inhibit the action of alloxan on isolated pancreatic cells (Fisher and Hamburger, 1980), and attenuate alloxan-induced hyperglycemia in intact animals (Cabbat and Heikkila, 1981). An ICRF-induced decrease in intracellular iron concentration could conceivably result in a reduction in the formation of hydroxyl radicals in pancreatic beta cells after alloxan or in myocardial cells after doxorubicin. In this case, ICRF-187 would not be acting as a free radical scavenger in the same manner as vitamin E or DMSO but instead would prevent the formation of free radicals.

The ability of ICRF-187 to alter toxic reactions such as elicited by alloxan is not an isolated event. A similar finding was obtained in studies utilizing acetaminophen. Liver alterations occur when high doses of acetaminophen (300 mg/kg) are given to Syrian golden hamsters on 2 consecutive days (El-Hage *et al.*, 1982). ICRF-187 (300 mg/kg) or DMSO (7.3 g/kg) given 1 hour prior to administration of acetaminophen markedly attenuated the increase in SGPT activity and reduced the incidence and severity of hepatocyte injury. The primary events in acetaminophen induced liver toxicity appear to be lipid peroxidation and the subsequent formation of toxic free radicals (Chiu and Bhakthan, 1978). Thus ICRF-187 could attenuate acetaminophen liver toxicity also by interfering with a free radical mechanism.

IX. Prospective Views

In this article, efforts have been made to summarize studies relating to the antineoplastic and other biological characteristics of bis(dioxopiperazine) derivatives. A concerted effort was made to explore the relationship of the structures to their antitumor and antimetastatic activities. From the information available it is apparent that the precise mechanism for the antineoplastic or antimetastatic actions remains to be resolved. This situation has hampered optimal clinical use of these agents.

The ability to ameliorate certain toxic effects of anthracycline antineoplastic drugs is also a potentially important property of the ICRF compounds. In this instance the mechanism of action may be related to the chelation of divalent metal cations. Since a number of essential cellular enzymes depend on these metals to function it is not surprising that the spectrum of activity of ICRF compounds has not been fully understood. The observed interactions with alloxan and acetaminophen indicate that ICRF compounds might modify the adverse effects of a variety of drugs. It is also anticipated that additional investigations could utilize ICRF compounds as probes to elucidate basic processes of normal and abnormal cells.

At present, a continued interest in the compounds centers around several major areas of research: (1) prevention of tumor metastasis; (2) radiosensitization of tumors; (3) synergism with other anticancer drugs; (4) protection from chronic toxicity of anticancer anthracyclines; (5) normalization of the tumor neovasculature; and (6) specific inhibition of dividing cells with no activity on nondividing cells.

Acknowledgments

Dr. Witiak gratefully acknowledges support of his work through U.S. Public Health Research Grant CA25445 from the National Cancer Institute.

References

Ahmann, D. L., O'Connell, K. H., Bisel, H. F., Edmonson, J. H., Hahn, R. G., and Frytak, S. (1977). *Cancer Treat. Rep.* **61,** 81.

Ahmann, D. L., Edmonson, J. H., Frytak, S., Kvols, L. K., Bisel, H. F., and Rubin, J. (1978). *Cancer Treat. Rep.* **62,** 151.

Atherton, A. (1975). *Eur. J. Cancer* **11,** 383.
Atherton, D. J., Wells, R. S., Laurent, M. R., and Williams, Y. F. (1980). *Br. J. Dermatol.* **202,** 307.
Bakowski, M. T. (1976). *Cancer Treat. Rev.* **3,** 95.
Bakowski, M. T., MacDonald, E., Mould, R. F., Cawte, P., Slowgen, J., Barret, A., Dalley, V., Newton, K. A., Westbury, G., James, S. E., and Hellmann, K. (1978). *Int. J. Radiat. Oncol. Biol. Phys.* **5,** 115.
Bakowski, M. T., Brearley, R. L., and Wrigley, P. F. M. (1979a). *Cancer Treat. Rep.* **63,** 2085.
Bakowski, M. T., Prentice, H. G., Lister, T. A., Malpas, J. S., McElwain, T. J., and Powles, R. L. (1979b). *Cancer Treat. Rep.* **63,** 127.
Bates, T. (1978). *Int. J. Radiat. Oncol. Biol. Phys.* **4,** 127.
Bellet, R. E., Mastrangelo, M. J., Dixon, L. M., and Yarbro, J. W. (1973). *Cancer Chemother. Rep.* **57,** 185.
Bellet, R. E., Rozencweig, M., Von Hoff, D. D., Penta, J. S., Wassermann, T. H., and Muggia, F. M. (1977). *Europ. J. Cancer* **13,** 1293.
Buettner, G. R., Oberly, L. W., and Chan-Leuthauser, S. (1978). *Photochem. Photobiol.* **28,** 693.
Burrage, K., Hellmann, K., and Salsbury, A. J. (1970). *Br. J. Pharmacol.* **39,** 205P.
Cabbat, F. S., and Heikkila, R. E. (1981). *Fed. Proc.* **40,** 741.
Camerman, A., and Camerman, N. (1981). Personal communication.
Chiu, S., and Bhakthan, N. M. G. (1978). *Lab. Invest.* **39,** 193.
Creaven, P. J., and Taylor, S. G. (1973). *Proc. Am. Assoc. Cancer Res.* **14,** 20.
Creaven, P. J., Cohen, M. H., Hansen, H. H., Selawry, O. S., and Taylor, S. G. (1974a). *Cancer Chemother. Rep.* **3,** 393.
Creaven, P. J., Allen, L. H., and Alford, D. A. (1974b). *J. Pharm. Pharmacol.* **12,** 914.
Creighton, A. M. (1970). *Progr. Antimicrob. Anticancer Chemotherap.* **1,** 167.
Creighton, A. M. (1971). Br. Patent 1,234,935.
Creighton, A. M. (1974). Br. Patent 1,374,979.
Creighton, A. M., Hellmann, K., and Whitecross, S. (1969). *Nature (London)* **222,** 384.
Creighton, A. M., and Birnie, G. D. (1969). *Biochem. J.* **114,** 58P.
Creighton, A. M., and Birnie, G. D. (1970). *Int. J. Cancer* **5,** 47.
Creighton, A. M., Jeffery, W. A., and Long, J. (1979). *Proc. Int. Med. Chem. Symp. 6th.*
Dawson, K. M. (1975). *Biochem. Pharmacol.* **24,** 2249.
Doolan, P. D., Schwartz, S. L., Hayes, J. R., Mullen, J. C., and Cummings, N. B. (1967). *Toxicol. Appl. Pharmacol.* **10,** 481.
Dubley, H.R., Ritchie, M. B., Schilling, A., and Baker, W. H. (1955). *New Engl. J. Med.* **252,** 331.
Eagan, R. T., Carr, D. T., Coles, D. T., Rubin, J., and Frytak, S. (1976). *Cancer Treat. Rep.* **60,** 947.
El-Hage, A., Herman, E. H., and Ferrans, V. J. (1981). *Res. Commu. Chem. Path. Pharmacol.* **23,** 509.
El-Hage, A., Herman, E., and Ferrans, V. (1982). *Proc. Am. Coll. Clin. Pharmacol.*
Fidler, I. J., and Nicolson, G. L. (1976). *J. Natl. Cancer Inst.* **57,** 1199.
Field, E. O., Mauro, F., and Hellmann, K. (1971). *Cancer Chemother. Rep.* **55,** 527.
Finkelstein, J. Z., Title, K., Meshnik, R., and Weiner, J. (1975). *Cancer Chemother. Rep. Part 1* **59,** 975.
Fisher, L. J., and Hamburger, S. A. (1980). *Diabetes* **29,** 213.
Flannery, E. P., Corder, M. P., Sheehan, W. W., Pajak, T. F., and Bateman, J. R. *Cancer Treat. Rep.* **62,** 465.

Forman, H. (1960). *In* "Metal-Binding in Medicine" (M. J. Seven and L. A. Johnson, eds.), pp. 82–94. Lippincott, Philadelphia.
Forman, H., Finnegan, C., and Lushbaugh, C. C. (1956). *J. Am. Med. Assoc.* **160,** 1042.
Gilbert, J. M., Hellmann, K., Evans, M., Cassell, P. G., Ellis, H., Wastell, C., and Stoodley, B. (1981). *In* "Adjuvant Therapy of Cancer III" (S. E. Salmon and S. E. Jones, eds.), pp. 519–526. Grune & Stratton, New York.
Gilbert, J. M., Hellmann, K., Evans, M., Cassell, P. G., Ellis, H., Wastell, C., and Stoodley, B. (1982). *Cancer Chemoth. Pharmacol.* (in press).
Giuliani, F., Casazza, A. M., DiMarco, A., and Savi, G. (1981). *Cancer Treat. Rep.* **65,** 267.
Gralla, E. J., Coleman, G. L., and Jonas, A. M. (1974). *Cancer Chemother. Rep.* **5,** 1.
Gram, T. E., Mimnaugh, E. G., Sikic, B. I., Drew, R., and Siddik, Z. H. (1978). *Proc. 7 Int. Congress Pharmacol. 7th,* 350.
Grieder, A., Maurer, R., and Stahalin, H. (1977). *Cancer Res.* **37,** 2998.
Hallowes, R. C., West, D. G., and Hellmann, K. (1974). *Nature (London)* **247,** 487.
Hellmann, K. (1972a). *In* "Advances in Antimicrobial and Antineoplastic Chemotherapy" (M. Hejzlav, M. Semonsky, and S. Mesak, eds.), Vol. II, p. 769. Univ. Park Press, Baltimore.
Hellmann, K. (1972b). *Chem. Br.* **8,** 69.
Hellmann, K., and Burrage, K. (1969). *Nature (London)* **224,** 273.
Hellmann, K., and Field, E. O. (1970). *J. Natl. Cancer Inst.* **44,** 539.
Hellmann, K., and Murkin, G. (1974). *Cancer* **34,** 1033.
Hellmann, K., and Murkin, G. (1978). Unpublished.
Hellmann, K., Newton, K. A., Whitemore, D. N., Hanham, I. W. F., and Bond, J. V. (1969). *Br. Med. J.* **1,** 822.
Hellmann, K., Salsbury, A. J., Burrage, K. S., LeServe, A. W., and James, S. E. (1973). *In* "Chemotherapy of Cancer Dissemination and Metastasis" (S. Garattini and G. Franchi, eds.), pp. 355–359. Raven, New York.
Hellmann, K., James, S. E., and Salsbury, A. S. (1974). *Br. J. Cancer* **30,** 179.
Hellmann, K., Grimshaw, M. B., and Hutchinson, G. E. (1978a). *Int. J. Radiat. Oncol. Biol. Phys.* **4,** 109.
Hellmann, K., Newton, K. A., and Humble, J. G. (1978b). *Br. J. Cancer* **37,** 479.
Herman, E., and Ferrans, V. (1981). *Cancer Res.* **41,** 3436.
Herman, E., and Ferrans, V. J. (1982). *Lab. Invest.* (submitted).
Herman, E., El-Hage, A., and Witiak, D. T. (1982). *Fed. Proc.* **41,** 1477.
Herman, E. H., Mhatre, R. M., Lee, I. P., and Waravdekar, V. S. (1972). *Proc. Soc. Exp. Biol. Med.* **140,** 234.
Herman, E. H., Mhatre, R. M., and Chadwick, D. (1974). *Toxicol. Appl. Pharmacol.* **27,** 517.
Herman, E., Ardalan, B., Bier, C., Waravdekar, V., and Krop, S. (1979). *Cancer Treat. Rep.* **63,** 89.
Herman, E. H., Ferrans, V. J., Jordan, W., and Ardalan, B. (1981). *Res. Commun. Chem. Pathol. Pharmacol.* **31,** 85.
Hoover, H. C., Jr., and Ketcham, A. S. (1975). *Cancer* **35,** 5.
James, S. E., and Salsbury, A. J. (1974). *Cancer Res.* **34,** 839.
Karrer, K., Humphreys, S. R., and Goldin, A. (1967). *Int. J. Cancer* **2,** 213.
Kline, I. (1974). *Cancer Chemother. Rep. Part 2* **4,** 33.
Krepler, O., and Pawlowsky, J. (1975). *Oesterr Z. Onkol.* **2,** 112.
Kvols, L. K., Eagan, R. T., and Myers, R. P. (1977). *Cancer Treat. Rep.* **61,** 311.
Landgrebe, J. A. (1981). *Chem. Eng. News.* **47.**
Lazo, J. S., Ingber, D. E., and Sartorelli, A. C. (1978). *Cancer Res.* **38,** 2263.
Lefrak, E. A., Pitha, J., Rosenheim, S., and Gottlieb, J. A. (1973). *Cancer* **34,** 302.

Lefrak, E. A., Pitha, J., Rosenheim, S., O'Bryan, R. M., Burgess, M. A., and Gottlieb, J. A. (1975). *Cancer Chemoth. Rep.* **6,** 203.

Leiter, J., Wodinsky, I., and Bourke, A. R. (1959). *Cancer Res.* **19** (Part II), 309.

LeServe, A. W. (1971). *Br. J. Pharmacol.* **43,** 457P.

LeServe, A. W., and Hellmann, K. (1972). *Br. Med. J.* **1,** 597.

Levine, B. S., Henry, M. C., Port, C. D., and Rosen, E. (1980). *Cancer Treat. Rep.* **64,** 1211.

Livingston, D. C., Creighton, A. M., and Fisher, S. W. (1972). *In* "Advances in Antimicrobial and Antineoplastic Chemotherapy" (M. Hejzlar, M. Semonsky, and S. Masak, eds.), Vol. II, pp 109. Univ. Park Press, Baltimore.

Mathé, G., Amiel, J. L., Hayat, M., de Vassal, F., Schwarzenberg, M., Schneider, M., Jasmin, C., and Rosenfeld, C. (1970). *Recent Results Cancer Res.* **30,** 52.

Mimnaugh, E. G., Siddik, Z. H., Drew, R., Sikic, B. I., and Gram, T. E. (1979). *Toxicol. Appl. Pharmacol.* **49,** 119.

Myers, C. E., McGuire, W. P., Liss, R. H., Ifrim, I., Grotzinger, K., and Young, R. C. (1977). *Science* **197,** 165.

Myers, C. E., Gianni, L., Simore, C. B., Klecker, R., and Greene, R. (1982). *Biochemistry* **21,** 1707.

Olweny, C. L., Sikyewunda, W., and Otim, D. (1980). *Oncology* **37,** 174.

Peters, L. J. (1975). *Brit. J. Cancer* **32,** 355.

Peters, L. J. (1976). *Br. J. Radiol.* **49,** 708.

Pimm, M. V., and Baldwin, R. W. (1975). *Br. J. Cancer* **31,** 62.

Pollard, M., Burleson, G. R., and Luckert, P. H. (1981). *The Prostate* **2,** 1.

Progress Report to Chemotherapy Program, National Cancer Institute (July 1973). Arthur D. Little, Inc.

Repta, A. J., Baltezor, M. J., and Bansal, P. C. (1976). *J. Pharm. Sci.* **65,** 238.

Rhomberg, W. U. (1978). *Int. J. Radiat. Oncol. Biol. Phys.* **4,** 121.

Ryall, R. D. (1978). *Int. J. Radiat. Oncol. Biol. Phys.* **4,** 133.

Ryall, R. D., Hanham, I. W., Newton, K. A., Hellmann, K., Brinkley, D. M., and Hjertaas, O. K. (1974). *Cancer* **34,** 1040.

Sadee, W., Staroscik, J., Finn, C., and Cohen, J. (1975). *J. Pharm. Sci.* **64,** 998.

Salsbury, A. J., Burrage, K., and Hellmann, K. (1970). *Br. Med. J.* **4,** 344.

Salsbury, A. J., Burrage, K., and Hellmann, K. (1974). *Cancer Res.* **34,** 843.

Sartorelli, A. C., and Johns, D. G. (1975). *In* "Antineoplastic and Immunosuppressive Agents Part II. Handbook of Experimental Pharmacology," Vol. XXXVIII/2, p. 885. Springer-Verlag, Berlin and New York.

Schroeder, H. A. (1960). *In* "Metal-Binding in Medicine" (M. J. Seven and L. A. Johnson, eds.), pp 59–67. Lipincott, Philadelphia.

Shah, M. K., Engstrom, P. F., Catalano, R. B., Paul, A. R., Bellet, R. E., and Creech, R. H. (1982). *Cancer Treat. Rep.* **66,** 557.

Sharpe, H. B., Field, E. O., and Hellmann, K. (1970). *Nature* (*London*) **226,** 524.

Spittle, N. F., Bush, N., James, S. E., and Hellmann, K. (1979). *Int. J. Radiat. Oncol. Biol. Phys.* **5,** 1649.

Spreafico, F., and Garattini, S. (1974). *Cancer Treat. Rev.* **1,** 239.

Stephens, T. C., and Creighton, A. M. (1974). *Br. J. Cancer* **29,** 99.

Tan, C., Tasaka, H., Yu, K.-P., Murphy, L., and Karnofsky, D. A. (1967). *Cancer* **20,** 333.

Taylor, I. W., and Bleehen, N. M. (1977). *Br. J. Cancer* **36,** 493.

Von Hoff, D. D., Howser, D., Lewis, B. J., Holcenberg, J., Weiss, R. B., and Young, R. C. (1981). *Cancer Treat. Rep.* **65,** 249.

Wampler, G. L., Speckhart, V. J., and Regelson, W. (1974). *Proc. Am. Soc. Clin. Oncol.* **15,** 189.

Ward; D. (1968). Unpublished.
Wang, G. M., and Finch, M. (1980). *Drug Chem. Toxicol.* **3,** 213.
Wang, G., Finch, M. D., Trevan, D., and Hellmann, K. (1981). *Br. J. Cancer* **43,** 871.
Wassermann, T. H., Friedman, M. A., Slavik, M., and Carter, S. K. (1973). *In* "(±)1,2-di(3,5-dioxopiperazin-1-yl)propane, ICRF-159, NSC-129943, Clinical Brochure." National Cancer Institute, Bethesda.
Witiak, D. T., Lee, H. J., Hart, R. W., and Gibson, R. E. (1977). *J. Med. Chem.* **20,** 630.
Witiak, D. T., Lee, H. J., Goldman, H. D., and Zwilling, B. S. (1978). *J. Med. Chem.* **21,** 1194.
Witiak, D. T., Trivedi, B. K., Campolito, L. B., Reiches, N. A., and Zwilling, B. S. (1981). *J. Med. Chem.* **24,** 1329.
Wolgemuth, R. L., Hagerman, L. M., Magliere, K. C., and Witiak, D. T. (1981). *Experientia* (submitted).
Woodman, R. J. (1971). Unpublished.
Woodman, R. J. (1974). *Cancer Chemother. Rep. Part 2* **4,** 45.
Woodman, R. J., Kline, I., and Venditti, J. M. (1972). *Proc. Am. Assoc. Cancer Res.* **13,** 31.
Woodman, R. J., Cysyk, R. L., Kline, I., Gang, M., and Venditti, J. M. (1975). *Cancer Chemother. Rep. Part 1* **59,** 689.
Zwilling, B. S., Campolito, L. B., Reiches, N. A., George, T., and Witiak, D. T. (1981). *Br. J. Cancer* **44,** 578.

NOTE ADDED IN PROOF. The biologic activity of a new diketopiperazine compound has been reported. This agent, Bimolane [bis-(N^4-morpholinomethyl-3,5-dioxopiperazinyl-1,2 ethane)] was found to be active, by both the oral and ip routes, against various experimental tumors (R. Yun-Feng, Shanghai Institute of Materia Medica, personal communication). The results of clinical studies indicate oral administration of Bimolane may be useful in the treatment of psoriasis, sympathetic ophthalmitis, uveitis, and malignant lymphomas (*Science* **213,** 1239, 1981). Two additional pharmocokinetic studies involving ICRF-187 have recently appeared. In mice iv administered radiolabeled ICRF-187 disappeared rapidly from plasma and was maximally concentrated in the kidney and liver (R. M. Mhatre, A. Rahman, S. Raschild, and P. Schein, *Proc. Am. Assn. Cancer Res.* **23,** 212, 1982). The amount of ICRF-187 detected in kidney, liver, and heart decreased to low levels within 2 hours. The second study was performed in 6 patients during a phase I trial (R. H. Earhart, K. Tutsch, J. M. Koeller, H. I. Robins, H. L. Davis, and D. C. Tormey, *Proc. Am. Assn. Cancer Res.* **23,** 128, 1982). Samples were collected during and following iv infusion of 1.0 g/m^2 by 3 different schedules (0.5, 8, and 48 hours). Serum kinetics followed a two compartment model. Renal clearances were not significantly different between schedules but nonrenal clearance was significantly greater with the 48 hour infusion. Greater biologic activity might be expected with the 48 hour infusion since this was the only schedule to achieve steady-state conditions. An attempt to demonstrate a possible correlation between biologic activities of the parent cyclic imides (ICRF-159 and 192) and the relative affinity of their hydrolysis products for one or more cations has been reported (Z. A. Huang, P. M. May, K. M. Quinlan, D. R. Williams, and A. M. Creighton, *Agents Actions* **12,** 1, 1982). Equilibrium constants for the main hydrolytic products with a number of biologically important cations have been measured and used in computer simulation models to assess the possible significance of *in vivo* chelation. It was found that the only difference in binding occurred with zinc, which was strongly chelated by the hydrolysis product of ICRF-192. How this effect could account for the difference in cytotoxicity exhibited by ICRF-159 and its inactive homolog ICRF-192 remains to be determined.

Index

A

Albendazole, chemistry and pharmacology, 70
Alkylating agents, effects on mononuclear phagocytes, 44–48
Antihelminthics
  activity, 140–141
  administration of, 141–144
  choice of, 144–146
  drug resistance and drug combinations, 146–147
  indications for, 136–137
  list of essential drugs, 138–140
  supportive treatment, 147
Antimetabolites, effects on mononuclear phagocytes, 41–44
Antimetastatic activity, of ICRF-159, 266–268
Antineoplastic therapy
  central nervous system toxicity
    chemotherapy, 218–225
    combined modality treatment, 225–229
    radiotherapy, 215–218
  in children
    chemotherapy, 212–215
    radiotherapy, 209–212
    surgery, 209
  endocrine organ toxicity
    gonadal, 233–236
    hypothalamic-pituitary, 230–232
    thyroid-parathyroid, 232–233
  psychosocial development and, 237–239
  skeletal growth and, 236–237

B

Benzimidazole carbamates
  in human medicine, 109–110
    cestode infections, 117–118
    nematode infections, 110–117
  in veterinary medicine, 82
    dogs and cats, 102–106
    domestic ruminants, 85–96
    equids, 83–85
    ovicidal activity, 107
    pig, 96–101
    poultry and birds, 101–102
    resistance to, 108–109
    rodents, 107–108
    wild and zoo animals, 106–107
Biodisposition, of chloroethylnitrosoureas, 20–25
Bis(dioxopiperazine) compounds, *see* ICRF-159

C

Cats, benzimidazole carbamates and, 102–106
Cell cycle, ICRF-159 and, 264–266
Central nervous system, toxicity of antineoplastic therapy and
  chemotherapy, 218–225
  combined modality treatment, 225–229
  radiotherapy, 215–218
Cestode infections, in humans, benzimidazole carbamates and, 117–118
Chemotherapeutic agents
  effects on mononuclear phagocytes
    agents affecting cytoskeleton, 52–54
    alkylating agents, 44–48
    antimetabolites, 41–44
    glucocorticosteroids, 37–41
    intercalating agents, 48–52
    overview, 54–56
  effects on tumor-associated macrophages, 56–57
Chemotherapy,
  in children, 212–215, 218–225
Childhood
  antihelminthic therapy in, 147–148
  antineoplastic therapy in
    chemotherapy, 212–215
    radiotherapy, 209–212
    surgery, 209

Chloroethylnitrosoureas
active species, 13–15
biodisposition, 20–25
chemicobiological interactions, 26
chemistry of, 5–9
mechanism of cytotoxicity, 15–20
new, development of, 1–5
reactive intermediates, 9–15
Ciclobendazole, chemistry and pharmacology, 70–72
Communities, antihelminthic therapy for, 148–150
Cytoskeleton, agents affecting, effects on mononuclear phagocytes, 52–54
Cytotoxicity
of chloroethylnitrosoureas, mechanism of, 15–20
of ICRF-159, 260–264

D

Dogs, benzimidazole carbamates and, 102–106

E

Electron affinity, of radiosensitizers, 163–167
Endocrine organs, toxicity of antineoplastic therapy and
gonadal, 233–236
hypothalamic-pituitary, 230–232
thyroid-parathyroid, 232–233
Equids, benzimidazole carbamates and, 83–85

F

Fenbendazole, chemistry and pharmacology, 72–74
Flubendazole, chemistry and pharmacology, 74–76

G

Glucocorticosteroids, effects on mononuclear phagocytes, 37–44
Gonads, antineoplastic therapy and, 233–236

H

Health, impact of intestinal helminths on, 132–135
Helminth(s)
of human intestinal tract, 131–132
intestinal, impact on human health, 132–135
Helminthiases
intestinal, symptoms of, 136
reinfection and, 137–138
therapeutic intervention
for communities, 148–150
for individuals, 147
treatment in childhood and during pregnancy, 147–148
Human medicine, benzimidazole carbamates in, 109–110
cestode infections, 117–118
nematode infections, 110–117
Hypothalamus-pituitary, antineoplastic therapy and, 230–232
Hypoxia, ways to overcome, 156–158

I

ICRF-159
biological characteristics
antimetastatic activity, 266–268
cell cycle specificity, 264–266
cytotoxicity, 260–264
chemistry and structure-activity relationships, 250–259
clinical aspects, 274–277
historical, 249–250
interactions with other agents, 278–286
pharmacology of, 269–270
radiosensitization and, 268–269
toxicology
clinical, 271
preclinical, 270–271
ICRF-187, toxicology
clinical, 274
preclinical, 272–273
Individuals, antihelminthic therapy for, 147
Intercalating agents, effects on mononuclear phagocytes, 48–52
Intestinal tract, human, helminths of, 131–132